Epidemiology, Pathogenesis, and Prevention of Head and Neck Cancer

Andrew F. Olshan
Editor

Epidemiology, Pathogenesis, and Prevention of Head and Neck Cancer

Springer

Editor
Andrew F. Olshan, Ph.D.
Professor and Chair
Department of Epidemiology
2101B McGavran-Greenberg Hall
Gillings School of Global Public Health CB#7435
University of North Carolina Chapel Hill, NC 27599
andy_olshan@unc.edu

ISBN 978-1-4419-1471-2 e-ISBN 978-1-4419-1472-9
DOI 10.1007/978-1-4419-1472-9
Springer New York Dordrecht Heidelberg London

Library of Congress Control Number: 2010921593

Printed on acid-free paper

Springer is part of Springer Science+Business Media (www.springer.com)

Preface

Head and neck cancer – defined here as cancers of the oral cavity, pharynx, and larynx – comprises a fascinating tumor model. With two well established risk factors – tobacco and alcohol – and the potential for screening, these tumors provide unique opportunities for prevention and control. Further, the known etiological factors also help frame studies of mechanisms and susceptibility. Finally, the role of the human papillomavirus (HPV) offers another cancer model to investigate the viral etiology of cancer.

This context has led to wonderful interdisciplinary research opportunities among clinicians, epidemiologists, and molecular biologists and geneticists. In that spirit, we have brought together the world's experts on the epidemiology, clinical aspects, and molecular biology of head and neck cancer. The book includes a spectrum of research foci from descriptive epidemiology to molecular biology. I hope that active researchers in the field of head and neck cancer will find these current summaries useful to guide their research as well as drawing in those not working on this cancer. The book illustrates much of what is known and also highlights the many unanswered questions.

I wish to thank the authors who worked so hard to develop their chapters. I also thank Rachel Warren of Springer Press for her editorial guidance.

Chapel Hill, NC — Andrew Olshan, Ph.D.

Contents

Contributors

Cristina Bosetti, Ph.D.
Istituto di Ricerche Farmacologiche "Mario Negri", via Giuseppe La Masa 19, 20156 Milan, Italy

Anil Chaturvedi, D.V.M., Ph.D.
Infections and Immunoepidemiology Branch, Division of Cancer Epidemiology and Genetics, 6120 Executive Boulevard, MSC 7242, Bethesda, Maryland 20892-7335

Susan S. Devesa, Ph.D.
Division of Cancer Epidemiology and Genetics, Department of Health and Human Services, National Cancer Institute, National Institutes of Health, 6120 Executive Blvd, Bethesda, MD 20892-7244, USA

Kimon Divaris, D.D.S.
Department of Epidemiology, Gillings School of Global Public Health, University of North Carolina, 2101B McGavran-Greenberg Hall, Chapel Hill, NC 27599, USA

Jacques Ferlay
Data Analysis and Interpretation Group, Section of Cancer Information, 150 cours Albert Thomas, Lyon 69008, France

Werner Garavello, M.D.
Istituto di Ricerche Farmacologiche "Mario Negri", via Giuseppe La Masa 19, 20156 Milan, Italy; Clinica Otorinolaringoiatrica, DNTB, Università Milano-Bicocca, via Donizetti 106, 20052 Monza, Italy

Maura L. Gillison, M.D., Ph.D.
Department of Internal Medicine, Division of Hematology & Oncology, Starling Loving Hall, 320 W. 10th Avenue, Columbus, OH 43210

Gloria Gridley, M.S.
Division of Cancer Epidemiology and Genetics, Department of Health and Human Services, National Cancer Institute, National Institutes of Health, 6120 Executive Blvd, Bethesda, MD 20892-7244, USA

Mia Hashibe, Ph.D.
Division of Public Health, Department of Family & Preventive Medicine, University of Utah School of Medicine, 375 Chipeta Way, Suite A, Salt Lake City, UT, 84108

Wayne M. Koch, M.D.
Department of Otolaryngology-Head & Neck Surgery, Johns Hopkins University School of Medicine, Baltimore, MD 21287, USA

Carlo La Vecchia, M.D.
Istituto di Ricerche Farmacologiche "Mario Negri", via Giuseppe La Masa 19, 20156 Milan, Italy; Istituto di Statistica Medica e Biometria, " G.A. Maccacaro", Università degli Studi di Milano, via Venezian 1, 20133 Milano, Italy

Guojun Li, M.D., Ph.D.
Department of Head and Neck Surgery and Department of Epidemiology, U. T. M. D. Anderson Cancer Center, 1515 Holcombe Blvd., Unit 0441, Houston, TX 77030, USA

Christopher H. Lieu, M.D.
Department of Thoracic/Head and Neck Medical Oncology, The University of Texas M. D. Anderson Cancer Center, 1515 Holcombe Blvd., Unit 432, Houston, TX 77030, USA

Scott M. Lippman, M.D.
Department of Thoracic/Head and Neck Medical Oncology, The University of Texas M. D. Anderson Cancer Center, 1515 Holcombe Blvd., Unit 432, Houston, TX 77030, USA

Ersilia Lucenteforte, Ph.D.
Istituto di Ricerche Farmacologiche "Mario Negri", via Giuseppe La Masa 19, 20156 Milan, Italy

Linda Morris Brown, M.P.H., Dr. P.H.
RTI International, 6110 Executive Blvd, Suite 902, Rockville, MD 20852-3907, USA

Melonie Nance, M.D.
Indiana University School of Medicine, 702 Barnhill Drive, RI0860 Indianapolis, IN 46202-5230

Andrew. F. Olshan, Ph.D.
Department of Epidemiology, Gillings School of Global Public Health, University of North Carolina, 2101B McGavran-Greenberg Hall, Chapel Hill, NC 27599, USA

Rengaswamy Sankaranarayanan, M.D.
Screening Group, Section of Early Detection and Prevention, International Agency for Research on Cancer, 150 cours Albert Thomas, Lyon 69008, France

Erich Sturgis, M.D., M. P. H.
Department of Head and Neck Surgery and Department of Epidemiology, U. T. M. D. Anderson Cancer Center, 1515 Holcombe Blvd., Unit 0441, Houston, TX 77030, USA

Li-E Wang, M.D.
Department of Epidemiology, U. T. M. D. Anderson Cancer Center, 1515 Holcombe Blvd., Unit 1365, Houston, TX 77030, USA

Qingyi Wei, Ph.D.
Department of Epidemiology, U. T. M. D. Anderson Cancer Center, 1515 Holcombe Blvd., Unit 1365, Houston, TX 77030, USA

William N. William, Jr., M.D.
Department of Thoracic/Head and Neck Medical Oncology, The University of Texas M. D. Anderson Cancer Center, 1515 Holcombe Blvd., Unit 432, Houston, TX 77030, USA

Classification, Clinical Features, and Molecular Genetic Models

Wayne M. Koch and Melonie Nance

Squamous cell carcinoma of the upper aerodigestive tract (head and neck squamous cell carcinoma, HNSCC) is often considered to be a single disease based on the cell of origin (mucosal epithelium) and histologic features. However, distinctive phenotypic patterns and genotypic correlates increasingly suggest that it might be more accurately thought of as consisting of different entities. These observations have been evolving in the context of the more traditional paradigms of tumor classification based on well established parameters such as primary tumor anatomical site, stage, and histologic features. Taken together, clinicians seek to use new and traditional tumor features to categorize tumors, predict their potential clinical course, and select appropriate strategies for their detection and treatment.

Traditional Concepts of Tumor Classification

Squamous cell carcinoma (SCCA) is the most common malignancy of the head and neck, accounting for 92% of cases [1]. In the head and neck, several types of SCCA present with different tumor behaviors, prognoses, and severities. Traditionally, tumors are classified by stage and anatomic site of origin. Patterns of tumor growth and invasion may vary predictably with the anatomic barriers or pathways that prevent or allow extension. Within the head and neck, these sites are classified based on established anatomic parameters. The upper aerodigestive tract is organized into the following site categories: Nasopharynx, Oral Cavity, Oropharynx, Hypopharynx, Larynx, and Trachea. Beyond the upper aerodigestive tract, the paranasal sinuses, skull base, salivary glands, endocrine glands, skin, ear, and temporal bones are other possible sites where primary SCCA tumors may arise.

W.M. Koch
Department of Otolaryngology - Head and Neck Surgery, Johns Hopkins University, 601N, Caroline St, Baltimore, MD 21287
e-mail: wkoch@jhmi.edu

M. Nance
Department of Otolaryngology - Head and Neck Surgery, Indiara University

A.F. Olshan (ed.), *Epidemiology, Pathogenesis, and Prevention of Head and Neck Cancer*,
DOI 10.1007/978-1-4419-1472-9_1, © Springer Science+Business Media, LLC 2010

Tumor Stage

Each anatomical site category has its own tumor staging system combining a numerical metric for the primary tumor, nodal basin, and distant metastatic field. The primary lesion stage (T stage) is based on size and location relative to important surrounding structures. The nodal (N) stage is determined by the size, the side (ipsilateral or contralateral to the primary) and the number of suspicious nodes. The distant metastasis (M) stage is generally a plus/minus dichotomy. The overall stage schema takes into account all three components and assigns a Roman numeral Stage I–IV. Staging may be clinical, based on physical examination and radiologic evaluation, or pathological, based on the size and extent of tumor judged after surgical resection. Staging systems as defined by the American Joint Committee on Cancer (AJCC)[1] and the United International Cancer Committee (UICC) have been widely adopted and used. Ideally, tumor stage categories are each distinctly predictive of outcome with poorer survival seen with each increment of advancing stage. This system is imperfect and undergoes periodic scrutiny with suggestions for revision. However, in many clinical outcome studies, stage remains one of the only valuable prognostic parameters.

Anatomical Categories

The boundaries of the oral cavity extend from the mucosal surface of the lips to the junction of the hard/soft palate (above), and the circumvillate papillae of the tongue (below). The oral cavity includes the lips, the gingivobuccal sulcus, the upper and lower alveolus ridges, buccal mucosa, floor of mouth, gingiva, retromolar trigone, and the hard palate. From the oral cavity, tumor may spread via the foramina of the hard or soft palate. Other avenues include circumventing the muscular sling of the floor of mouth, the buccopharyngeal fascia, which is just deep to the buccal mucosa, or into the mandible. Posteriorly, the retromolar trigone is contiguous with the mandibular mucosa, which is closely approximated to the bone; hence, cancer here often invades the periosteum. Lymphatic drainage is most often unilateral from the oral tongue and superficial floor of mouth, and bilateral from the deeper floor of mouth musculature and root of tongue. Tumor staging in the oral cavity is based on the size of the lesion and/or the presence of invasion into deeper structures. The depth of invasion has been shown to be an important prognostic factor as well; it is associated with the likelihood of metastatic nodal involvement, but is not currently included in staging.

The Nasopharynx is continuous with the nasal cavity through the choanae. It is bounded by the skull base superiorly and extends to the level of the soft palate inferiorly, where it is contiguous to the oropharynx. Laterally, the cartilage of the eustachian tube creates a bulge at its opening, the torus tubarius. Just posterior and

[1]AJCC Cancer Staging Manual, 6th edn. Springer-Verlag, New York, NY, 2003.

superior to the torus is the Fossa of Rosenmuller, the site of origin of most nasopharyngeal carcinoma (NPC). NPC is currently classified into three WHO subclassifications based on histologic differentiation: (I) keratinizing, (II) nonkeratinizing, and (III) undifferentiated.

The oropharynx extends from the soft palate to the epiglottis. It is continuous with the posterior oral cavity and demarcated by the circumvallate papillae at the posterior 1/3 of the oral tongue. Within the oropharynx, the tongue base and vallecula are anterior, glossoepiglottic folds are lateral, and the prevertebral pharyngeal wall is posterior.

Additional lymphoid tissue, the lingual tonsil, is located under the mucous membrane of the posterior third of the tongue. Together, the tonsillar tissues of the nasopharynx and oropharynx form a ring of lymphoid tissue that surrounds the entrances into the pharynx from the nose and the mouth known as Waldeyer's ring. The oropharynx is continuous with the hypopharynx below.

The Hypopharynx is a long mucosal region that extends from the epiglottis to the esophageal inlet at the level of C6, running posterior to and wrapping around the larynx. In this region, field cancerization and submucosal lymphatic spread are of paramount importance, and skip lesions are not uncommon. Tumors often spread beyond visible borders of lesion. The hypopharynx is continuous with the esophagus inferiorly, and with the larynx anteriorly through the laryngeal aditus, which is formed by the epiglottis and the aryepiglottic folds. On either side of these folds and medial to the thyroid cartilage are two pyramidal recesses, called the pyriform sinuses. Two-thirds of hypopharyngeal tumors start in the pyriform sinus. From there, tumors may spread laterally to the thyroid cartilage or the thyroid gland. Medial spread can involve the paraglottic space of the hemilarynx, crico-arytenoid joint, or recurrent laryngeal nerve leading to vocal fold immobility. The contralateral pyriform can become involved through spread across the posterior pharyngeal wall or postcricoid mucosa to the other side. The most common sites of metastases from the Hypopharynx are ipsilateral level II–IV nodes. Upon presentation, the incidence of nodal spread is very high: around 75%.

One-third of hypopharyngeal tumors arise from the posterior pharyngeal wall. From this site, tumor spread can affect the prevertebral fascia posteriorly. Retropharyngeal metastases to the nodes of Rouvier are common. Hypopharyngeal tumors that start in the postcricoid region are uncommon (5% of lesions). However, they pose a risk of circumferential spread along and into cricoid and cervical esophagus. They have the lowest rate of regional metastasis and tend to spread to paratracheal nodes first.

The Larynx extends from the epiglottis and the aryepiglottic folds to the cricoid cartilage. It communicates with the laryngopharynx above and the trachea below through the laryngeal aditus . Its lateral walls have two infoldings of mucous membrane, the vestibular folds above and the vocal folds below. The ventricle between the folds has a lateral extension, the saccule, between the vestibular fold and the thyroid cartilage. The mucous membrane of the larynx is primarily ciliated columnar epithelium. The larynx structurally consists of cartilages, muscles, and ligaments that are essential to its role in phonation.

One-third of laryngeal SCCA occurs in the supraglottis, which includes the epiglottis (lingual and laryngeal surfaces), false cords (including ventricle and saccule), arytenoids, and aryepiglottic folds. Tumors of the infrahyoid epiglottis have poorer prognosis due to the propensity of tumor spread inferiorly into the pre-epiglottic space. Lymphatic spread involves bilateral levels II–IV, with notably frequent involvement of IIB.

Most laryngeal SCCA starts in the Glottis which is comprised of the true vocal cords, ventricular floor, anterior commissure, interarytenoid region, and extends inferiorly to a variable distance below true cords. Clinical presentation usually includes dysphonia. Regional metastases from here are very rare in early-stage disease. However, in advanced lesions (T3-4), metastases are more common and may first involve level VI nodes, before moving laterally. The subglottis is the area from 10 mm below the anterior commissure and 5 mm below posterior true cords and extends to inferior border of cricoid. This region is the most infrequent primary site of the larynx cancer at <5% incidence. Disease in the subglottis most often presents with stridor or shortness of breath. From here, regional metastases are generally seen in levels II–IV and IV of the neck.

Histologic Features

While SCCA has traditionally been categorized by its anatomic site of occurrence, other factors may also be important in determining prognosis. Over the years, several different types of SCCA have been described. Some histopathologic findings have been shown to have prognostic significance. Certain tumor characteristics, such as keratin production; level of differentiation; nuclear appearance; mitoses; and host factors, such as inflammation, desmoplastic reaction, patterns of invasion, and vascular invasion, have been described as adjuncts to clinical staging for predicting outcome. Though this information may be useful, no firm and consistent evidence supports including histologic features in formal cancer classification outside of the nasopharynx. Staging remains based solely on clinical examination and diagnostic imaging.

Histopathologically, SCCA is classified as squamous proliferation that is either keratinizing or nonkeratinizing in nature. Some variants, including basaloid and adenosquamous CA are known to have more aggressive tumor behavior. They are characterized by their small cells with scant cytoplasm, high mitotic rate, and comedonecrosis. Histologic grade is judged according to the degree the squamous cells have departed from their normal appearance. Characteristics that contribute to higher grade malignancy include pleomorphism, hyperchromatism, and increased mitotic activity (especially abnormal mitosis). The presence of keratin is an important determinant, indicating better differentiated lesions (lower grade). Keratin is found within the cytoplasm of well-differentiated cells and scattered throughout many invasive carcinomas in the form of pink-staining, rounded, lamellated "pearls." These epithelial pearls are not characteristic of carcinoma in situ; however, they are seen in some other forms of cancer such as basal cell carcinoma.

Cells present at the deep invasive tumor front have different molecular and morphological characteristics than those in superficial areas of the tumor. For this reason, several studies have shown that the deep invasive tumor front is the most important area of the tumor for prognostication [2, 3]. Bryne et al. proposed a scoring system that excludes the evaluation of luminal areas of the tumor, demonstrating the prognostic value of grading the deep invasive front. They found that the most important events pertaining to invasion and distant spread occur in this area, and devised a scoring system with high prognostic value. This scoring system assesses cell differentiation, pattern of invasion, and host immune response expressed by peritumoral inflammation [4]. Byrne et al. reported a strong correlation between the total malignancy grade and prognosis in glottic carcinoma. Subsequently, Kurokawa et al. and others used multivariate analysis to support the predictive value of invasive front grading (IFG) in association with the prognosis and survival rates in oral squamous cell carcinoma [5–7]. IFG was shown to provide useful prognostic information when selecting the most appropriate treatment modalities in both glottic and oral cavity squamous cell carcinoma studies [6].

Risk Factors

Etiologic factors and other pathologic agents have been implicated and have an important role in prognosis. Tobacco use, especially in conjunction with alcohol abuse has been the best supported etiologic factor in HNSCCA in the oral cavity and larynx. Over 75% of head and neck squamous cell carcinoma (HNSCC) patients are long-time tobacco users, and many of them ingest alcoholic beverages regularly [8]. The fact that alcohol promotes the carcinogenic effects of tobacco is well established. Numerous studies have found that smoking confers a several fold increased risk of developing HNSCC. Blot and colleagues found a 1.9-fold risk in males and 3.0-fold risk in females [9]. For HNSCC, the cancer risk is directly proportional to the amount of tobacco consumed, measured in pack-years. Compared with nondrinkers, males who consume 1–2 drinks per day have a 1.7-fold HNSCC cancer risk. This risk for heavy drinkers is more than 3.0-fold. Individuals who smoke (2 packs per day) and drink (4 units of alcohol per day) have a multiplicative increase in risk with an odds ratio of 35 for the development of HNSCC, compared to controls [9]. Smokeless tobacco confers approximately a 4.0-fold risk of oral cavity SCCA. When HNSCC is caused by these factors, resulting tumors are often very invasive and can respond poorly to even the most aggressive trimodal therapies, including surgery, radiation, and chemotherapies.

An increasing number of studies suggest that comorbidity is an important prognostic indicator of mortality among head and neck cancer patients [10]. Reid et al. used the American Society of Anesthesiologists'(ASA) class to measure comorbidity for research and clinical purposes and in comparison to the previously validated Charlson index [11]. The ASA class had comparable or even greater prognostic ability for mortality as assessed by multivariate analyses and retained prognostic ability well beyond the peri-operative period. Their study supported the use of the ASA class as a measure of comorbidity and prognostic factor for elderly patient undergoing surgical therapy for HNSCCA.

Some tumors may be described as more indolent due to their relatively predictable response to standard therapies. In 1999, Koch et al. identified distinctive clinical categories in HNSCC patients when comparing groups of nonsmokers with smokers [8]. They found that nonsmokers were more likely to present at extremes of age (old or young), to be female, and to have oral cavity tumors. In this study, they noted that most tumors of the larynx and hypopharynx arose in smokers or former smokers. Additionally, molecular alteration patterns in the tumors of smokers have been found to be distinct from those of nonsmokers. Smokers were more likely to have tumors with p53 mutation, LOH at chromosomes 3p, 4q, and 11q13, and a higher overall percentage of chromosomal microsatellite alterations [8].

The human papilloma virus (HPV) is an epitheliotropic virus detected in samples of oropharyngeal squamous cell carcinoma. Infection alone is not sufficient for malignant conversion; however, results of multiple studies have shown that HPV has an etiologic role in a subset of head and neck squamous cell carcinoma. The rate of HPV DNA presence is slightly higher in the tumors of nonsmokers. Patients with HPV-related tumors are more likely to be nonsmokers and of younger age than the traditional smoker-drinker HNSCC patient. Detailed analyses of tumors for HPV genomic DNA and viral oncogene expression in case–control studies have indicated that HPV infection is nearly exclusively associated with HNSCC of the oropharynx, where it is observed in 40–60% of patients. HPV-positive oropharyngeal tumors are clinically and molecularly distinct.

Analyses of retrospective case series have consistently demonstrated that patients with HPV-positive tumors have a better prognosis than patients whose tumors are HPV negative. This subject is more fully developed in a subsequent chapter. Retrospective survival assessment, though, may be limited by relatively poor quality of collected data and the absence of information on confounding factors of known prognostic value. Recently, Fakhry et al. reported their evaluation of the effect of tumor HPV status on treatment response and survival outcomes among a prospectively collected series of patients with oropharyngeal or laryngeal squamous cell carcinoma [12]. The study participants were uniformly treated with induction chemotherapy and chemoradiation as participants in a phase II trial conducted by the Eastern Cooperative Oncology Group (ECOG). They reported improved survival outcomes for patients with HPV-positive HNSCC and increased tumor sensitivity to chemotherapy and chemoradiation. Several hypotheses have been proposed to explain these differences, including the absence of field cancerization, effective immune surveillance to viral-specific tumor antigens, and an intact apoptotic response to radiation. Because of this distinct tumor behavior, some researchers have proposed a reduction in the intensity of standard therapy in HPV positive disease to reduce the comorbidities caused by chemotherapy and external been radiation therapy. They also propose a modification to the current staging system to include HPV status. These concepts are currently under investigation.

Other proposed etiologic influences include the proximity of tissue to mechanical irritation, thermal injury, and/or chemical exposure. Environmental ultraviolet light exposure has been associated with the development of lip cancer as well as skin SCCA. Solar exposure has been implicated in the pathogenesis of squamous cell carcinomas arising on the vermilion border of the lower lip, and skin of the nose, scalp, and upper auricles. Other entities associated with SCCA include Plummer–Vinson syndrome (achlorhydria; iron deficiency anemia; and mucosal atrophy of the mouth, pharynx, and esophagus), chronic infection with syphilis, ill-fitting dentures, and long-term immunosuppression (30-fold increase with renal transplant).

Within the oral cavity various benign appearing lesions have some propensity for premalignancy. Leukoplakia, a white mucosal lesion, may occur due to hyperkeratosis and dysplasia. These changes have been estimated to have a variable malignant transformation rate. Erythroplakia is a red appearing lesion of the mucosal surface. The red color is due to increased vascularity due to angiogenesis, which portends a higher likelihood of malignancy than leukoplakia.

A separate class of white lesion, which is a distinct entity, is lichen planus. This is a common affliction, likely of autoimmune inflammatory or multifactorial origin. It has been described as either being (1) induced by drugs or dental materials; (2) associated with chronic liver or other disorders; or (3) idiopathic with immunopathogenesis involving T-cells in particular [13]. The characteristic lesions are most commonly found on the lateral tongue and the buccal mucosa. Lesions are classified as reticular, plaque-like, atrophic, papular, erosive, and bullous. They are characterized by white or gray strands forming a linear or reticular pattern on a violaceous background. Erosive lesions have a shallow, red, ulcerative center. Lichen planus has been found to have a 1% risk of malignant transformation overall, however, rates have been found to be higher in men [14, 15].

Nodal Basin Involvement

Regional metastasis to cervical lymph nodes (LN) occurs commonly, and is often the location of treatment failure or recurrence in HNSCC. At the time of primary tumor presentation the presence and size of cervical LN metastases, quantified by N-stage, is the most accurate predictor of cancer-related outcome (in the absence of distant metastases). The presence of LN metastases reduces disease-related survival per primary site and stage by 50% [1]. Lymph node metastases are undetectable using any means for the first month or even for years. Undetectable nodal disease is termed "occult". Because of the high propensity and danger of occult disease in cervical nodes, standard regimens for all but the earliest cancers include some form of treatment for the neck. Depending on tumor site and likely location of metastases, treatment may be therapeutic or elective and include neck dissection or radiation. When LN metastases are clinically evident, (N+ disease), the path of disease spread is obvious and treatment can be tailored accordingly.

Radiographic imaging is limited with respect to the ability to identify occult metastases in the cN0 setting. Imaging modalities, including MRI and PET/CT are increasingly more sensitive, but may sacrifice specificity. They are not as accurate as histologic evaluation of malignancy. Neck palpation alone has reported error rate of 20–50%. Analysis of the neck dissection specimen is the most definitive determination of nodal status of the neck. END (Elective neck dissection) provides pathologic staging of the neck, which permits better estimates of patient prognosis. Without clinical or radiologic evidence of cervical LN metastasis the patient is staged as clinically N0 (cN0). In this setting, lymphatic metastases may exist but are too small for radiological or clinical detection. In cN0 cases, there are three therapeutic options; (1) clinical observation; (2) elective neck dissection; and (3) elective neck irradiation. Clinical observation, sometimes referred to as watchful waiting, is the active process of repeated clinical examinations at regularly scheduled intervals. In that paradigm, surgical neck dissection is reserved for those who subsequently develop regional metastases.

Extensive literature exists indicating the likelihood of occult involvement of lymph nodes based on the site and stage of the primary lesion. These estimates are derived from studies of the rate of nodal involvement at the time of neck dissection or after long-term follow-up [16–18]. Anatomic, radiologic, and pathologic investigations of neck dissection specimens have corroborated the classical clinical study by Lindberg published in 1972 [19, 20]. These studies and others have shown that, for example, neck levels II, III, and IV are at greatest risk for metastases from carcinomas of the oropharynx, larynx, and hypopharynx. In addition, the prevalence of level V involvement is low (2–7%), and always lower in a clinically N0 neck compared with a clinically positive neck. In supraglottic and subglottic HNSCC, the risk for regional metastasis is around 50%. This risk is even higher for hypopharyngeal carcinomas. Conversely, this risk in glottic HNSCC is only 25–40%, even for advanced stage (T4) tumors. In addition to surveillance for ipsilateral spread, an appropriate level of suspicion for contralateral metastatic disease must be maintained. Sites such as the soft palate, tongue base, and supraglottis have the highest density of crossing lymph channels. Because of this, approximately 20% of patients with soft palate or tongue base disease already have contralateral cervical lymph node metastases at the time of presentation. Based on anatomic site, tumor stage, and histopathologic characteristics of the primary, a cervical metastatic risk of at least 15–20% is generally accepted as an indication for treatment. For clinically N0 disease, this criterion includes all stages of T3 and some T2 supraglottic and hypopharyngeal carcinomas, T3 and many T2 oral cavity carcinomas, and carcinomas of the tongue thicker than 3 mm.

In light of the estimated risk, elective treatment may be planned for the clinically negative neck. (END) is not only therapeutic, but also a part of the staging process. Pathologic examination of the neck dissection specimen allows for meticulous investigation of each cervical node to understand the extent of disease spread and predict prognosis. Subclinical or occult metastases may be detected on pathologic examination of neck dissection specimens. This is perhaps the most important type of discordance between the clinical and pathologic nodal stages (Koch et al.).

Elective neck irradiation (ENI) is another option that delivers therapy to all possibly affected neck levels. It is often undertaken when radiation is chosen as treatment modality for the primary tumor. These active forms of treatment have expected sequelae such as postoperative pain, stiffness and numbness, or postradiation xerostomia. For many years these management options have been debated among head and neck surgeons. As significant advances in imaging, surgical technique, radiation methods, and innovative chemotherapy options continue, controversy about their best applications persists. Even the most basic questions, such as when to use elective neck dissection in cN0 disease are not wholly agreed upon. As recently as 2003 and 2004, large surveys among board certified otolaryngologist in the US demonstrate great differences in the preferred treatment for cN0 cases.

Multiple factors contribute to the controversy over management of the N0 neck. Studies that compare END to observation of cN0 patients are limited to retrospective reviews not suitable for meta-analysis. Prospective studies with adequate statistical power do not exist, thus preventing the demonstration of statistically significant survival differences among patients managed with END and those not treated. Due to clinical constraints of the very large sample size needed to show statistically significant differences, it is unlikely that prospective randomized trials will ever conclusively resolve the controversy.

Molecular Biology Basics

Cancer is a genetic disease. This does not imply inheritance, but rather that agents that bring about malignant transformation of a cell in the foundational step of tumorigenesis do so by affecting change in the tumor DNA. This may be by alteration in the base sequence (through mutation, deletion, insertion, or rearrangement), change in copy number of a chromosomal segment (through duplication, larger segment deletion, and loss of heterozygosity) alterations in the level at which a gene is transcribed through rearrangements that bring the gene into new association with promoter regions, or through epigenetic events, including hypermethylation of promoter regions, which block expression of mRNA into protein. In order for a genetic or epigenetic alteration to contribute to the malignant state, it must permanently confer some behavior intrinsic to the cancer phenotype while not triggering immune surveillance, apoptosis, or cell cycle arrest leading to correction of the aberrant phenomenon.

Genetic alterations that convey a survival and/or proliferation advantage to a single cell facilitate a phenomenon called "clonal expansion". In clonal expansion, a more altered cell is able to divide, producing daughter cells sharing the same growth advantages. Eventually, the population of altered cells arising from the original cell and sharing its DNA (clonal population) constitutes the predominate proportion of the cells in an area. With the loss of control on polarity of orientation and cell–cell inhibition through contact with neighbors, the clonal population begins to develop an unusual arrangement of cells that will eventually be recognizable as tumor through phenotypic phenomena such as mass effect or thickness.

Clonal expansion can be used to explain a well-known clinical phenomenon called "field cancerization". This concept is attributed to Slaughter, who in the 1950s pointed out that many HNSCC patients develop second cancers within the upper aerodigestive tract [22]. The intervening mucosa may have dysplastic changes even when it appears to be uninvolved on visual inspection. Biopsies of normal mucosa around oral malignancies have been shown to display genetic and epigenetic alterations that are also found within the nearby cancer, but not present in tissue from a distant site in the body. Again, the relative growth advantage conferred by early alterations in a cell along with increased motility allows the partially transformed cell to overtake its neighbors and replace the population found at distance around an index cancer with clonally related precancerous cells. In clonal expansion, early DNA alterations may also predispose the cell to accumulate additional alterations, rendering it a fertile ground for more rapid progress toward a more malignant appearance and behavior. Additional alterations add further malignant characteristics such as angiogenesis, invasive capability, and motility for migration.

Since the earliest days of molecular biologic investigation of cancer, it has been hypothesized that many genetic alterations are required to produce a fully transformed tumor cell. Knudsen's hypothesis proposed that at least two alterations were required, altering both copies of key genes such as the Retinoblastoma (Rb) gene [23]. In cases of inherited cancer, one aberrant DNA copy came from a carrier parent. Early in life a second event results in the loss or alteration of the second copy initiating the malignant transformation cascade. The discovery of oncogenes (which add to the malignant phenotype through increased activity or expression) and tumor suppressor genes (the loss of whose function contributes to tumorigenesis through the removal of controls) followed with identification of a number of tumor-specific candidates such as p53, PTEN, ras, myc, BRAF, DCC, etc. A lull in discovery of well characterized tumor-related genes turned attention toward surrogate markers of genetic change such as tumor-specific loss of critical portions of DNA (loss of heterozygosity, LOH) presumed to include key tumor suppressor genes. Recent efforts in the laboratory of Bert Vogelstein, to sequence the entire genome of breast and colon cancer have reinforced earlier estimates of multiple tumor-specific alterations selected from over 100 candidates in individual cancers. Some of these alterations are common to many tumors in the population (so called "hills" of alterations in the sequencing histograms) and others are less commonly altered "mounds". This large number of alterations provides ample opportunity for phenotypic heterogeneity to account for the observed variation in tumor appearance and behavior within and between clinical categories [24].

Genetic alterations are maintained within a tumor, and can be used as markers for tumor detection and surveillance. Genetic alterations accumulate within the clonal population, producing ever-more altered subpopulations within the region of the initial event. Heterogeneity within a tumor can be analyzed by sampling different regions, amplifying DNA through PCR and comparing the profile of changes present. Alterations that produce more marked phenotypic change contributing to tumor appearance will be present in biopsies of the tumor, while those conveying less obvious change may be present in the normal appearing periphery.

In a similar fashion, epigenetic alterations may be tumor-specific and may be maintained throughout the process of clonal expansion and tumorigenesis, contributing to the cancer phenotype by the abrogation of tumor-suppressor function. Microarray technology permits the screening of the entire spectrum of promoter regions within the genome with a resultant assessment of the "methylome" that is present within cancer. A large scale screening of the methylome of various types of cancer cell lines and primary tumors has been reported recently. Some 200 methylated candidate genes were identified of which cancer-specific methylation was confirmed by sequencing in 28. A panel of 8 of these targets was used to probe 300 primary tumors and at least one altered target was present in each sample [25].

Another approach to the global assessment of genetic alterations present in a tumor is comparative genomic hybridization (CGH). CGH detects large-scale DNA sequence copy number aberrations through the hybridization of chromosomal material from tumor compared with normal reference DNA. Regions of amplification and deletion are tabulated. Noutomi and colleagues have used CGH to describe two distinct types of oral SCC and surrounding dysplasia, those with small and large numbers of DNA sequence copy number aberrations. They postulate that the underlying events that determine this feature are early and formative, representing distinct genetic pathways [26].

Several viruses that infect humans have been implicated in tumorigenesis with unique and specific clinical features in the upper aerodigestive tract. The Human Papillomavirus (HPV) and particularly its oncogenic strains (HPV-16, 18 and others) when integrated into epithelial cells in the lymphoepithelium of the lingual and palatine tonsils contributes to the development of HPV-related SCC demonstrating basaloid squamous histology and a propensity for early metastasis often with cystic lymph nodes. HPV DNA encodes two proteins, E6 and E7 which bind and inactivate critical tumor suppressor gene products, p53 and Rb, respectively. This binding abrogates the function of p53 and Rb acting in lieu of their mutation or deletion to contribute to the cancer phenotype. The downstream ramification of HPV infection may be less disruptive than mutation to the network of pathways in which p53 and Rb play a role, resulting in a somewhat better clinical response to therapy and outcome for cancers arising in the setting of HPV infection as compared to genetic disruption associated with alcohol and tobacco use [27]. Similarly, Epstein Barr Virus (EBV) is present in many cases of nasopharyngeal cancer world-wide.

The reason for the distinctive site specificity for HPV and EBV related HNSCC is unknown. The fact that the vast majority of HPV-related cancers arise in the tonsils (lingual and palatine) and that these tumors have other distinctive clinical features is the strongest rationale to date to support the concept that HNSCC is actually comprised of several distinctive pathophysiologic entities. In our series investigating the presence of HPV in HNSCC, several cases originally classified as oral cavity and laryngeal in origin could be correctly reclassified as base of tongue or palatine tonsil tumors when further investigation uncovered data from previous outside records. This observation further strengthened the impression of the uniformity of clinical correlates in HPV tonsil cancer.

There are other distinctive subforms of HNSCC that can be partially defined by patient demographics and exposure history. Perhaps most obvious of these is the formation of lateral tongue cancer in younger, nonsmoking patients. This phenom enon has been recognized for many years, but is becoming, perhaps, more obvious with the relative decline of the once-common presentation of oral cancer in the smoker–drinker. Efforts to demonstrate a molecular correlate in the nonsmoker-lateral tongue CA group have thus far been met with frustration. Using single-nucleotide polymorphism chip analysis, no significant differences were demonstrated between tongue tumors from young nonsmokers and older smokers [28]. Young nonsmokers with tongue cancer tend to do either very well with simple excision, or to have very aggressive and persistent disease with poor prognosis. A small fraction of the cases with progressive disease may have Fanconi's anemia [29]. Elderly (>75 years of age) patients with HNSCC also demonstrate unique clinical themes. Cancers of the buccal mucosa and maxillary alveolus are more common in these individuals than in their younger counterparts.

Comparative Profiles of Phenotype and Genotype Contribute to Tumor Progression Models

Estimating the relative timing of genetic alteration accumulation: The specific profile of accumulated genetic, epigenetic, and viral disruptions in a clonal population of cells may result in variations in tumor virulence and behavior. While some alterations may produce conditions favorable to the accumulation of further disruptions, the relative order of accumulated alterations may also be somewhat variable. Comparison of populations of tumors looking at the spectrum of alterations supports this idea in that not all tumors of the same histology display even the most common genetic alterations. For example, only slightly more than one half of all HNSCC have a mutation in TP53 while 90% or more have alterations in p16.

An understanding of the relative order of genetic and epigenetic alterations seen in the general population of HNSCC may be useful in several ways. First, it may provide clues to the mechanism by which clonal progression occurs on the way to eventual full-blown malignancy. Early alterations that provide clonal growth advantage are also likely to produce susceptibility to further disruption. In addition, early alterations may be the most common and thereby serve as the best target for chemoprevention or early therapeutic intervention. Moreover, early alterations are likely the best candidates for strategies aimed at the early detection of cancer. Later alterations, on the other hand, are more likely to be found in some but not all cancers, and may account for variations in clinical presentation and behavior. Later alterations may serve as better prognostic factors and targets for therapeutic intervention aimed at a particular subset of tumors.

One approach to estimate the relative order in which tumor-specific alterations occur within a population of tumors is to compare the relative frequency of the alterations in groups of lesions clustered along the clinical progression pathway. In general, then, HNSCC which affects the upper aerodigestive tract mucosa may begin with clinically unapparent change in the mucosa, moving on to hyperplasia, dysplasia, carcinoma in situ, and eventually invasive cancer. Laboratory investigation of genetic alterations using a variety of methods may contribute to a data set that can be used to produce a molecular tumor progression model for HNSCC. Alterations that occur frequently in early lesions, without becoming increasingly more common in advanced cases are likely to have occurred early in the course of tumorigenesis. Other alterations that occur infrequently in early lesions and become progressively more common in later cases represent later events in a tumorigenesis model. Several factors enhance the value of data from investigations of this sort. The larger the number of specimens examined using the same approach and technique, the more useful the results were . Lesions that are clinically well characterized and clearly categorized are of the greatest value. Premalignant regions surrounding an invasive cancer may be used, but may be misleading compared to truly independent premalignant lesions. That is because clonal expansion and field cancer change could result in a tail or rim of a subclone around an invasive lesion that is not actually the original earliest clonal population.

Studies investigating the frequency of specific genetic alterations in HNSCC and premalignant lesions from the upper aerodigestive tract include those focused on p53 protein staining and gene mutation, microsatellite alterations (loss of heterozygosity or shift), cytogenetic alterations, and epigenetic changes (promoter hypermethyaltion). Lippman et al. showed p53 protein stained by IHC in 90% cases of oral leukoplakia, compared with no staining in normal oral mucosa [30] Lesions that stained with p53 in the parabasal layer had a higher likelihood of progression to cancer [31]. The correlation between p53 protein overexpression and gene mutation is good, but not 100%. Boyle et al. have shown that gene mutation also increases as tumors progress from premalignant to invasive phenotype [32]. They compared the percentage of lesions containing mutations in 65 primary invasive carcinomas and 37 noninvasive specimens consisting of 13 severe dysplasias and 24 carcinoma in situ lesions. The incidence of p53 mutations in noninvasive lesions was 19% (7/37) and increased to 43% (28/65) in invasive carcinomas. These studies suggest that p53 overexpression occurs early in H&N tumorigenesis, but gene mutation appears to be an intermediate to late event.

Mutations of the TP53 gene have been used to further categorize HNSCC patients. The spectrum of base pair change in TP53 mutation was noted to be different between smoker and nonsmoker groups with more G–C transitions at CpG islands in the nonsmokers [33]. This finding was interpreted as arising from different mutational pressure with spontaneous mutation occurring, albeit infrequently, in nonsmokers without the presence of the more common carcinogenic effects of cigarette smoke. Recent analysis of a large ($n = 420$) cohort of HNSCC patients enrolled in a cooperative group study demonstrated that TP53 mutation could be meaningfully categorized as "disruptive" (of protein function) and "nondisruptive" on the basis of the biochemical effect of the resulting amino acid substitution and its location within the p53 protein. Mutations that resulted in amino acid change from polar to nonpolar, or charged to noncharged moieties, occurring within the DNA binding domain, or that resulted in truncation or complete abrogation of protein production were classified as disruptive. The clinical outcome (overall and disease-free survival) of cases with disruptive TP53 mutation was significantly poorer (HR = 1.87) than that of patients with wild-type and nondisruptive mutant

TP53 [34]. These mutation-based categories may be helpful in the future as attempts are made to deliver tumor-specific tailored therapy.

The Epidermal growth factor receptor (EGFR) is overexpressed in most (up to 90%) HNSCC. It is a member of the ErbB/HER family of receptor tyrosine kinases, and acts in signal transduction, playing a key role in a number of cancer phenotypic functions including growth, invasion, angiogenesis, and metastasis. The genetic mechanism behind EGFR overexpression in HNSCC is incompletely understood. Production of mRNA for EGFR is elevated in most cancers, while protein overexpression occurs in somewhat less than one half of the cases [35]. The degree of expression increases in general from dysplasia to invasive cancer [36]. Several factors seem to contribute to increased EGFR mRNA synthesis, including amplification and polymorphisms in dinucleotide repeats in intron 1 of the EGFR gene, but mutation of EGFR is rare [37]. While an important factor in HNSCC activity, the place of EGFR in molecular epidemiology is not well understood.

Mitochondria contain a genome separate from that of the host nuclear material and can display tumor-associated alterations which may play a role in tumorigenesis as well as serving as markers for malignant cells. A recent report indicates that nearly 50% of a population of 83 HSCC lesions contained MtDNA mutations in noncoding D loop and coding regions. Margins of dysplasia around invasive cancers showed identical mitochondrial mutations. Furthermore, the presence of mitochondrial mutations correlated with p53 mutations in the population [38]. When the mitochondrial genome from 137 premalignant head and neck lesions from 93 patients was studied, a hot-spot of alteration was discovered in the C-tract. There was an increase in the incidence of C-tract alterations from hyperplasia to dysplasia to carcinoma in situ. Mitochondrial alterations found in synchronous and metachronous lesions from the same patients showed a clonal relationship in most cases [39]. Subsequently, simply the overall content of mitochondrial DNA present in premalignant and malignant HNSCC was found to vary. The mean CoxI/β-actin DNA ratio for mild, moderate, and severe dysplasia progressed from 0.0529 to 0.0607 and then to 0.1201, while invasive cancers showed a mean ratio of 0.1667. These differences were modestly significant ($p = 0.04$). The authors admit that this may be a measure of relative DNA injury rather than of genetic alteration [40].

Loss of heterozygosity of DNA in regions of putative tumor suppressor genes in HNSCC was intensely investigated in the 1990s. Califano and colleagues showed that an increased rate of 10 LOH loci correlated with histopathologic tumor progression [41] with more histopathologically advanced areas exhibiting additional genetic alterations. Others subsequently showed that LOH of markers on chromosomal arms 3p and 9p were particularly indicative of increased risk of malignant transformation [42, 43]. 3p and 9p loss carried a 3.8-fold increased risk of tumor progression. The presence of additional LOH at any of a number of other loci increased the likelihood of progression markedly, to a relative risk of 33 for malignant transformation. This data is perhaps the most powerful example of molecular prognostic potential in HNSCC. The presence of LOH of key loci indicates a high degree of likelihood of tumor progression independent of the histologic grade of the epithelium. Furthermore, less aggressive types of HNSCC (verrucous, papillary, and well-differentiated) have lower levels of LOH of key chromosomal segments compared with more aggressive histologic types (basaloid, sarcomatoid, and poorly-differentiated) [44].

Similar results were found when premalignant and invasive lesions were examined for the presence of microsatellite shifts (instability) (MSI). Two of 34 hyperplasias studied (6%) had MSI compared to 2/12 mild dysplasias (17%), 7/26 high grade dyplasias (27%), and 6/18 invasive cancers (33%) [45].

Regions of dysplasia that surround or abut invasive upper aerodigestive tract cancers are common. These areas of less advanced disease are part of the field effect well known to exist in HNSCC. El–Naggar and associates report shared foci of MSI between invasive lesions and surrounding dysplasia. Similar to Ha's findings, dysplastic regions showed one half the rate of MSI (15 vs. 30%) compared to related invasive cancer [46]. LOH and MSI are also found in the stroma surrounding invasive HNSCC as demonstrated when stromal elements were isolated by laser capture microdissection [47].

Chromosome 9p is the loci containing the putative tumor suppressor gene p16, which plays a critical role in the Rb cell cycle control pathway. Most HNSCC samples have a loss of p16 activity, either through LOH, mutation, or hypermethylation of the p16 promoter region [48]. Promoter hypermethylation is an epigenetic mechanism that abrogates the function of genes through inactivation of transcription. This occurs when CpG-rich regions of certain gene promoters are methylated altering histone complexes. For example, methylation of RAR-β2 has been shown to be present in over 50% of oral leukoplakic lesions [49], perhaps contributing to tumor progression.

New approaches (microarrays) to assess entire genome-patterns: Powerful tools such as microarrays have been developed to screen the entire genome for molecular alterations. One of these is cDNA microarrays, platforms that can be used to compare samples from similar tumors looking for differences in the genetic expression profile of each in order to identify potential markers or patterns of difference between them. Sophisticated statistical methods have been developed to detect clustering of altered expression in an attempt to make sense of the vast array of data derived from this approach. Primary cultures of dysplasias, invasive cancers, and normal epithelium have been studied using Affymetrix U133A and B chips and results analyzed using spectral clustering, singular value decomposition, and other techniques showing that invasive cancers display transcriptional changes not found in associated areas of dysplasia. High grade dysplasias more closely resemble invasive cancers [50]. Studies such as these require very sophisticated statistical methods and defy attempts to draw inferences based on intuitively transparent simple comparison. The chosen comparative paradigm must be derived using a training set of samples followed by application to an independent test set in order to validate the findings.

Carinci et al. compared the genetic expression profile of dysplastic tongue lesions compared with tumors with and without metastases and normal controls [51]. Hierarchical agglomerative clustering methods were applied to data from 6,026 clones in their microarray. 105 clones were found to have significantly different levels of expression between dysplastic lesions and tumors without metastases, while 570 clones differed between invasive tumors with and without metastases. In silico analysis sought genes that coded for known oncogenes, transcription factors and cell cycle regulators as potential markers of progression and metastases. Studies such as these are exploratory, and much further work is required to validate the different levels of expression and further evaluate the candidate genes identified to strengthen the level of interest that exists for in depth study of each. Other approaches using microarrays have been used to try to develop a profile indicative of metastatic phenotype. In one such study, differential expression of 301 genes was identified comparing primary tumors with cervical node metastases [52].

Another approach to genome-wide screening to identify differences between categorized HNSCC and premalignant lesions uses comparative genomic hybridization, a sophisticated DNA hybridization technique. This approach can detect large scale DNA copy number aberrations. Once again, additional genetic alterations are typically seen in fully invasive regions of tumor samples compared with adjacent premalignant (dysplastic) regions [26]. Microarray CGH has been used to compare tumors with and without HPV16. Four regions had alterations in HPV-negative tumors that were absent in HPV-positive lesions, including losses at 18q, 3p, and 9p as well as gains at 11q [53]. This result coincides with other studies comparing tumors arising from environmental carcinogen exposure with those attributed to HPV-16 with a common theme of greater genetic alteration complexity in the HPV-negative population.

Prognosis and Genetic Profile

The presence of tumor-specific genetic and epigenetic alterations in various tissue samples can serve as a means to detect the presence of cancer or precancerous lesions. Molecular detection using saliva and serum have been investigated extensively. Saliva contains sloughed epithelial cells as well as naked DNA released when tumor cells undergo apoptosis. Serum also can contain circulating tumor cells as well as naked tumor DNA. These different compartments may contain differing profiles of normal DNA. Lymphocytic DNA can serve as a normal control for both, but the presence of very early genetic and epigenetic alterations may be indicative of field cancerization rather than of the presence of cancer, making the interpretation of molecular detection results somewhat problematic.

Using a panel of 23 microsatellite alterations as genetic markers, we were able to identify cancer-specific signals in oral rinse samples harvested before treatment, from the great majority of cancer patients. 86% of cases had at least one microsatellite alteration present from the panel in tumor samples, and of those with alterations in the tumor, 90% could be detected in the saliva rinse [54]. Presence of tumor-specific microsatellite alterations in serum from advanced-staged cancer patients was detected in a subset and was associated with a higher rate of distant metastasis and death due to disease [55].

However, microsatellite analysis is labor intensive, and for this reason efforts to develop a high-throughput platform for molecular detection of cancer has progressed to the use of promoter hypermethylation. Hypermethylation can be detected using a PCR based fluorescent release assay, quantitative methylation-specific PCR (QMSP). We have developed a panel of methylation targets that can detect cancer cells in oral rinses of the majority of HNSCC patients but are not present in cells sloughed from the oral cavity of healthy control subjects [56]. These panels show promise for the early detection of recurrent cancer in patients during surveillance after initial treatment for cancer, and may, in time, permit wide-spread de novo screening of populations at risk for cancer. The use of a molecular screening paradigm for cancer will require low cost, high sensitivity, and very high specificity. Furthermore, the signal must be associated with some clinically detectable mucosal change in order for screening to result in early cancer detection. If, instead, a positive cancer signal may be found from persons with very early, occult pre-cancer, the only course of action would be more careful serial surveillance studies (physical exam, PET scanning).

Microarray analysis of saliva from HNSCC patients compared with controls was able to identify over 1,500 RNA species that were differentially present in the tumor population. Further study focused on seven cancer-related mRNA markers that displayed at least a 3.5-fold elevation in the cancer group, which serve as potential biomarkers for further evaluation [57].

Conclusion

Traditional methods for cancer detection, evaluation and staging, prognostication, and treatment selection remain the most reliable and consistently useful. The advent of molecular evaluation of cancer promised revolutionary enhancements in these endeavors, but with the exception of HPV detection, molecular markers have yet to prove of substantial utility in tumor management. It appears that the complexity of the inner workings of a cancer cell as well as the complex series of interactions of the cancer cell with its host are sufficient to frustrate the application of single gene alterations in paradigms of clinical cancer management. Ever more sophisticated tools permit more in depth and increasingly broad assessment of the cancer molecular milieu, allowing hope to grow that clinically relevant breakthroughs are forthcoming.

References

1. Bailey BJ, Johnson JT, Newlands S (2006) Head and neck surgery – otolaryngology, 3rd edn. Lippincot, Williams, and Wilkins, Philadelphia
2. Bryne M, Koppang HS, Lilleng R, Stene T, Bang G, Dabelsteen E (1989) New malignancy grading is a better prognostic indicator than broders' grading in oral squamous cell carcinomas. J Oral Pathol Med 18:432–437

3. Bryne M, Jenssen N, Boysen M (1995) Histological grading in the deep invasive front of T1 and T2 glottic squamous cell carcinomas has high prognostic value. Virchows Arch 427:277–281
4. Fonseca I, Pereira T, Rosa-Santos J, Soares J (2001) Expression of CD44 isoforms in squamous cell carcinoma of the border of the tongue: a correlation with histological grade, pattern of stromal invasion, and cell differentiation. J Surg Oncol 76:115–120
5. Bankfalvi A, Piffko J (2000) Prognostic and predictive factors in oral cancer: the role of the invasive tumour front. J Oral Pathol Med 29:291–298
6. Kurokawa H, Zhang M, Matsumoto S et al (2005) The high prognostic value of the histologic grade at the deep invasive front of tongue squamous cell carcinoma. J Oral Pathol Med 34:329–333
7. Piffko J, Bankfalvi A, Ofner D et al (1997) Prognostic value of histobiological factors (malignancy grading and AgNOR content) assessed at the invasive tumour front of oral squamous cell carcinomas. Br J Cancer 75:1543–1546
8. Koch WM, Lango M, Sewell D, Zahurak M, Sidransky D (1999) Head and neck cancer in nonsmokers: a distinct clinical and molecular entity. Laryngoscope 109:1544–1551
9. Blot WJ, McLaughlin JK, Winn DM et al (1988) Smoking and drinking in relation to oral and pharyngeal cancer. Cancer Res 48:3282–3287
10. Piccirillo JF, Wells CK, Sasaki CT, Feinstein AR (1994) New clinical severity staging system for cancer of the larynx. five-year survival rates. Ann Otol Rhinol Laryngol 103:83–92
11. Reid BC, Alberg AJ, Klassen AC, Koch WM, Samet JM (2001) The american society of anesthesiologists' class as a comorbidity index in a cohort of head and neck cancer surgical patients. Head Neck 23:985–994
12. Fakhry C, Westra WH, Li S et al (2008) Improved survival of patients with human papillomavirus-positive head and neck squamous cell carcinoma in a prospective clinical trial. J Natl Cancer Inst 100:261–269
13. Chuang TY, Stitle L, Brashear R, Lewis C (1999) Hepatitis C virus and lichen planus: a case–control study of 340 patients. J Am Acad Dermatol 41:787–789
14. Chuang T, Sittle L. Lichen Planus. http://www.emedicine.com/DERM/topic233.htm#section~References.
15. Scully C, Beyli M, Ferreiro MC et al (1998) Update on oral lichen planus: etiopathogenesis and management. Crit Rev Oral Biol Med 9:86–122
16. Byers RM, Weber RS, Andrews T, McGill D, Kare R, Wolf P (1997) Frequency and therapeutic implications of "skip metastases" in the neck from squamous carcinoma of the oral tongue. Head Neck 19:14–19
17. Cummings CW, Flint PW (2005) Otolaryngology head & neck surgery, 4th edn. Mosby, Philadelphia, p 2614
18. Clayman GL, Frank DK (1998) Selective neck dissection of anatomically appropriate levels is as efficacious as modified radical neck dissection for elective treatment of the clinically negatice neck in patients with squamous cell carcinoma of the upper respiratory and digestive tracts. Arch Otolaryngol Head Neck Surg 124:348–352
19. Barkley HT Jr, Fletcher GH, Jesse RH, Lindberg RD (1972) Management of cervical lymph node metastases in squamous cell carcinoma of the tonsillar fossa, base of tongue, supraglottic larynx, and hypopharynx. Am J Surg 124:462–467
20. Lindberg R (1972) Distribution of cervical lymph node metastases from squamous cell carcinoma of the upper respiratory and digestive tracts. Cancer 29:1446–1449
21. Kutler DI, Wong RJ, Schoder H, Kraus DH (2006) The current status of positron-emission tomography scanning in the evaluation and follow-up of patients with head and neck cancer. Curr Opin Otolaryngol Head Neck Surg 14:73–81
22. Slaughter DP, Southwick HW, Smejka W (1953) "Field cancerization" in oral stratified squamous epithelium. Cancer 6:963–968
23. Knudsen A (1971) Mutation and cancer: statistical study of retinoblastoma. Proc Natl Acad Sci U S A 68(4):820–823

24. Wood LD, Parsons DW, Jones S, Lin J, Sjöblom T, Leary RJ, Shen D, Boca SM, Barber T, Ptak J, Silliman N, Szabo S, Dezso Z, Ustyanksky V, Nikolskaya T, Nikolsky Y, Karchin R, Wilson PA, Kaminker JS, Zhang Z, Croshaw R, Willis J, Dawson D, Shipitsin M, Willson JK, Sukumar S, Polyak K, Park BH, Pethiyagoda CL, Pant PV, Ballinger DG, Sparks AB, Hartigan J, Smith DR, Suh E, Papadopoulos N, Buckhaults P, Markowitz SD, Parmigiani G, Kinzler KW, Velculescu VE, Vogelstein B (2007) The genomic landscapes of human breast and colorectal cancers. Science 318(5853):1108–1113
25. Hoque MO, Kim MS, Ostrow KL, Liu J, Wisman GB, Park HL, Poeta ML, Jeronimo C, Henrique R, Lendvai A, Schuuring E, Begum S, Rosenbaum E, Ongenaert M, Yamashita K, Califano J, Westra W, van der Zee AG, Van Criekinge W, Sidransky D (2008) Genome-wide promoter analysis uncovers portions of the cancer methylome. Cancer Res 68(8): 2661–2670
26. Noutomi Y, Oga A, Uchida K, Okafuji M, Ita M, Kawauchi S, Furuya T, Ueyama Y, Sasaki K (2006) Comparative genomic hybridization reveals genetic progression of oral squamous cell carcinoma from dysplasia via two different tumourigenic pathways. J Pathol 210:67–74
27. Gillison ML, Koch WM, Capone RB, Spafford M, Westra WH, Wu L, Zahurak ML, Daniel RW, Vigiolone M, Symer DE, Shah KV, Sidransky D (2000) Evidence for a causal association between human papillomavirus and a subset of head and neck cancers. J Natl Cancer Inst 92:709–720
28. Tong BC, Dhir K, Ha PK, Westra WH, Alter BP, Sidransky D, Koch WM, Califano JA (2004) Use of single nucleotide polymorphism arrays to identify a novel region of loss on chromosome 6q in squamous cell carcinoma of the oral cavity. Head Neck 26:345–352
29. Kutler DI, Auerbach AD, Satagopan J, Giampietro PF, Batish SD, Huvos AG, Goberdhan A, Shah JP, Singh B (2003) High incidence of head and neck squamous cell carcinoma in patients with Fanconi anemia. Arch Otolaryngol Head Neck Surg 129(1):106–112
30. Lippman SM, Shin DM, Lee JJ, Batsakis JG, Lotan R, Tainsky MA, Hittelman WN, Hong WK (1995) p53 and retinoid chemoprevention of oral carcinogenesis. Cancer Res 55(1):16–19
31. Cruz IB, Snijders PJ, Meijer CJ, Braakhuis BJ, Snow GB, Walboomers JM, van der Waal I (1998) p53 expression above the basal cell layer in oral mucosa is an early event of malignant transformation and has predictive value for developing oral squamous cell carcinoma. J Pathol 184(4):360–368
32. Boyle JO, Hakim J, Koch W, van der Riet P, Hruban RH, Roa RA, Corio R, Eby YJ, Ruppert JM, Sidransky D (1993) The incidence of p53 mutations increases with progression of head and neck cancer. Cancer Res 53:4477–4480
33. Brennan JA, Boyle JO, Koch WM, Goodman SN, Hruban RH, Eby Y, Couch M, Forastiere AA, Sidransky D (1995) Association between cigarette smoking and mutation of the p53 gene in squamous-cell carcinoma of the head and neck. N Engl J Med 332:712–717
34. Poeta ML, Manola J, Goldwasser MA, Forastiere A, Benoit N, Califano JA, Ridge JA, Goodwin J, Kenady D, Saunders J, Westra WH, Sidransky D, Koch WM (2007) TP53 mutations and clinical outcome in head and neck squamous carcinoma. N Engl J Med 357:2552–2561
35. Ongkeko WM, Altuna X, Weisman RA, Wang-Rodriguez J (2005) Expression of protein tyrosine kinases in head and neck squamous cell carcinomas. Am J Clin Pathol 124(1):71–76
36. Shin DM, Ro JY, Hong WK, Hittelman WN (1994) Dysregulation of epidermal growth factor receptor expression in premalignant lesions during head and neck tumorigenesis. Cancer Res 54(12):3153–3159
37. Kalyankrishna S, Grandis JR (2006) Epidermal growth factor receptor biology in head and neck cancer. J Clin Oncol 24(17):2666–2672
38. Zhou S, Kachap S, Sun W, Wu G, Chuang A, Poeta L, Grumbine L, Mithani SK, Chatterjee A, Koch W, Westra WH, Maitra A, Glazer C, Carducci M, Sidransky D, McFate T, Verma A, Califano JA (2007) Frequency and phenotypic implications of mitochondrial DNA mutations in human squamous cell cancers of the head and neck. Proc Natl Acad Sci U S A 104(18): 7540–7545

39. Ha PK, Tong BC, Westra WH, Sanchez-Cespedes M, Parrella P, Zahurak M, Sidransky D, Califano JA (2002) Mitochondrial C-tract alteration in premalignant lesions of the head and neck: a marker for progression and clonal proliferation. Clin Cancer Res 8:2260–2265
40. Kim MM, Clinger JD, Masayesva BG, Ha PK, Zahurak MK, Westra WH, Califano JA (2004) Mitochondrial DNA quantity increases with histopathologic grade in premalignant and malignant head and neck lesions. Clin Cancer Res 10:8512–8515
41. Califano J, van der Riet P, Westra W, Nawroz H, Clayman G, Piantadosi S, Corio R, Lee D, Greenberg B, Koch W, Sidransky D (1996) A genetic progression model for head and neck cancer: implications for field cancerization. Cancer Res 56:2488–2492
42. Zhang L, Cheung KJ, Lam WL, Cheng X, Poh C, Priddy R, Epstein J, Le ND, Rosin MP (2001) Increased genetic damage in oral leukoplakia from high risk sites: potential impact on staging and clinical management. Cancer 91(11):2148–2155
43. Mao L, Lee JS, Fan YH, Ro JY, Batsakis JG, Lippman S, Hittelman W, Hong WK (1996) Frequent microsatellite alterations at chromosomes 9p21 and 3p14 in oral premalignant lesions and their value in cancer risk assessment. Nat Med 2(6):682–685
44. Choi HR, Roberts DB, Johnigan RH, Sturgis EM, Rosenthal DI, Weber RS, Luna MA, Batsakis JG, El-Naggar AK (2004) Molecular and clinicopathologic comparisons of head and neck squamous carcinoma variants. Am J Surg Pathol 28(10):1299–1310
45. Ha PK, Pilkington TA, Westra WH, Sciubba J, Sidransky D, Califano JA (2002) Progression of microsatellite instability from premalignant lesions to tumors of the head and neck. Int J Cancer 102:615–617
46. El-Naggar AK, Hurr K, Huff V, Clayman GL, Luna MA, Batsakis JG (1996) Microsatellite Instability in preinvaive and invasive head and neck squamous carcinoma. Am J Pathol 148(6):2067–2072
47. Weber F, Xu Y, Zhang L, Patoes A, Shen L, Platzer P, Eng C (2007) Microenvironmental genomic alterations and clinicopathological behavior in head and neck squamous cell carcinoma. JAMA 297(2):187–195
48. Reed AL, Califano J, Cairns P, Westra WH, Jones RM, Koch W, Ahrendt S, Eby Y, Sewell D, Nawroz H, Bartek J, Sidransky D (1996) High frequency of p16 (CDKN2/MTS-1/INK4A) inactivation in head and neck squamous cell carcinoma. Cancer Res 56: 3630–3633
49. Youssef EM, Lotan D, Issa JP, Wakasa K, Fan YH, Mao L, Hassan K, Feng L, Lee JJ, Lippman SM, Hong WK, Lotan R (2004) Hypermethylation of the retinoic acid receptor-beta(2) gene in head and neck carcinogenesis. Clin Cancer Res 10(5):1733–1742
50. Hunter KD, Thurlow JK, Fleming J, Drake PJ, Vass JK, Kalna G, Higham DJ, Herzyk P, Macdonald DG, Parkinson EK, Harrison PR (2006) Divergent routes to oral cancer. Cancer Res 66(15):7405–7413
51. Carinci F, Lo Muzio L, Piattelli A, Rubini C, Chiesa F, Ionna F, Palmieri A, Maiorano E, Pastore A, Laino G, Dolci M, Pezzetti F (2005) Potential markers of tongue tumor progresion selected by cDNA microarray. Int J Immunopathol Pharmacol 18(3):513–524
52. Liu CJ, Liu T-Y, Kuo L-T, Cheng H-W, Chu T-H, Chang KW, Lin SC (2008) Differential gene expression signature between primary and metastatic head and neck squamous cell carcinoma. J Pathol 214:489–497
53. Smeets SJ, Braakhuis BJM, Abbas S, Snidjers PJF, Ylstra B, van de Wiel MA, Meijer GA, Leemans CR, Brakenhoff RH (2006) Genomic-wide DNA copy number alterations in head and neck squamous cell carcinomas with or without oncogene-expressing human papillomavirus. Oncogene 25:2558–2564
54. Spafford M, Koch WM, Reed AL, Xu L, Eisenberger CF, Yip L, Leong PL, Wu L, Liu SX, Geronimo C, Westra WH, Sidransky D (2001) Detection of head and neck squamous cell carcinoma in saliva by microsatellite analysis. Clin Cancer Res 7:607–612
55. Nawroz H, Koch W, Anker P, Stroun M, Sidransky D (1996) Microsatellite alterations in plasma DNA of head and neck cancer patients. Nat Med 2:1035–1037

56. Carvalho AL, Jeronimo C, Kim MM, Henrique R, Zhang Z, Hoque MO, Chang S, Brait M, Nayak CS, Jiang WW, Claybourne Q, Tokumaru Y, Lee J, Goldenberg D, Garrett-Mayer E, Goodman S, Moon CS, Koch W, Westra WH, Sidransky D, Califano JA (2008) Evaluation of promoter hypermethylation detection in body fluids as a screening/diagnosis tool for head and neck squamous cell carcinoma. Clin Cancer Res 14(1):97–107
57. Li Y, St John MAR, Zhou X, Kim Y, Sinha U, Jordan RCK, Eisele R, Abemayor E, Elashoff D, Park NH, Wong DT (2004) Salivary transcriptome diagnostics for oral cancer detection. Clin Cancer Res 10:8442–8450

Descriptive Epidemiology: U.S. Patterns

Linda Morris Brown, Gloria Gridley, and Susan S. Devesa

Abbreviations

US	United States
HN	head and neck
SEER	Surveillance, Epidemiology, and End Results
HPV	Human Papillomavirus
ICD-O-3	International Classification of Diseases for Oncology, third edition
API	Asian/Pacific Islander
AI/AN	American Indian/Alaskan Native

Overview

According to 2009 estimates provided by the American Cancer Society, approximately 35,160 men and 12,850 women are expected to be diagnosed with cancers of the oral cavity, pharynx, and larynx in the United States, and approximately 8,140 men and 3,120 women are expected to die from these cancers [1]. This chapter reviews the descriptive patterns of squamous cell carcinomas of the oral cavity, pharynx, and larynx. Tabulations of cancers of the oral cavity and pharynx usually include those of the lip, tongue, gums, floor of the mouth, hard and soft palate, salivary glands, tonsils, oropharynx, hypopharynx, and nasopharynx. For this analysis, we have excluded cancers of the lip, salivary glands, and nasopharynx since salivary

L.M. Brown (✉)
RTI International, 6110 Executive Blvd, Suite 902, Rockville, MD, 20852-3907, USA
e-mail: lindabrown@rti.org

G. Gridley and S.S. Devesa
Division of Cancer Epidemiology and Genetics, National Cancer Institute,
National Institutes of Health, Department of Health and Human Services, 6120 Executive Blvd, Bethesda, MD, 20892-7244, USA
e-mail: devesas@mail.nih.gov; gridleyg@aol.com

A.F. Olshan (ed.), *Epidemiology, Pathogenesis, and Prevention of Head and Neck Cancer*,
DOI 10.1007/978-1-4419-1472-9_2, © Springer Science+Business Media, LLC 2010

gland cancers are primarily adenocarcinomas, and tumors of the lip and nasopharynx have etiologic profiles that differ from those of the other head and neck (HN) cancers. We also excluded sarcomas, lymphomas, and other nonsquamous cell carcinomas because it is likely that they are also etiologically distinct.

Methods

Data from population-based registries in the National Cancer Institute's Surveillance, Epidemiology, and End Results (SEER) program [2] were used to calculate incidence and survival rates. Primary site and histologic type have been coded according to the International Classification of Diseases for Oncology, third edition [ICD-O-3] [3]. We selected all cases of invasive squamous cell carcinoma (morphology codes 8050-8084) of the oral cavity (topography codes C019-C069), pharynx (codes C090-C109, C129-C148), and larynx (codes C320-C329). For selected analyses, we divided cancers of the oral cavity and pharynx into three categories based on human papillomavirus (HPV) status: HPV-related cancers (codes C019 – base of tongue, C024 – lingual tonsil, C090-C109 – tonsil and oropharynx, C142 – Waldeyer ring), HPV-unrelated cancers (codes C020-C023 and C025-069 – other tongue except lingual tonsil, gum, floor of mouth, palate, other and unspecified parts of mouth), and HPV role unknown (C129-C140, C148 – pyriform sinus, hypopharynx, pharynx, overlapping oral cavity and pharynx) [4].

Age-adjusted incidence rates (using the 2000 U.S. standard) and age-specific rates (5-year age groups) per 100,000 person-years were calculated separately for each site and for all three sites combined by sex and race using SEER*Stat [5]. Five-year relative survival rates were calculated by time period of diagnosis (1975–1984, 1985–1994, and 1995–2003, with follow-up through 2004) and stage (localized, regional, distant, and unknown using SEER historic stage A). Relative survival rates take into account the expected mortality for a comparable race-, sex-, age- and time period-specific cohort and are expressed as percentages. Data from the original nine SEER registries (SEER 9) were utilized for analysis of long-term incidence and survival rates among whites and blacks; these nine registries account for approximately 10% of the U.S. population and are located in the metropolitan areas of Atlanta, Detroit, San Francisco-Oakland, and Seattle-Puget Sound and the states of Connecticut, Hawaii, Iowa, New Mexico, and Utah [6]. The SEER program was expanded in 1992 to include four additional registries for a total of 13 registries (SEER 9 plus the California metropolitan areas of San Jose-Monterey and Los Angeles, several counties in rural Georgia, and the Alaska Native Tumor Registry) [7]. The populations in these 13 areas account for 14% of the U.S. population and include substantial numbers of Asian/Pacific Islanders (APIs) and Hispanics.

National vital statistics data for 1950–2004 from the National Center for Health Statistics were used to calculate long-term mortality rates for each site by race and sex. We selected all deaths due to oral cavity cancer (excluding lip and salivary glands), pharynx cancer (excluding nasopharynx), and larynx cancer; all histologic types are included because histology is generally not reported on the death certificate and is not coded even if specified.

Only data points representing populations with at least 10 cases were presented. All temporal trends were plotted such that a slope of 10° represented a change of 1% per year (i.e., 40 years on the horizontal axis is the same length as one logarithmic cycle on the vertical axis) [8].

Demographic Patterns

Incidence

During the period 1992–2004, more than 48,000 HN cancers were diagnosed among residents of the 13 SEER registries (Table 1). Forty-three percent of HN tumors occurred in the oral cavity, 34% in the larynx, and 24% in the pharynx. The tongue and tonsil were the predominant specific sites in the oral cavity and pharynx, respectively. Among laryngeal cancers, the glottis was more frequent than the supraglottis among males but not among females. All HN cancers combined occurred 3–4 times more frequently among men than women. Among white non-Hispanics, the male/female rate ratios ranged from 2.2 for oral cavity to 3.4 for pharynx and 4.5 for larynx cancers. The male/female rate ratios were all larger among blacks, ranging from 3.2 for oral cavity to 4.4 for pharynx and 5.0 for larynx; the ratios among APIs and Hispanics, frequently, were even greater due to relatively low rates among the women. Incidence rates were higher among blacks than white non-Hispanics for most sites, especially among males. The black/white non-Hispanic rate ratio among males was 1.52 for all HN cancers combined and ranged from 1.21 for oral cavity to 1.70 for pharynx and 1.72 for larynx cancers. The highest rate among white non-Hispanic men was for cancer of the oral cavity (7.1), whereas the highest rate for black men was for cancer of the larynx (11.5). Rates for American Indian/Alaska Native (AI/AN), API, and Hispanic men were generally 33–50% lower than for white non-Hispanic men. Among females, oral cavity rates were 18% lower among blacks than white non-Hispanics due primarily to the higher rates of tongue cancer among white non-Hispanic women; in contrast, pharynx and larynx cancer rates were 31% and 53% higher among blacks than white non-Hispanics, respectively. Rates for AI/AN, API, and Hispanic women were considerably lower than for white non-Hispanic women.

Age-Specific Patterns

Age-specific incidence rates in the SEER 13 registries during 1992–2004 rose exponentially among males and females of each racial/ethnic group for all three sites until at least the age of 60 (Fig. 1). Among males, oral cavity cancer rates

Table 1 Incidence rates of squamous cell carcinoma of the oral cavity, pharynx, and larynx by race/ethnicity, sex, and site, 1992–2004, SEER 13[a,b,c]

	White non-Hispanic		Black		American Indian/ Alaska Native[d]		Asian/ Pacific Islander		Hispanic–Latino[e]	
	Count	Rate	Count	Rate	Count	Rate	Count	Rate	Count	Rate
Males										
All three sites	26,118	18.2	4,760	27.6	136	10.7	1781	9.1	2,356	12.0
Oral cavity	10,175	7.1	1,534	8.6	56	4.2	707	3.6	773	3.8
Tongue	5,837	4.0	756	4.3	30	2.0	435	2.2	410	2.0
Floor of mouth	1,860	1.3	348	1.9	13	1.2	70	0.4	169	0.8
Gum and other mouth	2,478	1.8	430	2.5	13	1.0	202	1.0	194	1.0
Pharynx	6,351	4.4	1,333	7.5	38	3.2	462	2.3	619	3.0
Tonsil	3,236	2.2	560	3.1	13	1.0	201	1.0	288	1.3
Oropharynx	659	0.5	193	1.1	3	–	24	0.1	69	0.3
Hypopharynx	1,903	1.3	464	2.7	20	1.8	211	1.1	215	1.2
Other oral cavity and pharynx	553	0.4	116	0.7	2	–	26	0.1	47	0.2
Larynx	9,592	6.7	1,893	11.5	42	3.3	612	3.2	964	5.2
Glottis	5,820	4.1	956	6.0	24	1.9	389	2.1	606	3.3
Supraglottis	2,803	1.9	617	3.7	11	0.8	149	0.8	230	1.2
Other and unspecified	969	0.7	320	1.9	7	–	74	0.4	128	0.7
Females										
All three sites	10,608	6.1	1,519	6.7	52	3.5	691	2.9	720	3.0
Oral cavity	5,921	3.3	618	2.7	36	2.4	503	2.1	428	1.8
Tongue	2,863	1.7	288	1.2	15	1.0	313	1.3	237	0.9
Floor of mouth	911	0.5	116	0.5	11	0.7	36	0.2	53	0.2
Gum and other mouth	2,147	1.2	214	1.0	10	0.7	154	0.7	138	0.6
Pharynx	2,158	1.3	386	1.7	9	–	96	0.4	122	0.5
Tonsil	1,017	0.6	165	0.7	2	–	58	0.2	75	0.3
Oropharynx	271	0.2	52	0.2	0	–	7	–	13	0.1
Hypopharynx	617	0.4	124	0.5	6	–	29	0.1	29	0.1
Other oral cavity and pharynx	253	0.1	45	0.2	1	–	2	–	5	–
Larynx	2,529	1.5	515	2.3	7	–	92	0.4	170	0.7
Glottis	953	0.6	136	0.6	1	–	41	0.2	81	0.3
Supraglottis	1,295	0.8	299	1.3	5	–	40	0.2	65	0.3
Other and unspecified	281	0.2	80	0.4	1	–	11	0.0	24	0.1

[a]Rates are per 100,000 person-years and age-adjusted to the 2000 US Standard Population (19 age groups)

[b]Excludes lip, salivary gland, and nasopharynx cancers

[c]Rate subtotals may differ from the sum of the components due to rounding and/or suppression

[d]Contract Health Service Delivery Area (CHSDA) counties only

[e]12 SEER areas (excluding Alaska)

[–]Rate not shown because fewer than 10 cases

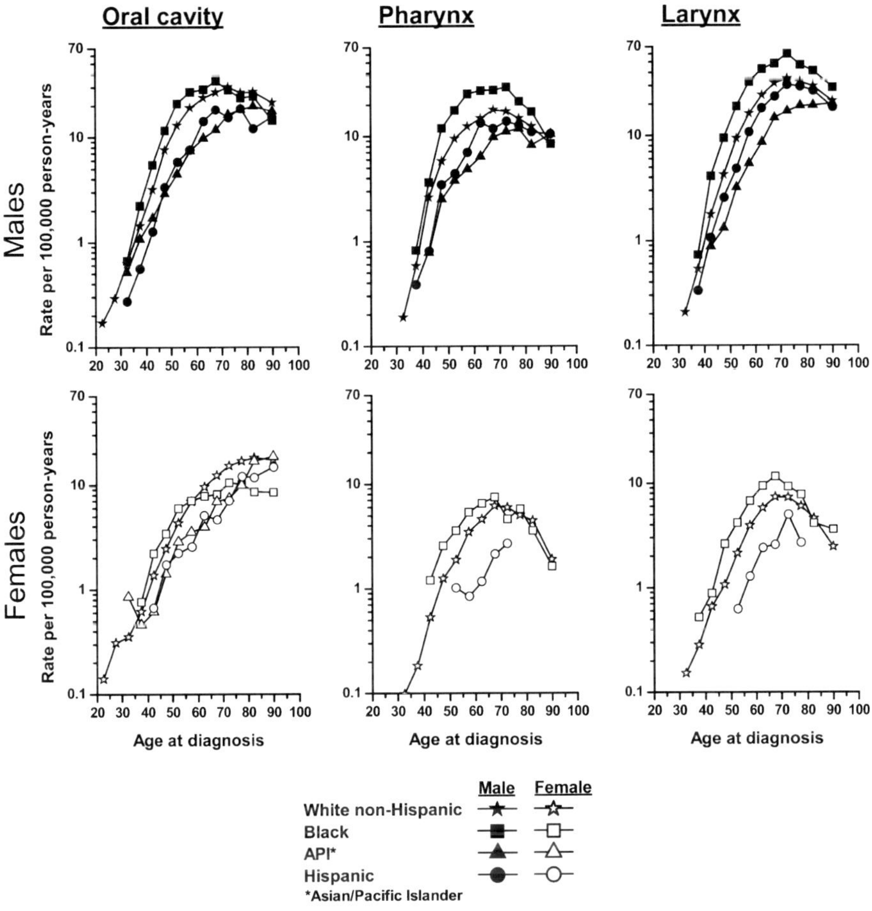

Fig. 1 Age-specific incidence rates of oral cavity, pharynx, and larynx squamous cell carcinoma by sex and race/ethnicity during 1992–2004, SEER 13 (excludes lip, salivary gland, and nasopharynx cancers)

dropped off at the older ages but were higher among blacks than white non-Hispanics at all but ages 70 and older. Rates among API and Hispanic men were similar at all ages but were lower than those among white non-Hispanics. Similar to cancer of the oral cavity, pharynx and larynx cancer rates among males rose with age before dropping off at the older ages. Blacks had the highest pharynx cancer rates, followed by white non-Hispanics, at all ages except for the oldest (85+). API males had the lowest rates at virtually all ages. The declines in incidence rates with age were especially pronounced among blacks and white non-Hispanics for both pharynx and larynx cancers and among Hispanics for larynx cancer. The black/white non-Hispanic differences were most pronounced across the middle age groups for pharynx cancer and the least for oral cavity cancer.

Among females, oral cancer rates generally increased with age for all race groups (Fig. 1). In contrast to males, blacks had the highest rates only at younger ages (<60) and white non-Hispanics had the highest rates at ages 60–84. Oral cancer rates plateaued at older ages among blacks and white non-Hispanics but continued to rise with age among APIs and Hispanics. As a result, rates among Hispanics and APIs were higher than those among blacks at the older ages. The patterns for larynx and pharynx cancers were distinctly different, with the highest rates among white non-Hispanics and blacks at ages 65–69, followed by dramatic declines at older ages. Rates were notably higher among blacks than white non-Hispanics at virtually all ages for larynx cancer but only at ages <70 years for pharynx cancer. Hispanic women had the lowest rates for these two cancers. The numbers of pharynx and larynx cases among API women were too small to graph.

Time Trends

The temporal incidence trends for the HN cancers varied considerably by site, sex, and race/ethnicity (Fig. 2). Age-adjusted incidence rates per 100,000 for oral cavity cancer among black men peaked at 13.3 in 1980–1984 and then began a marked 45% decline, reaching 7.3 in 2000–2004. Rates among white men also peaked in 1980–1984 at 8.1 per 100,000 but had a more gradual 17% decline to 6.7 and 6.8 in 1995–1999 and 2000–2004, respectively. Rates among API, AI/AN, and Hispanic men all declined between 1995–1999 and 2000–2004. Although rates of oral cavity cancer were much lower among females than males, they similarly declined from highs during the time period 1980–1984. The decline was more rapid in black females, resulting in lower rates among black than white females during 1985–2004. Small declines were also observed for API, AI/AN, and Hispanic females during recent years. Pharynx cancer rates among black men peaked in 1985–1989 at 11.0/100,000 and then declined 39.5% to 6.7 in 2000–2004. From 1980–1984 to 2000–2004, rates declined 44% among black women, from 2.7 to 1.5, and 31% among white women, from 1.6 to 1.1. Rates among white men decreased much less rapidly, and rates among the other ethnic groups all declined between 1995–1999 and 2000–2004. In contrast to the trends for cancers of the oral cavity and pharynx, the greatest decline in larynx cancer rates occurred among white men (a 36% decrease) from 9.4 in 1980–1984 to 6.0 in 2000–2004. Larynx cancer rates peaked during the late 1980s among black males and females and among white females; rates declined in recent years among virtually all gender and race/ethnic groups.

Differences in the temporal incidence patterns for HPV-related and -unrelated cancers of the oral cavity and pharynx were most pronounced among white males (Fig. 3). In contrast to the relatively stable oral cavity and pharynx cancer rates shown in Fig. 2, rates for HPV-related cancer among white men increased 47% from 3.4 in 1975–1979 to 5.0 in 2000–2004, rates of HPV-unrelated cancer peaked at 6.6 in 1980–1984 and then declined 32% to 4.5 in 2000–2004, and rates for

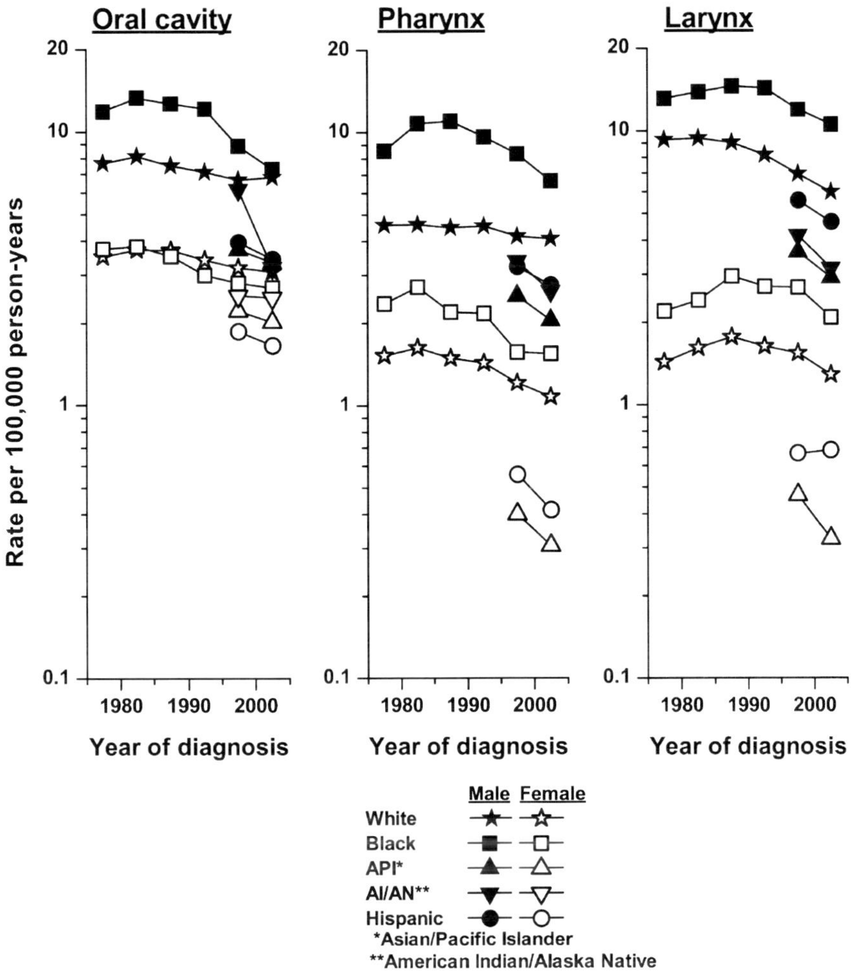

Fig. 2 Temporal trends in oral cavity, pharynx, and larynx squamous cell carcinoma incidence by sex during 1975–1979 to 2000–2004 among whites and blacks in SEER 9 and during 1995–1999 to 2000–2004 among Asian/Pacific Islanders and Hispanics in SEER 12 and among American Indian/Alaska Natives in SEER 13 (rates age-adjusted using 2000 U.S. population standard; excludes lip, salivary gland, and nasopharynx cancers)

cancers with unknown HPV role decreased 44% from 2.5 to 1.4. Among black men, rates for HPV-related cancer peaked at 8.8 in 1985–1989 and then declined 26% to 6.5 in 2000–2004; rates for HPV-unrelated and HPV role unknown declined even more rapidly (52% and 55%, respectively), from highs of 10.1 and 6.0 in 1980–1984 to lows of 4.8 and 2.7 in 2000–2004. Among both white and black females, all rates decreased following highs in the early 1980s, but the rate of decline was greater for black females. Rates of HPV-unrelated cancers were

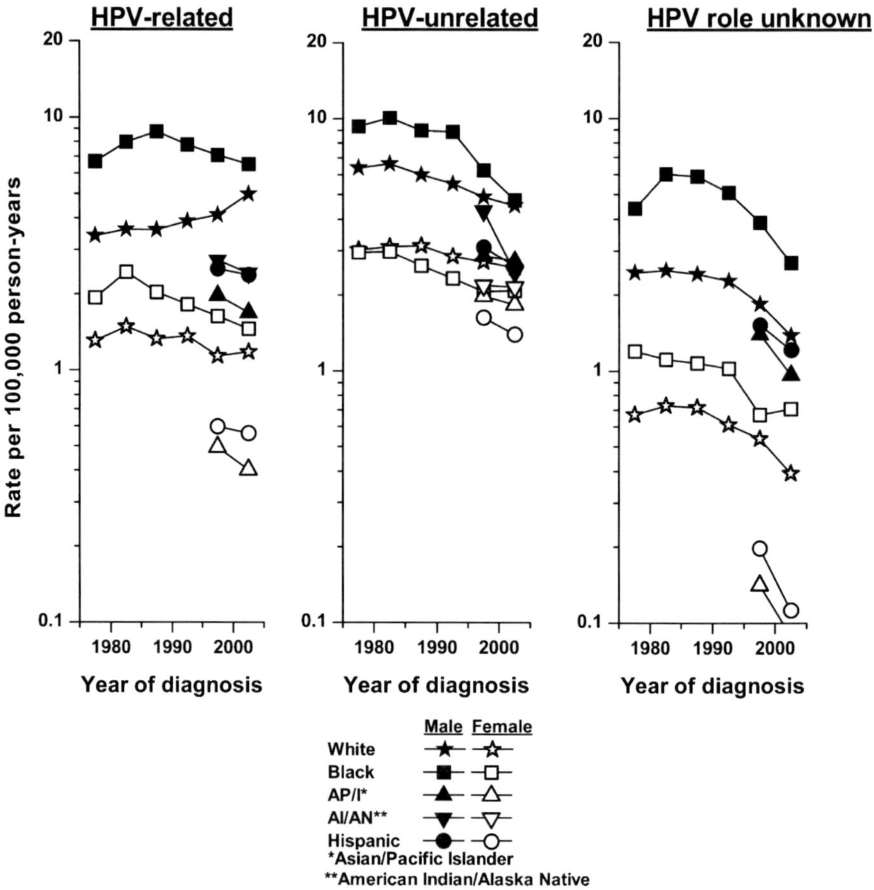

Fig. 3 Temporal trends in oral cavity and pharynx squamous cell carcinoma incidence by sex according to HPV-relationship during 1975–1979 to 2000–2004 among whites and blacks in SEER 9 and during 1995–1999 to 2000–2004 among Asian/Pacific Islanders and Hispanics in SEER 12 and among American Indian/Alaska Natives in SEER 13 (rates age-adjusted using 2000 U.S. population standard; excludes lip, salivary gland, and nasopharynx cancers)

higher in white than black females, whereas rates of HPV-related and HPV role unknown cancers were higher in black females. Rates generally decreased among API, AI/AN, and Hispanic males and females between 1995–1999 and 2000–2004. Thus, HPV-related cancer rates rose notably among white males while declining in recent years among all other race/ethnic/sex groups. HPV-unrelated cancer rates decreased among all groups, more rapidly among blacks than whites. In fact, the black/white HPV-unrelated cancer rate ratio declined from 1.5 in 1975–1979 to 1.1 in 2000–2004 among men, and from 1.0 in 1975–1979 to 0.8 in 2000–2004 among women.

Mortality

Time Trends

National mortality rates are available for the time period 1950–1954 to 2000–2004 for nonwhites and whites, 1970–1974 to 2000–2004 for blacks, and 1995–1999 to 2000–2004 for APIs, AI/ANs, and Hispanics by site and sex (Fig. 4). Rates specifically for blacks have been higher than for all nonwhite populations combined, with the differences increasing over time as the Asian population, with lower rates, grew. Rates for all three cancers among nonwhite and black males and females rose notably before peaking during the 1980s, earlier for oral cavity and pharynx cancers than for larynx cancers, and they have declined 30–60% since then. Rates for all three cancers among white males, which had been higher than those among nonwhites during the 1950s, declined steadily over the last 55 years – about 56% for oral cavity cancer, 36% for pharynx cancer, and 32% for larynx cancer. In contrast, rates among white females rose modestly until peaking in the early 1970s for oral cancer, the late 1970s for pharynx cancer, and the early 1990s for larynx cancer, and declining thereafter. Mortality rates among the other three racial/ethnic groups declined during the recent decade for larynx and oral cancers among all except API females, whereas they rose for pharynx cancer among all except Hispanic males.

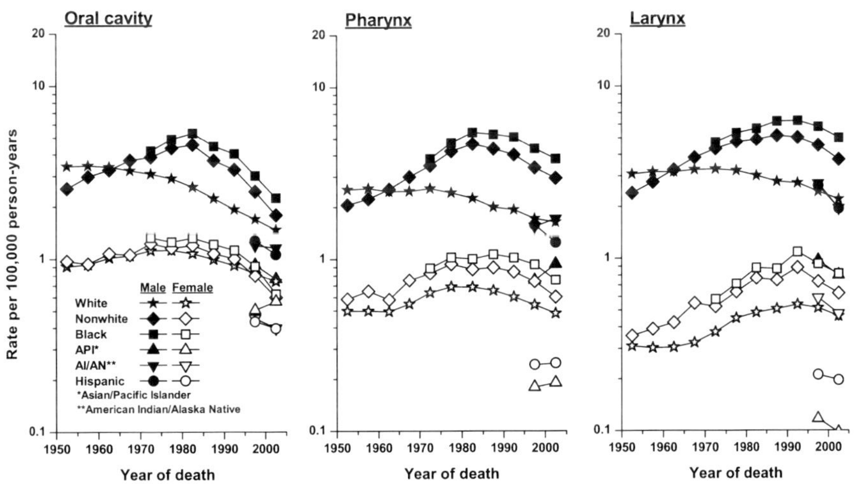

Fig. 4 Temporal trends in oral cavity, pharynx, and larynx cancer mortality by sex during 1950–1954 to 2000–2004 among whites and nonwhites, during 1970–1974 to 2000–2004 among blacks, and during 1995–1999 to 2000–2004 among Asian/Pacific Islanders, American Indian/Alaska Natives, and Hispanics (rates age-adjusted using 2000 U.S. population standard; excludes lip, salivary gland, and nasopharynx cancers)

Geographic Variation

Maps showing age-adjusted mortality rates by state economic area for white men and women during the 25-year period 1980–2004 are presented in Fig. 5a and b, respectively. This is the first time that maps for cancers of the oral cavity and pharynx have been presented separately. Oral cavity cancer rates were high along the East coast among white males and in the Southeast among white females. Rates for females also were elevated in areas of the Northeast, in Nevada, and along the Pacific coast. Rates were low across the Central, Plains, and Rocky Mountain states in both sexes. The clustering of excess mortality among white females in the Southeast was even more prominent during 1950–1969 [9] and was attributed to snuff dipping among women in the rural South [10]. Although the prevalence of snuff dipping has declined in recent decades [11], patches of elevated oral cancer rates still remain in parts of the Carolinas, Georgia, and Florida. Rates of pharynx cancer among white males were elevated across broad stretches of the Southeast, particularly along the East coast and across the Gulf coast into Texas. Rates among females tended to cluster along both the Northern and Southern Atlantic coasts and most of the Pacific coast. Rates were relatively low in the Rocky Mountain and Plains states, more so among males than females. Larynx cancer rates among white men and, to a lesser extent, white women were elevated in scattered areas of the eastern third of the country and in southern Louisiana, but they tended to be low in central and western regions. The clustering of high rates across the eastern part of the country was more pronounced in 1980–2004 than in the period 1950–1979 (data not shown). The geographic patterns of pharynx and larynx cancers are quite similar to those of lung cancer, consistent with the patterns of cigarette smoking, which is a major risk factor [9, 12].

Survival

Recent Patterns and Time Trends

Five-year relative survival rates among patients diagnosed during 1995–2003 with oral cavity, pharynx, or larynx cancer were highest among white males and females – 59% and 57% – and lowest among black males – 39% (Table 2). Within each race/sex group, survival rates were highest for patients with larynx cancer (ranging from 46 to 68%), intermediate among patients with oral cavity cancer (34–58%), and lowest among patients with pharynx cancer (26–51%). For all three sites combined, 5-year relative survival rates improved over the past three decades among whites but not blacks. Rising survival rates were notable among patients with pharynx cancer, except black females; oral cancer patient survival also improved among whites, especially males. In contrast, survival among larynx cancer patients did not improve and even appeared to decline except among white males. When oral cavity and pharynx cancers were divided into presumed HPV-related or not categories,

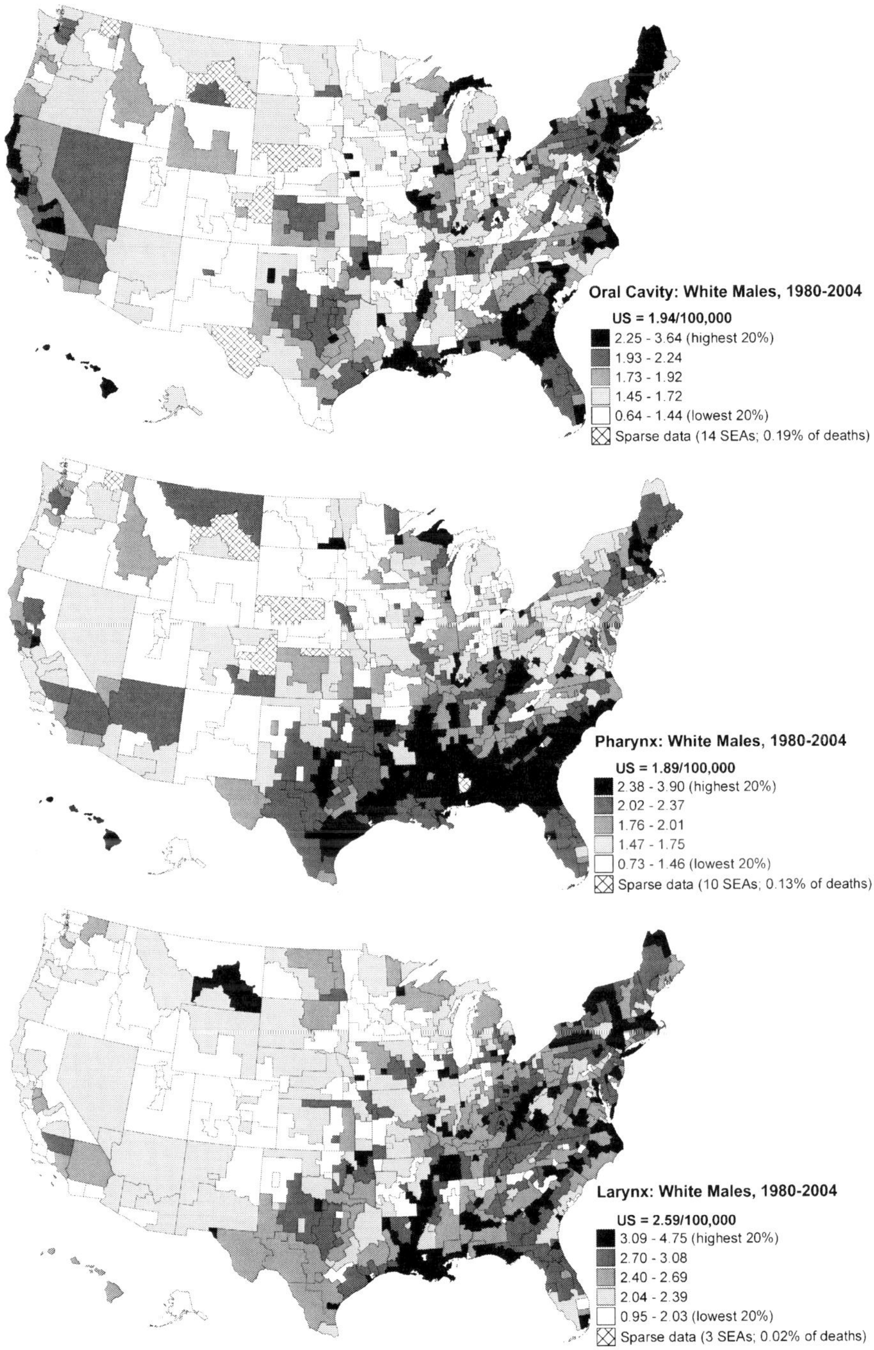

Fig. 5 (**a**) Oral cavity, pharynx, and larynx cancer mortality rates among white males during 1980–2004 by State Economic Area (SEA) (rates age-adjusted using 2000 U.S. population standard; excludes lip, salivary gland, and nasopharynx cancers)

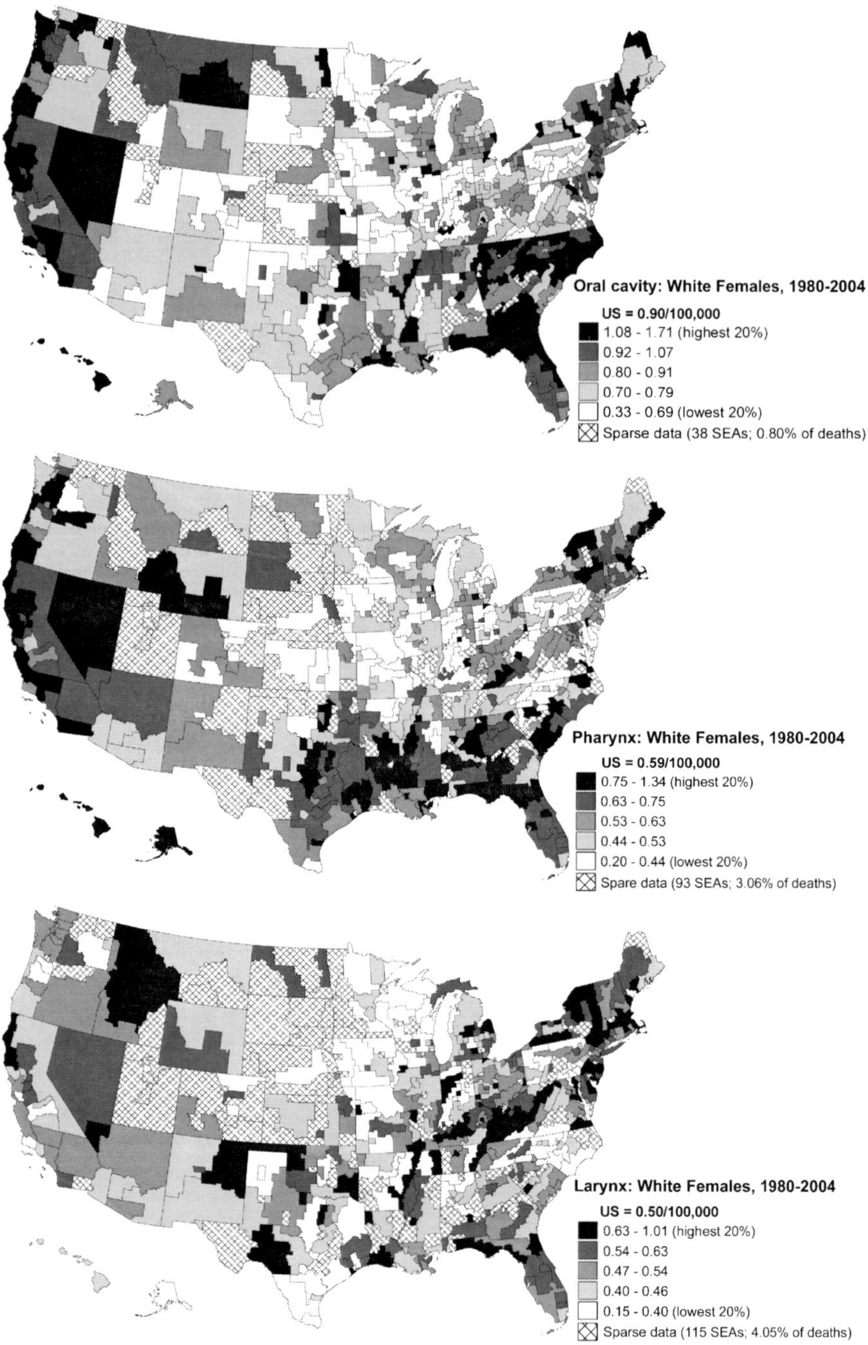

Fig. 5 (continued) (**b**) Oral cavity, pharynx, and larynx cancer mortality rates among white females during 1980–2004 by State Economic Area (SEA) (rates age-adjusted using 2000 U.S. population standard; excludes lip, salivary gland, and nasopharynx cancers)

Table 2 Five-year relative survival rates among patients diagnosed with squamous cell carcinoma of the oral cavity, pharynx, or larynx during 1975–2003 by race, gender, and time period, SEER 9[a]

Site	Year of diagnosis	White males Count	White males Rate	White females Count	White females Rate	Black males Count	Black males Rate	Black females Count	Black females Rate
All three sites	1975–1984	14,313	52.9%	5,166	53.3%	2,028	38.0%	587	42.8%
	1985–1994	13,930	55.3%	5,394	55.8%	2,404	36.8%	672	41.7%
	1995–2003	11,860	59.2%	4,410	56.5%	1,934	38.7%	615	41.9%
Oral cavity	1975–1984	5,054	46.3%	2,757	55.0%	693	31.8%	255	43.0%
	1985–1994	4,886	50.2%	2,822	58.4%	788	28.9%	248	39.0%
	1995–2003	4,480	56.1%	2,426	58.1%	599	33.8%	242	44.6%
Pharynx	1975–1984	2,974	30.3%	1,210	37.2%	533	17.0%	169	28.8%
	1985–1994	3,000	36.4%	1,176	40.2%	678	22.6%	187	29.9%
	1995–2003	2,904	50.5%	868	45.5%	566	26.2%	139	29.3%
Larynx	1975–1984	6,285	68.9%	1,199	65.6%	802	57.9%	163	56.8%
	1985–1994	6,044	69.1%	1,396	63.7%	938	54.5%	237	54.0%
	1995–2003	4,476	68.1%	1,116	61.8%	769	52.0%	234	46.4%
Oral cavity and pharynx									
HPV-related	1975–1984	2,283	34.8%	1,048	40.4%	411	18.1%	153	29.0%
	1985–1994	2,533	43.5%	1,050	46.0%	547	25.0%	152	31.9%
	1995–2003	3,219	59.3%	880	55.8%	518	32.1%	143	36.5%
HPV-unrelated/ unknown	1975–1984	5,745	42.6%	2,919	52.8%	815	29.1%	271	41.8%
	1985–1994	5,353	45.7%	2,948	55.5%	919	26.5%	283	36.8%
	1995–2003	4,165	49.8%	2,414	54.1%	647	28.4%	238	40.5%

[a]Excludes lip, salivary gland, and nasopharynx cancers; includes follow-up through 2004

survival rates improved markedly among patients with HPV-related cancers for all four race/sex groups. During the most recent time period, survival rates were higher among patients with HPV-related than HPV-unrelated/unknown status cancers, except among black females.

Stage-Specific Patterns

Stage of disease at diagnosis has a dramatic effect on subsequent survival among all patients with HN cancer (Table 3). Among patients diagnosed with oral cavity cancer during 1995–2003, 5-year relative survival rates ranged from 57 to 74% for localized disease to 28–51% for regional disease and 25–38% for distant-stage disease. The corresponding ranges for patients with pharynx cancer were 46–64% for localized, 29–53% for regional, and 10–25% for distant-stage disease; and for patients with larynx cancer, they were 61–86%, 40–50%, and 20–29%, respectively. The largest numbers of patients were diagnosed with regional stage disease for all three cancers among all four race/gender groups, except oral cavity cancer among white females and larynx cancer among whites, where the number localized was the largest. The proportion with distant-stage disease was modest for oral cavity and larynx cancers, but for pharynx cancer, the number of patients with distant-stage disease exceeded the number with localized disease for all except white females. Among white males, the stage distribution at diagnosis was less favorable for HPV-related cancers than not; however, the relative survival rates among patients with regional or distant-stage disease were each notably better among HPV-related cases than not. These figures suggest the improvement in overall survival rates that might be achieved by public health measures aimed at increasing early detection through cancer surveillance programs.

Discussion

Both tobacco and alcohol are well established risk factors for HN cancers regardless of the type of alcoholic beverage consumed or form of tobacco used [13, 14]. For most race/sex groups, the declines in HN cancer incidence and mortality parallel the reduction in cigarette smoking prevalence and may also reflect decreases in alcohol consumption, especially the use of hard liquor [15, 16]. The recent declines in incidence rates for these three squamous cell carcinomas (except for oral cavity and pharynx cancers among white males) are remarkably similar to the declines in squamous cell carcinoma of the lung [17] and esophagus [16, 18]. HPV infection has recently been identified as a risk factor for a subset of oral and pharyngeal cancers arising in the oropharynx, tonsil, and base of tongue, which are also characterized by an improved prognosis [4, 14]. The much smaller declines in the incidence of cancers of the oral cavity and pharynx among white men are probably due to the increased incidence of HPV-associated cancers [15]. The increasing incidence of

Table 3 Five-year relative survival rates among patients diagnosed with squamous cell carcinoma of the oral cavity, pharynx, or larynx during 1995–2003 by race, gender, and stage of disease at diagnosis, SEER 9[a]

		White males		White females		Black males		Black females	
Site	Stage	Count	Rate	Count	Rate	Count	Rate	Count	Rate
All three sites	Localized	4,228	79.9%	1,742	73.9%	457	64.1%	166	63.1%
	Regional	6,226	51.3%	2,122	48.7%	1,128	33.7%	346	35.5%
	Distant	1,024	26.2%	349	24.6%	285	22.2%	82	25.8%
	Unstaged	382	51.2%	197	41.3%	64	21.3%	21	28.2%
Oral cavity	Localized	1,562	73.5%	1,062	74.4%	106	56.8%	60	69.8%
	Regional	2,362	50.6%	1,049	48.5%	378	27.6%	143	34.3%
	Distant	384	25.1%	183	27.3%	90	37.9%	34	30.6%
Pharynx	Localized	307	63.9%	134	59.0%	53	45.9%	13	47.1%
	Regional	2,140	53.3%	595	47.5%	383	29.0%	97	31.4%
	Distant	370	24.9%	107	21.1%	107	10.0%	23	17.8%
Larynx	Localized	2,359	86.0%	546	76.0%	298	70.0%	93	61.2%
	Regional	1,724	49.8%	478	50.4%	367	45.1%	106	39.7%
	Distant	270	29.3%	59	20.4%	88	21.3%	25	25.5%
Oral cavity and pharynx									
HPV-related	Localized	332	70.1%	147	65.4%	41	61.9%	17	53.3%
	Regional	2,440	62.2%	604	58.3%	355	34.2%	97	36.0%
	Distant	374	33.0%	97	29.3%	107	17.4%	25	29.5%
HPV-unrelated/unknown	Localized	1,537	72.2%	1,049	73.7%	118	50.8%	56	69.5%
	Regional	2,062	39.8%	1,040	41.9%	406	22.8%	143	31.1%
	Distant	380	16.9%	193	22.9%	90	27.9%	32	22.5%

[a]Excludes lip, salivary gland, and nasopharynx cancers; includes follow-up through 2004

these tumors, many with an improved prognosis, may also have contributed to the dramatic improvement in survival seen for white men in the most recent time period, 1995–2003. The decreased survival for patients with larynx cancer has been noted previously and is possibly due to the increase in nonsurgical management (i.e., radiation and chemoradiation) instead of the more invasive laryngectomy [19]. Dietary factors, particularly consumption of fruits and vegetables, have been consistently associated with a reduced risk of HN cancers [13, 14]. Per capita consumption of fresh fruits and vegetables increased 31% and 24%, respectively, from the early 1970s to the late 1990s, which may have contributed to the downward incidence trends observed for these tumors in recent years [16, 18, 20]. Occupational exposures probably play only a minor role in the etiology of HN cancers and are unlikely to explain any of the observed descriptive patterns [13, 14].

The temporal trends and race/sex patterns observed most likely reflect the impact of exposure to tobacco (particularly cigarettes) and alcohol (particularly hard liquor), diet (especially intake of fruits and vegetables), and more recently, HPV (often through oral sex practices [21]). Although it has been suggested that rates of oral cavity and pharynx cancer could be reduced if HPV vaccination were widespread among boys as well as girls [22, 23], it would take many years before such a reduction was evident in the temporal trends. Finding explanations for some anomalous observations, including the decreasing black/white rate ratios for HPV-unrelated cancers among females, may help clarify the roles of known and as yet unidentified risk factors.

Acknowledgments This research was supported by the Intramural Research Program of the Division of Cancer Epidemiology and Genetics, order should by Intramural Research Program of the DCEG, NCI, NIH, National Cancer Institute, National Institutes of Health. The authors thank Mr. John Lahey and Mr. David Castenson, Information Management Services, Inc., Rockville, MD and Mr. David Check, Biostatistics Branch, DCEG, NCI, Rockville, MD for data tabulation and preparation of figures.

References

1. Jemal A, Siegel R, Ward E, Hao Y, Xu J, Thun MJ (2009) Cancer Statistics, 2009. CA Cancer J Clin 54:225–249
2. Ries LAG, Melbert D, Krapcho M, Mariotto A et al (eds) (2007) SEER cancer statistics review, 1975–2004. National Cancer Institute, Bethesda, MD. http://seer.cancer.gov/csr/1975_2004/, based on November 2006 SEER data submission, posted to the SEER web site, 2007
3. World Health Organization (2000) International classification of diseases for oncology, 3rd edn. World Health Organization, Geneva (Switzerland)
4. Chaturvedi AK, Engels EA, Anderson WF, Gillison ML (2008) Incidence trends for human papillomavirus-related and unrelated oral squamous cell carcinomas in the United States. J Clin Oncol 26:612–619
5. SEER*Stat (2007) Surveillance Research Program, National Cancer Institute SEER*Stat software (www.seer.cancer.gov/seerstat) version 6.3.6. Accessed 25 Feb 2008

6. Surveillance, Epidemiology, and End Results (SEER) Program (www.seer.cancer.gov) SEER*Stat Database: Incidence – SEER 9 Regs Limited-Use, Nov 2006 Sub (1973–2004) – Linked To County Attributes – Total U.S., 1969–2004 Counties, National Cancer Institute, DCCPS, Surveillance Research Program, Cancer Statistics Branch, released April 2007, based on the November 2006 submission
7. Surveillance, Epidemiology, and End Results (SEER) Program (www.seer.cancer.gov) SEER*Stat Database: Incidence – SEER 13 Regs Limited-Use, Nov 2006 Sub (1973–2004) – Linked To County Attributes – Total U.S., 1969–2004 Counties, National Cancer Institute, DCCPS, Surveillance Research Program, Cancer Statistics Branch, released April 2007, based on the November 2006 submission
8. Devesa SS, Donaldson J, Fears T (1995) Graphical presentation of trends in rates. Am J Epidemiol 141:300–304
9. Devesa SS, Grauman DJ, Blot WJ, Pennello GA, Hoover RN, Fraumeni JF Jr (eds) (1999) Atlas of cancer mortality in the United States 1950–94. National Institutes of Health, National Cancer Institute, NIH Publication No. 99-4564
10. Winn DM, Blot WJ, Shy CM, Pickle LW, Toledo A, Fraumeni JF Jr (1981) Snuff dipping and oral cancer among women in the southern United States. N Engl J Med 304:745–749
11. Giovino GA, Schooley MW, Zhu BP et al (1994) Surveillance for selected tobacco-use behaviors-United States, 1900–1994. MMWR CDC Surveill Summ 43:1–43
12. Devesa SS, Grauman DJ, Blot WJ, Fraumeni JF Jr (1999) Cancer surveillance series: changing geographic patterns of lung cancer mortality in the United States, 1950 through 1994. J Natl Cancer Inst 91:1040–1050
13. Olshan AF (2006) Cancer of the larynx. In: Schottenfeld D, Fraumeni JF Jr (eds) Cancer epidemiology and prevention, 3rd edn. New York, Oxford
14. Mayne ST, Morse DE, Winn DM (2006) Cancers of the oral cavity and pharynx. In: Schottenfeld D, Fraumeni JF Jr (eds) Cancer epidemiology and prevention, 3rd edn. New York, Oxford
15. Sturgis EM, Cinciripini PM (2007) Trends in head and neck cancer incidence in relation to smoking prevalence – an emerging epidemic of human papillomavirus-associated cancers? Cancer 110:1429–1435
16. Brown LM, Devesa SS (2002) Epidemiologic trends in esophageal and gastric cancer in the United States. Surg Oncol Clin N Am 11:235–256
17. Devesa SS, Bray FB, Vizcaino AP, Parkin DM (2005) International lung cancer trends by histologic type: male:female differences diminishing and adenocarcinoma rates rising. Int J Cancer 117:294–299
18. Brown LM, Devesa SS, Chow W-H (2008) Incidence of adenocarcinoma of the esophagus among white Americans by sex, stage, and age. J Natl Cancer Inst 100:1184–1187
19. Hoffman HT, Porter K, Karnell LH (2006) Laryngeal cancer in the United States: changes in demographics, patterns of care, and survival. Laryngoscope 116(Suppl. 111):1–13
20. Putnam JJ, Allshouse JE (1999) Food consumption, prices, and expenditures, 1970–97. In: Statistical Bulletin – Economic Research Service (USA) no. 965, USDA, Economic Research Service, Washington, DC
21. Gillison ML (2007) Current topics in the epidemiology of oral cavity and oropharyngeal cancers. Head Neck 29:779–792
22. D'Souza G, Kreimer AR, Viscidi R et al (2007) Case-control study of human papillomavirus and oropharyngeal cancer. N Engl J Med 356:1944–1956
23. Closmann JJ (2007) The human papilloma virus, the vaccines, and oral and oropharyngeal squamous cell carcinoma: what every dentist should know. Gen Dent 55:252–254

Descriptive Epidemiology: International Patterns

Mia Hashibe, Jacques Ferlay, and Rengaswamy Sankaranarayanan

Head and neck cancers (HNC) are a group of neoplasms common in several regions of the world where the prevalence of tobacco habits and alcohol consumption in the population is high. These cancers accounted for 420,000 new cases among males and 142,000 incident cases among females in 2002 around the world (Table 1) [1]. They are responsible for 8% of male (257,779/3,092,119) and 4% of female cancers (101,654/2,735,386) in the developing world. In developed countries, they account for 6% of male (163,377/2,698,175) and 2% of female cancers (40,762/2,317,939). The incidence rate of HNC and the distribution of cancers in head and neck anatomical subsites vary greatly in different geographical regions. The variation in cancer distribution by subsites is most likely due to differences in the relative distribution of the known risk factors such as tobacco chewing, smoking, and alcohol consumption. Misclassification of subsites is also a possibility due to the difficulties in assigning the primary site of origin, especially due to the anatomical proximity between the various subsites (for example, cancers of the supraglottic larynx and hypopharynx). However, patterns of disease distribution provide valuable clues for disease prevention and control. We will review the global geographical distribution and trends in incidence and mortality of HNC.

M. Hashibe (✉),
Division of Public Health, Department of Family & Preventive Medicine,
University of Utah School of Medicine, Salt Lake City, Utah
e-mail: mia.hashibe@utah.edu

J. Ferlay
Data Analysis and Interpretation Group, Section of Cancer Information,
International Agency for Research on Cancer, Lyon, France

R. Sankaranarayanan
Screening Group, Section of Early Detection and Prevention,
International Agency for Research on Cancer, Lyon, France

A.F. Olshan (ed.), *Epidemiology, Pathogenesis, and Prevention of Head and Neck Cancer*,
DOI 10.1007/978-1-4419-1472-9_3, © Springer Science+Business Media, LLC 2010

Table 1 Head and neck cancer cases and deaths by world region for men and women, 2002

	Male		Female	
Head and neck cancers[a]	Cases	Deaths	Cases	Deaths
World total	421,369	227,331	142,463	74,078
Eastern Africa	7,092	4,752	4,572	2,821
Middle Africa	2,001	1,365	1,270	861
Northern Africa	4,474	3,244	1,479	977
Southern Africa	2,885	1,765	820	482
Western Africa	3,567	2,346	1,232	794
Africa total	20,019	13,472	9,373	5,935
Caribbean	2,950	1,638	912	487
Central America	4,236	1,992	1,326	667
South America	23,170	11,469	5,195	2,871
Northern America	36,015	9,121	13,290	3,661
Americas total	66,371	24,220	20,723	7,686
Eastern Asia	32,766	15,922	11,105	5,369
South-Eastern Asia	17,832	11,030	8,016	4,661
South Central Asia	157,543	100,304	65,659	38,831
Western Asia	7,918	4,533	2,825	1,535
Asia total	216,059	131,789	87,605	50,396
Eastern Europe	41,517	28,502	6,804	3,575
Northern Europe	8,669	3,504	3,456	1,359
Southern Europe	27,394	11,187	4,432	1,684
Western Europe	37,965	13,503	8,605	2,890
Europe total	115,545	56,696	23,297	9,508
Australia/New Zealand	2,666	750	1,008	283
Oceania total	3,375	1,154	1,465	553

[a]Includes salivary glands. Source: GLOBOCAN 2002

Sources of Data

For this review, HNC consists of those cancer sites classified in the International Classification of Diseases (O_2 edition) [2] categories C00–C06, C09–C14, and C32 (lip, tongue, gingiva, floor of mouth, palate, cheek mucosa, oropharynx, hypopharynx, pharynx unspecified, and larynx). Salivary gland and nasopharyngeal tumors were excluded when possible since the etiologic pattern is different [3, 4]. Age standardized incidence rates for these categories were extracted from volumes XI of the series Cancer Incidence in Five Continents and the GLOBOCAN 2002 program [1, 5]. Population-based survival data were obtained from publications of the Surveillance, Epidemiology, and End Results (SEER) program of the National Cancer Institute of USA [6], which collects cancer data on a routine basis from selected cancer registries in various regions of the United States of America, and from the European Cancer Registry-based Study of Survival and Care of Cancer Patients (EUROCARE) project [7, 8] involving survival data from 21 European countries and the on-going multinational collaborative project on survival from developing countries, co-ordinated by the International Agency for Research on Cancer (IARC) [9]. Mortality data for selected countries were obtained from the World Health Organization (WHO) mortality data bank [10]. Results from the mortality data included salivary gland tumors and nasopharyngeal tumors since they could not be separated. Figures from GLOBOCAN 2002 included salivary gland since they could not be separated.

Incidence Patterns

The majority of head and neck cancer cases and deaths occur in Asia for both men and women (Table 1). Within Asia, South Central Asia carries the heaviest burden of head and neck cancer. Following Asia, Europe and North America are the regions with the greatest number of HNC cases and deaths.

The highest reported incidence rate of HNC cancer among males around 2002 is that reported from Somme, France, an age standardized rate (ASR) of 46.2/100,000; the highest incidence of HNC among females is reported from South Karachi, Pakistan (23.9/100,000) (Table 2) [5]. There are great differences in the distribution of cancers by other subsites between geographical regions. In select regions of France, the highest incidence rates among men were observed for cancers of the tongue, other oropharynx, and hypopharynx. Among women, the highest incidence rates were observed for cancers of the tongue, mouth, and hypopharynx in South Karachi, Pakistan. The lowest incidence rates of head and neck cancer among both men and women was in Valdivia, Chile.

For most of the HNC sites, the highest incidence rate among men was at least twofold greater than the corresponding rate for women, with almost a sixfold difference for laryngeal cancer (men in Spain vs. Black women in the US). An exception was for tongue and mouth cancers, where the rates among Pakistani women were close to the highest incidence rate reported among men.

Figures 1 and 2 show the world map with ASRs for HNC in males and females, respectively [1]. High rates of HNC (above 22.6/100,000) in men are found in France, Spain, Germany, Central and Eastern Europe, the Indian sub-continent, Botswana, Gabon, and Papua New Guinea. For women, high rates of HNC (above 5.6/100,000) are found in France, the Indian subcontinent, Sudan, Ethiopia, Tanzania, Zimbabwe, Madagascar, Phillipines, Papua New Guinea, and Australia.

Figures 3 and 4 show select ASRs for HNC within geographic regions for males and females, respectively [5]. ASRs were particularly high among men in Sao Paolo (Brazil), black men in the US, South Karachi (Pakistan), Basque Country (Spain), Somme (France), and the Northern Territory (Australia). The greatest contrast among men appeared to be in Asia, where the ratio of the high incidence to low incidence rates was nearly tenfold. Similarly for women, the ratio of the high incidence to low incidence was the greatest in Asia.

Figures 5–12 show the ASRs for the oral cavity (mouth, lip, and tongue), oropharynx, hypopharynx, and larynx for men and women separately. About one third of the highest ASR among males in Somme, France, was due to oral cavity cancer while another one third was due to hypopharyngeal cancer. About half of the

Table 2 Range of variation in head and neck cancer age standardized incidence rates (ASR) by sex around 1998–2002

	Male (ASR)		Female (ASR)	
Site (ICD-10 code)	Highest	Lowest	Highest	Lowest
Lip (C00)	9.8 (Spain, Granada)	0.1 (Costa Rica)	2.6 (Australia, Northern Territory)	0.1 (Costa Rica)
Tongue (C01–02)	7.0 (France, Somme)	0.2 (Algeria, Setif)	6.6 (Pakistan, South Karachi)	0.1 (Algeria, Setif)
Mouth (C03–06)	15.3 (Pakistan, South Karachi)	0.2 (Chile, Valdivia)	12.3 (Pakistan, South Karachi)	0.1 (Algeria, Setif)
Tonsil (C09)	5.5 (Australia, Northern Territory)	0.1 (Oman: Omani)	1.6 (Australia, Northern Territory)	0.1 (Uganda, Kyadondo)
Other oropharynx (C10)	4.4 (France, Calvados)	0.1 (Costa Rica)	1.0 (Germany, Hamburg)	0.1 (Brazil, Goiania)
Pharynx unspecified (C14)	3.5 (Brazil, Cuiaba)	0.1 (Algeria, Setif)	1.1 (Brazil, Cuiaba)	0.1 (Algeria, Setif)
Hypopharynx (C12–13)	10.2 (France, Somme)	0.1 (Zimbabwe, Harare: African)	1.8 (Pakistan, South Karachi)	0.1 (Zimbabwe, Harare: African)
Larynx (C32)	16.1 (Spain, Basque Country)	1.1 (China, Jiashan)	2.7 (USA, Pennsylvania: Black)	0.1 (Algeria, Setif)
Head and neck (C00, C01–02, C03–06, C09, C10, C14, C12–13, C32)	46.2 (France, Somme)	2.7 (Chile, Valdivia)	23.9 (Pakistan, South Karachi)	0.2 (Chile, Valdivia)

Source: Curado, M.P., Edwards, B., Shin. H.R., Storm. H., Ferlay. J., Heanue. M., Boyle. P., eds (2007) Cancer Incidence in Five Continents, Vol. IX. IARC Scientific Publications No. 160, Lyon, IARC

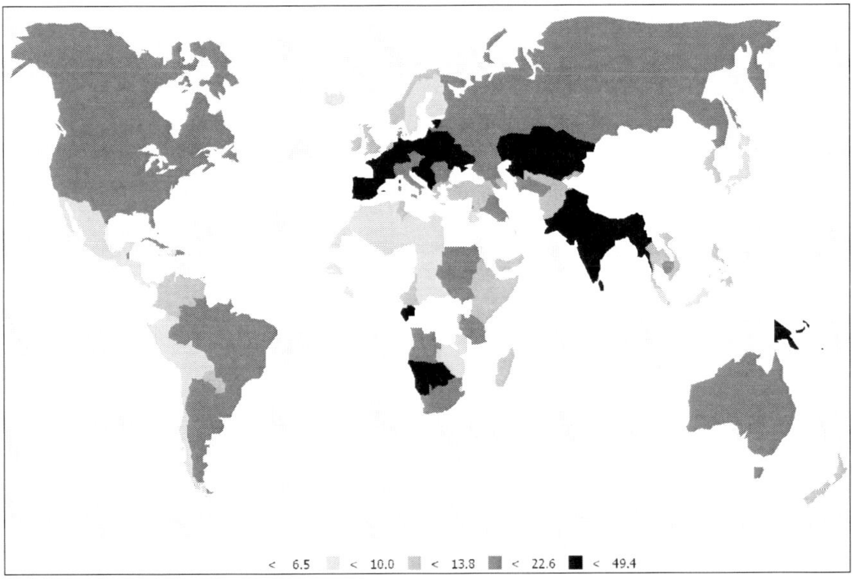

Fig. 1 Age-standardized incidence rates (ASR) of head and neck cancers, men. Includes salivary glands. Source: GLOBOCAN 2002

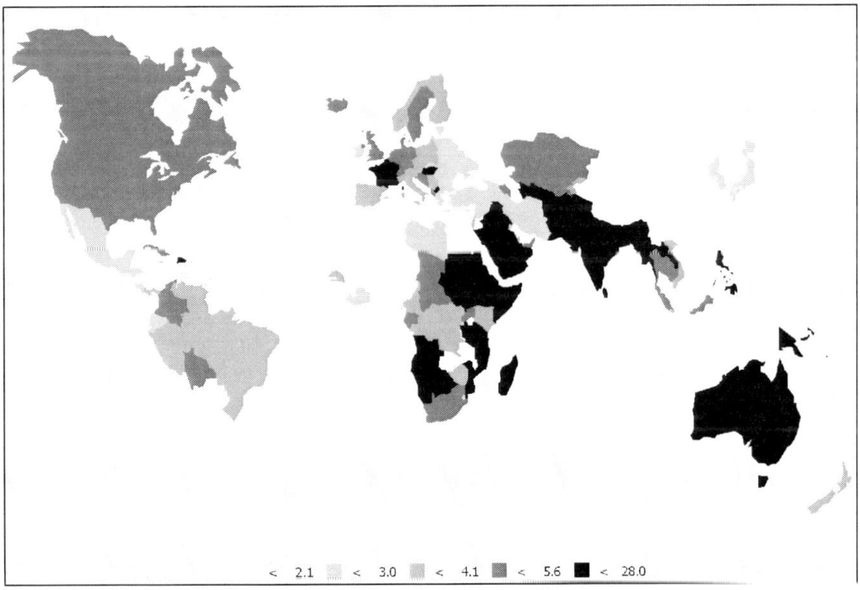

Fig. 2 Age-standardized incidence rates (ASR) of head and neck cancers, women. Includes salivary glands. Source: GLOBOCAN 2002

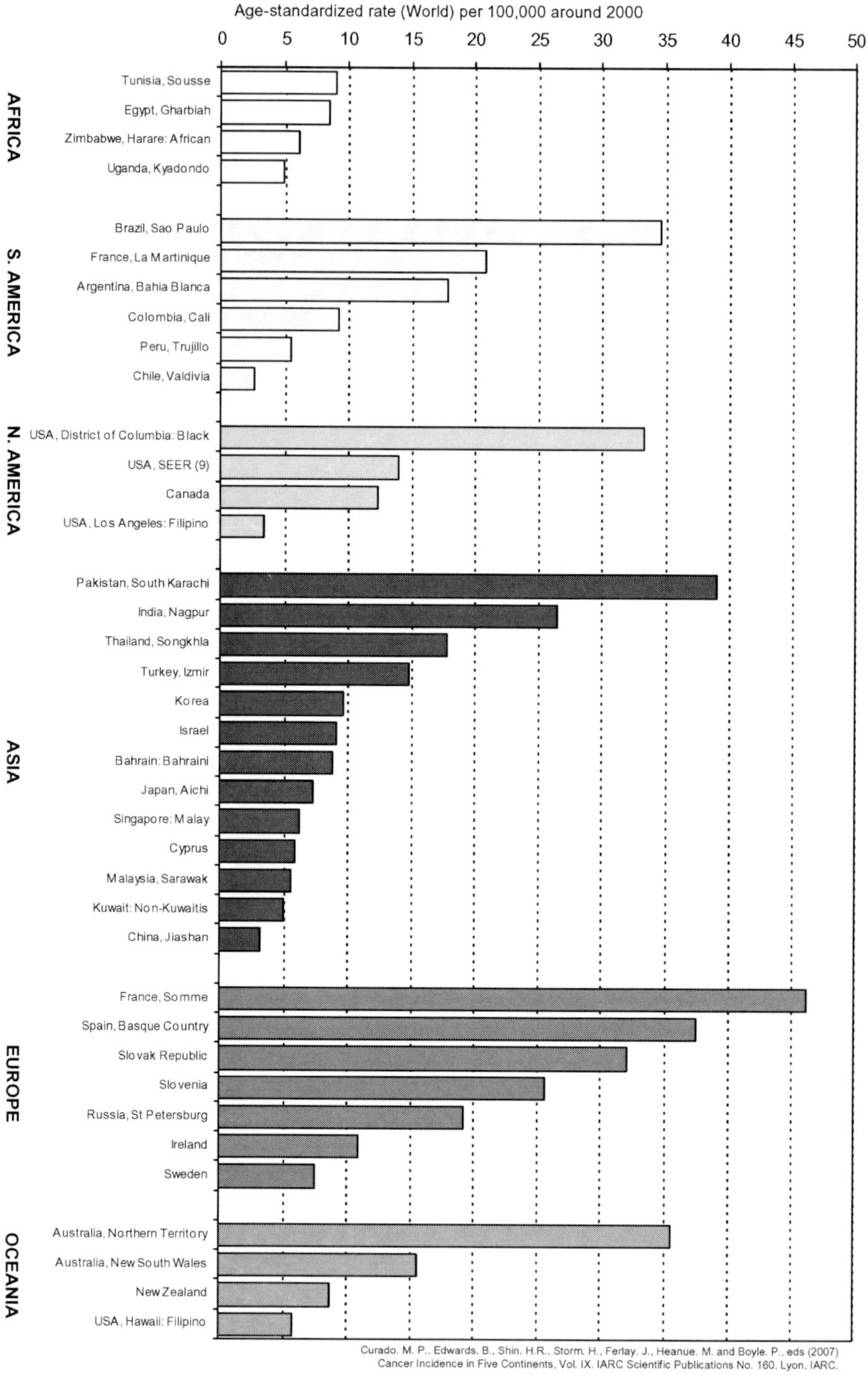

Fig. 3 Head and neck cancers in males, all ages

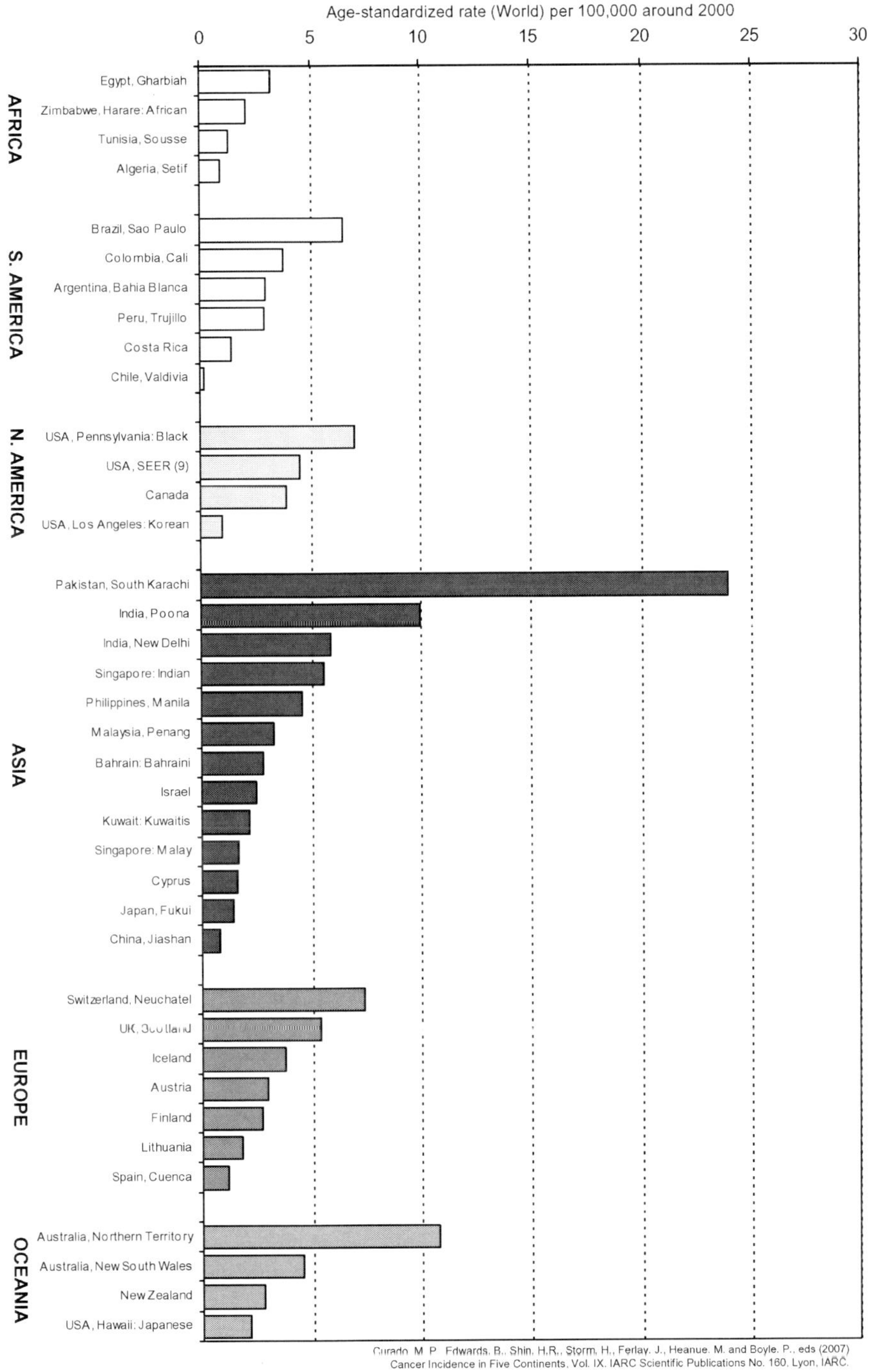

Fig. 4 Head and neck cancers in females, all ages

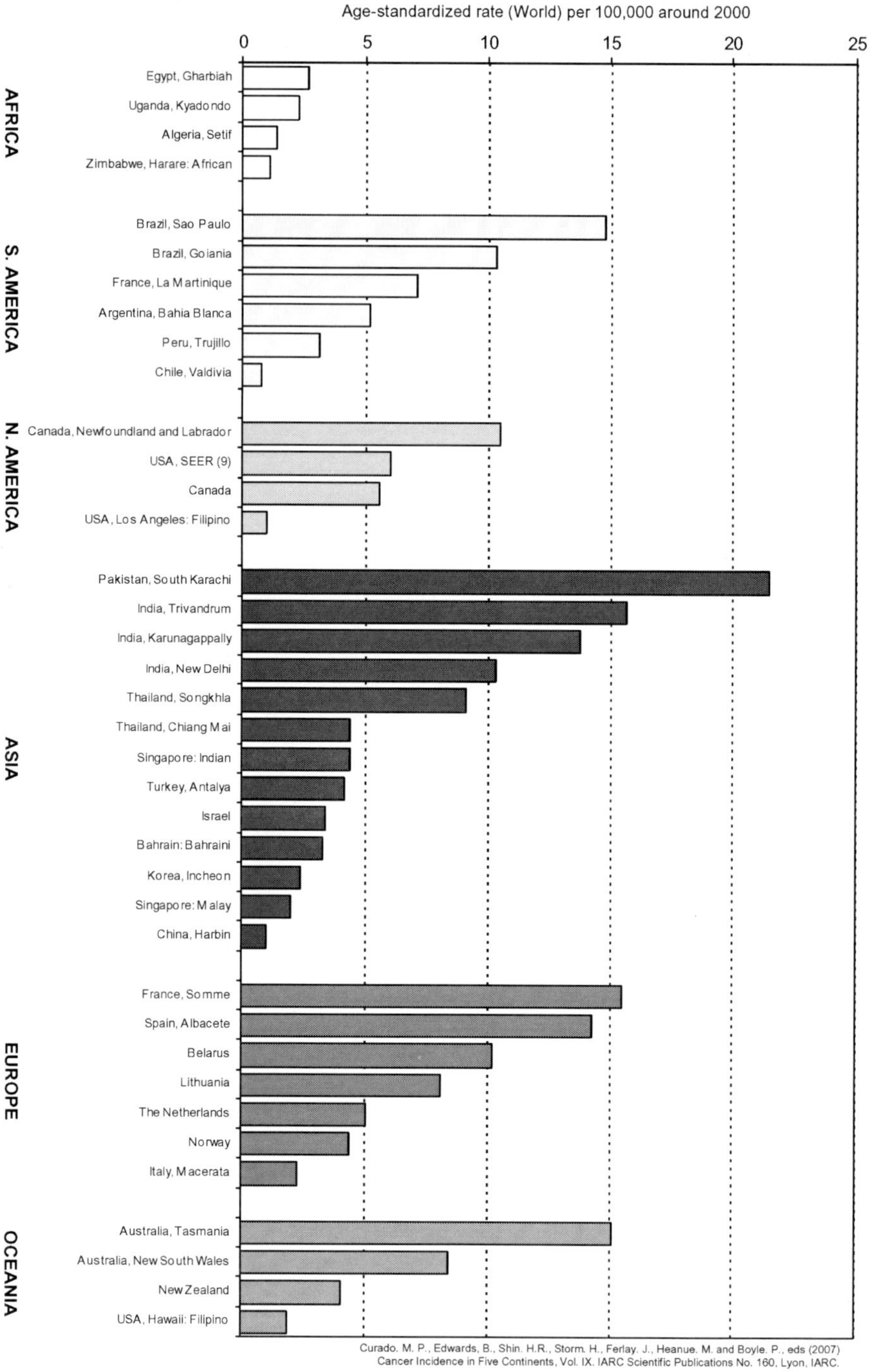

Fig. 5 Lip, tongue and mouth (C00–06) cancer in males, all ages

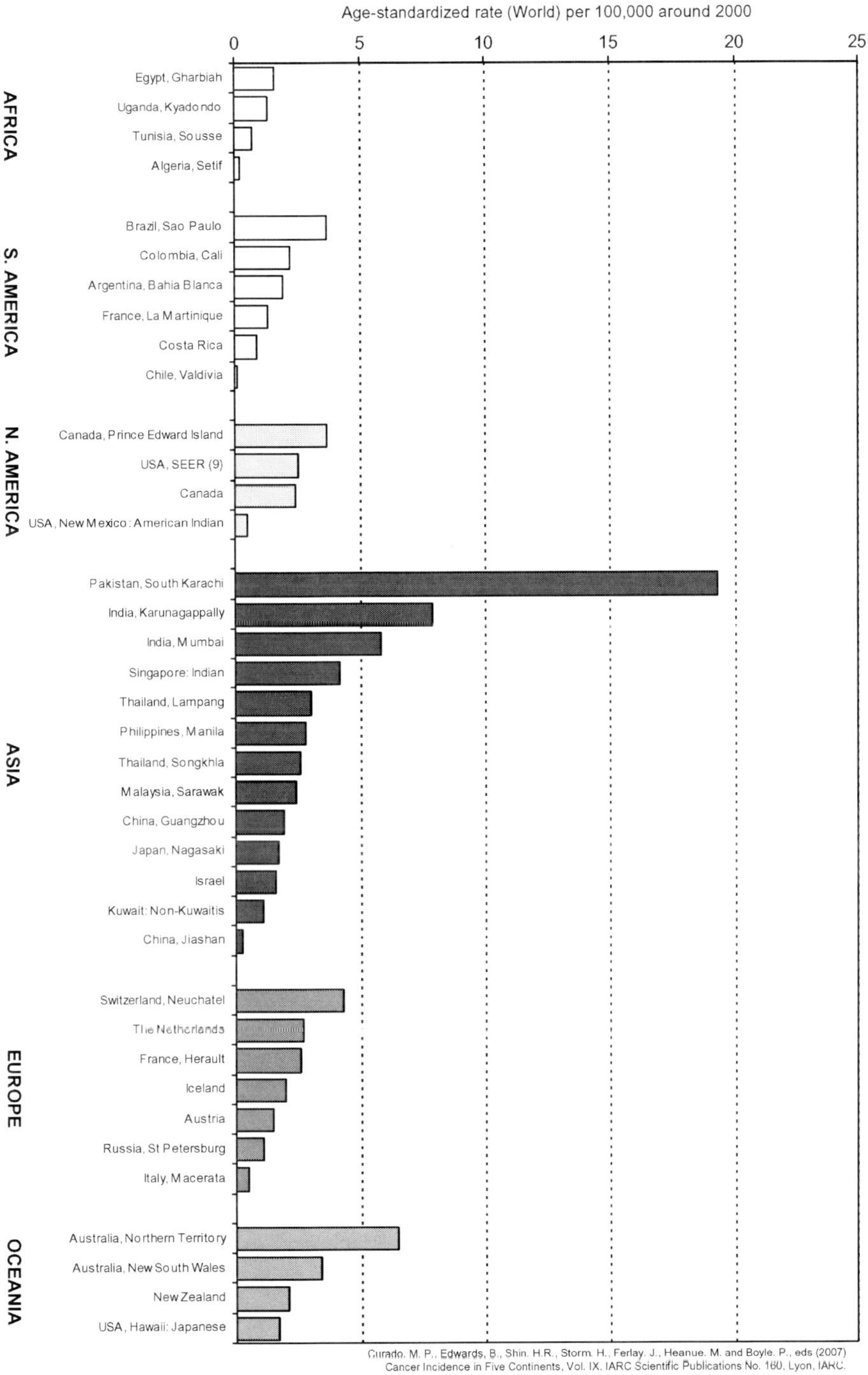

Fig. 6 Lip, tongue and mouth (C00–06) cancer in females, all ages

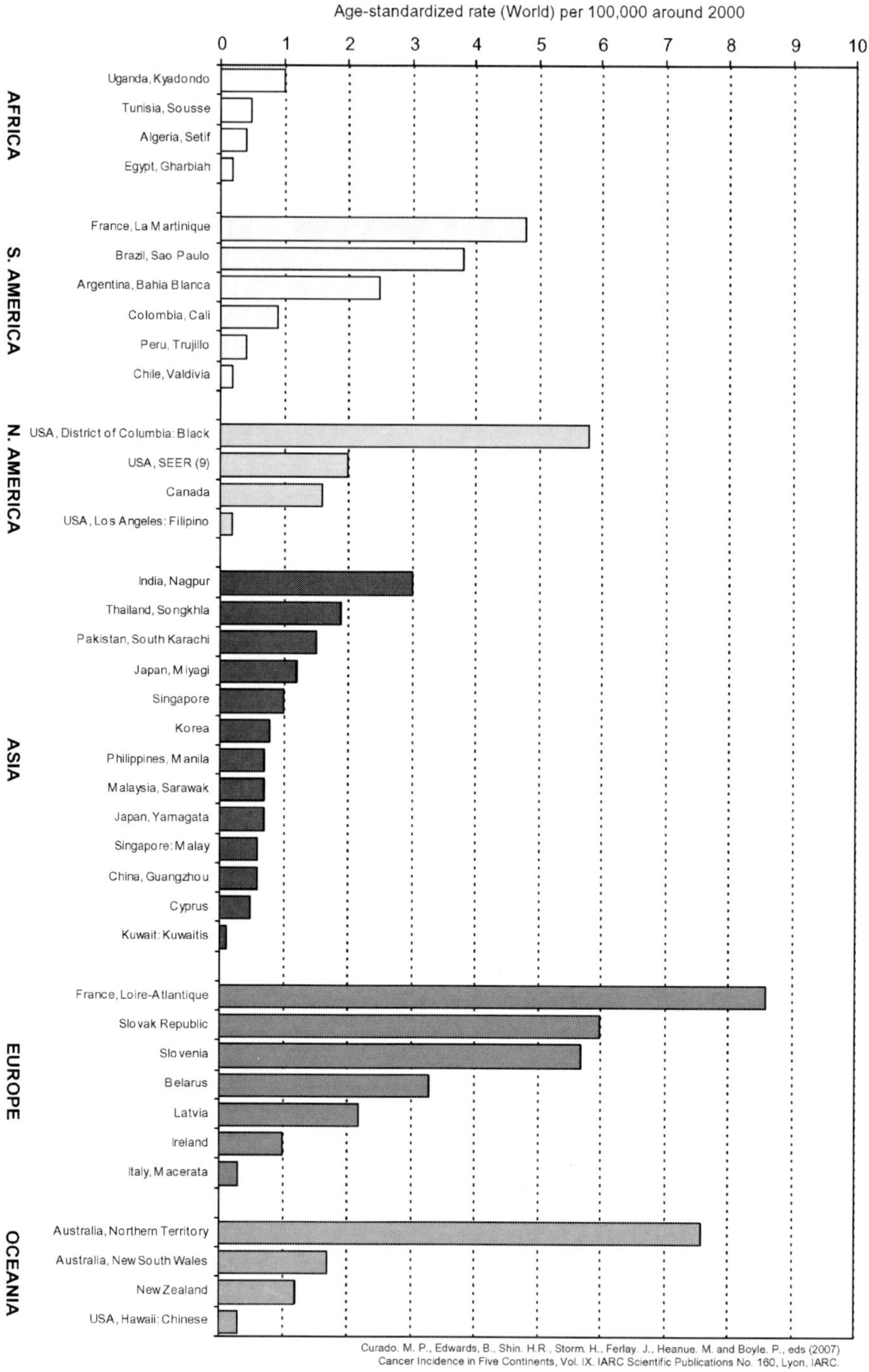

Fig. 7 Oropharynx (C09–10) cancer in males, all ages

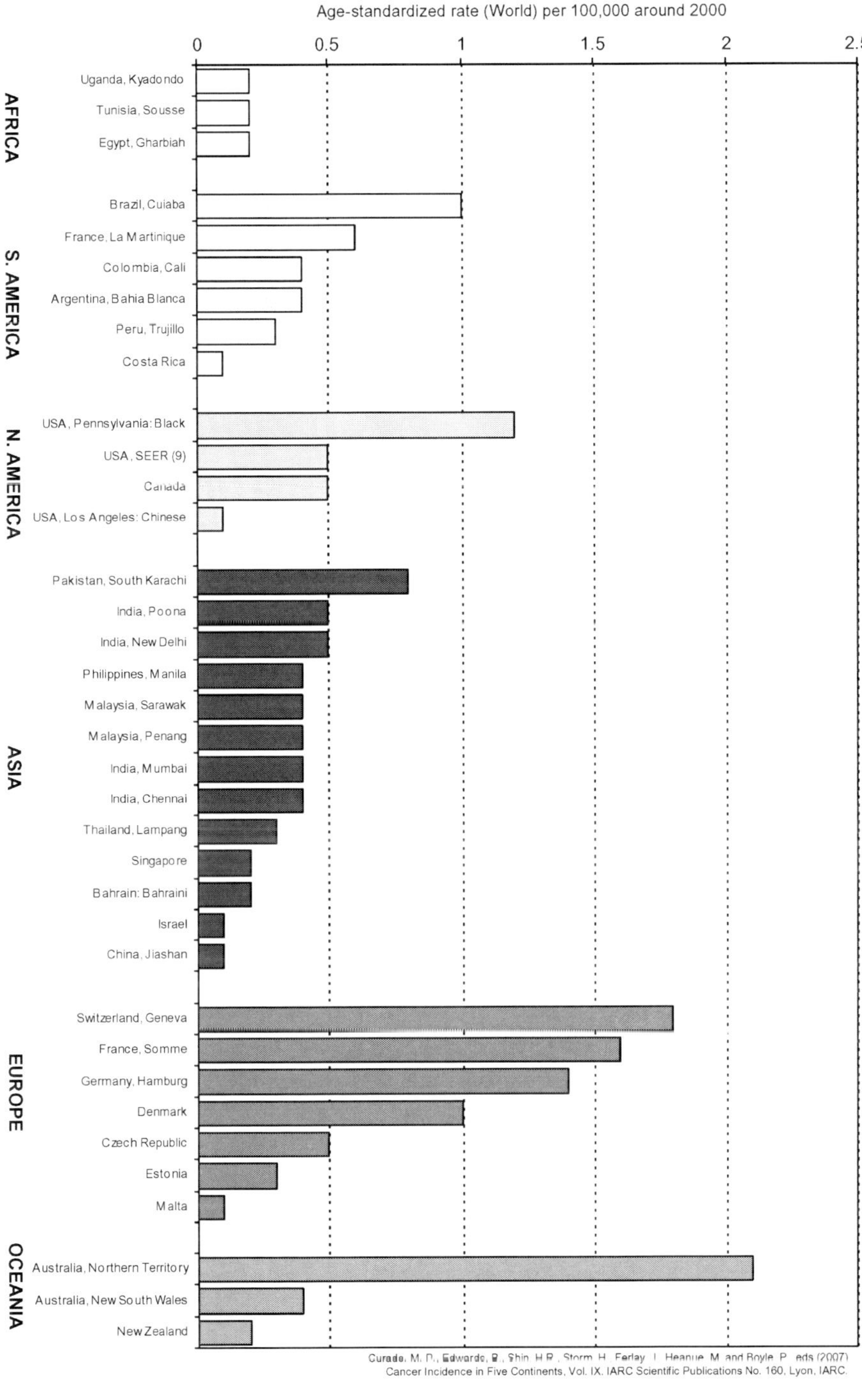

Fig. 8 Oropharynx (C09–10) cancer in females, all ages

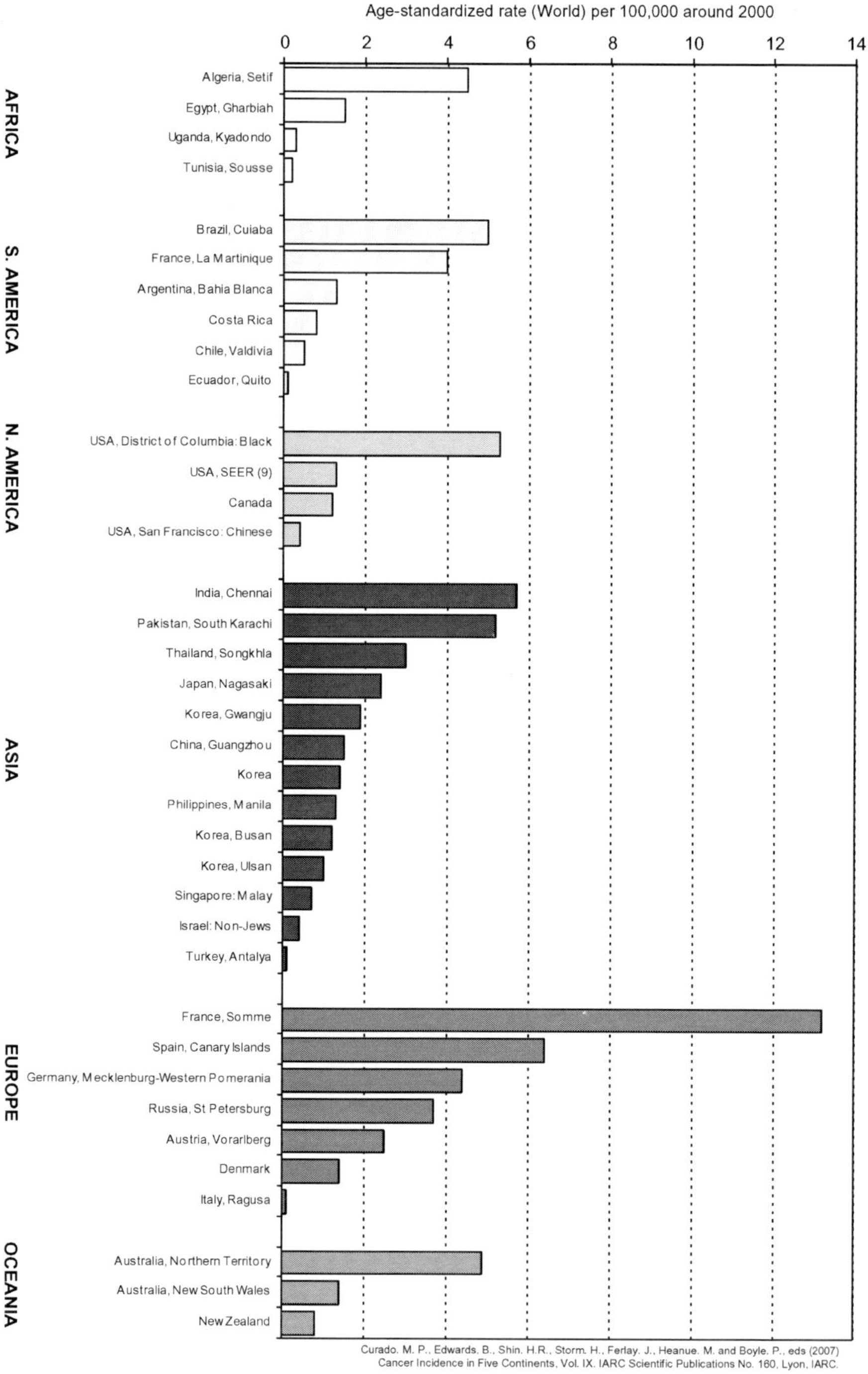

Fig. 9 Hypopharynx (C12–14) cancer in males, all ages

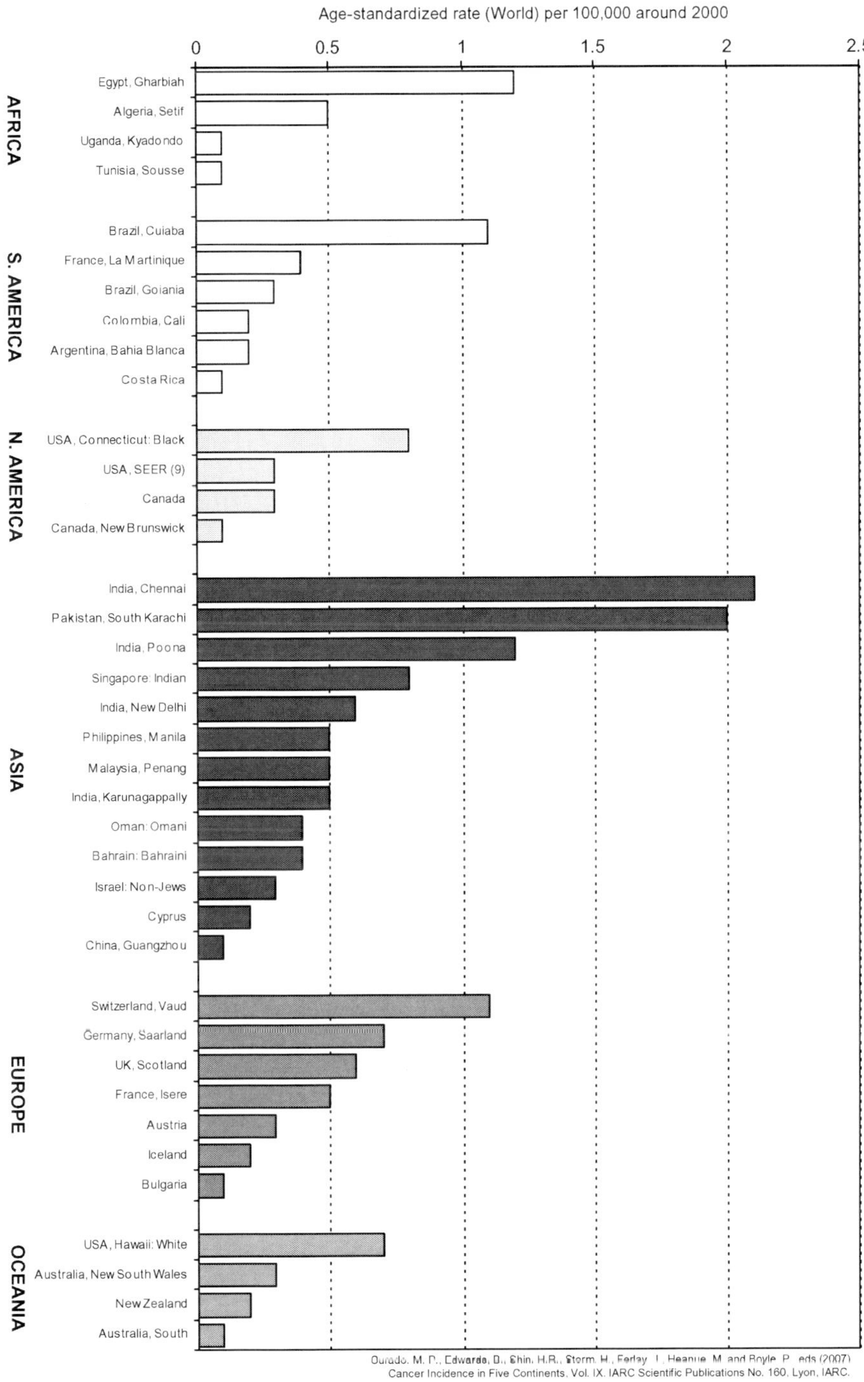

Fig. 10 Hypopharynx (C12–14) cancer in females, all ages

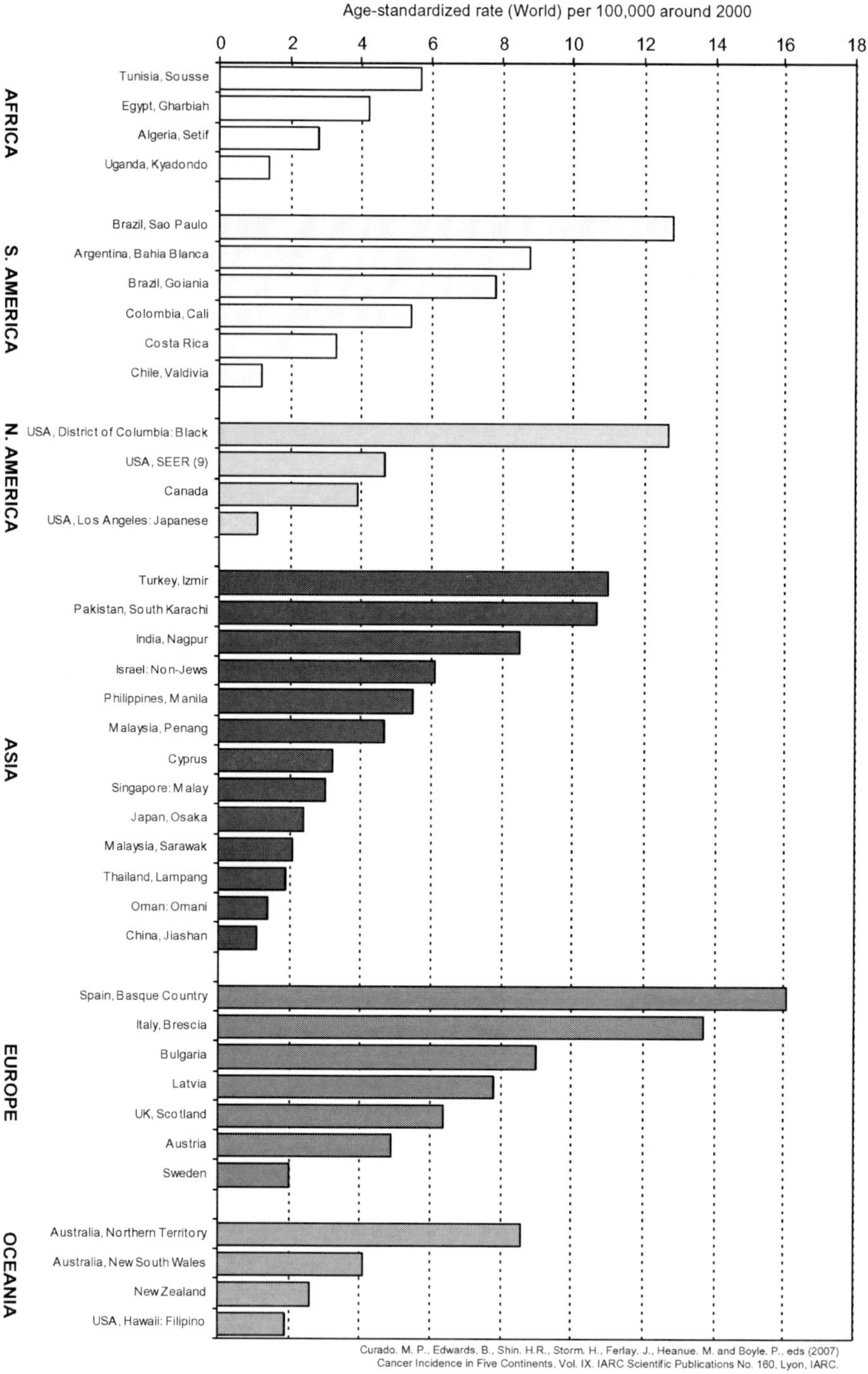

Fig. 11 Larynx (C32) cancer in males, all ages

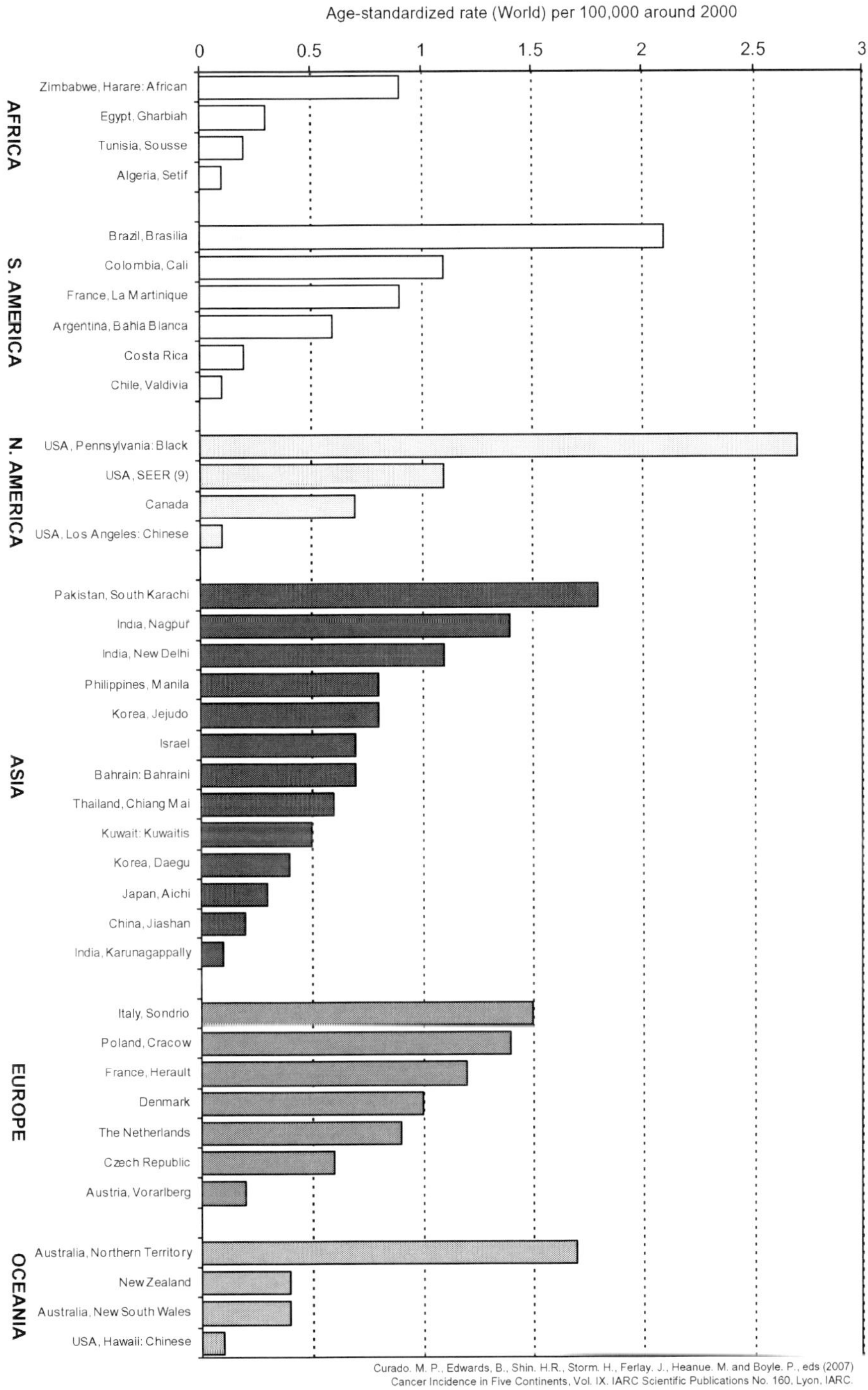

Fig. 12 Larynx (C32) cancer in females, all ages

high incidence of head and neck cancer among men in South Karachi was due to oral cavity cancer while another quarter was laryngeal cancer. Among women in South Karachi, the majority of the head and neck cancer incidence was due to oral cavity cancers.

Trends

Aggregate HNC incidence rates have been slowly declining in the Indian subcontinent, East Asia, Western Europe, and the United States for men. On the other hand, the rates are rising in males in Central Europe. Figures 13–15 reveal the incidence trends among men in ASR of HNC in selected regions of the world. The greatest decline in incidence rates among Asian men was observed in India and China, while the rates in Australia and Singapore were slowly decreasing. In Europe, a substantial decrease in incidence among men was observed in France. The incidence rates in Spain and Slovakia were rising through the 1970s and 1980s and show some decline in the 1990s. In Scotland, the incidence rate for men appears to be increasing very gradually. In the Americas, both the United States and South American incidence rates among men were gradually declining. The data from Africa is available more recently, thus trends are difficult to assess.

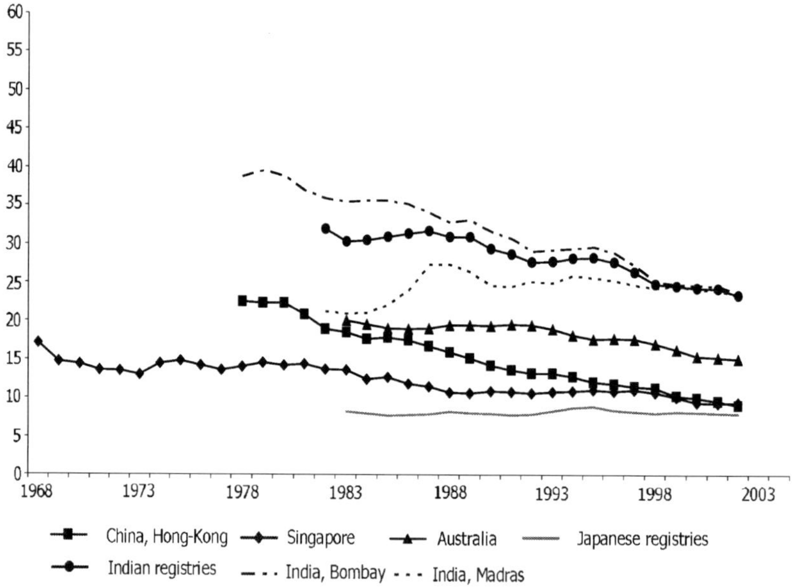

Fig. 13 Trends in age-standardized incidence rates (ASR) of head and neck cancers in selected Asia-Pacific regions, men. Rates have been smoothed using 3 years average

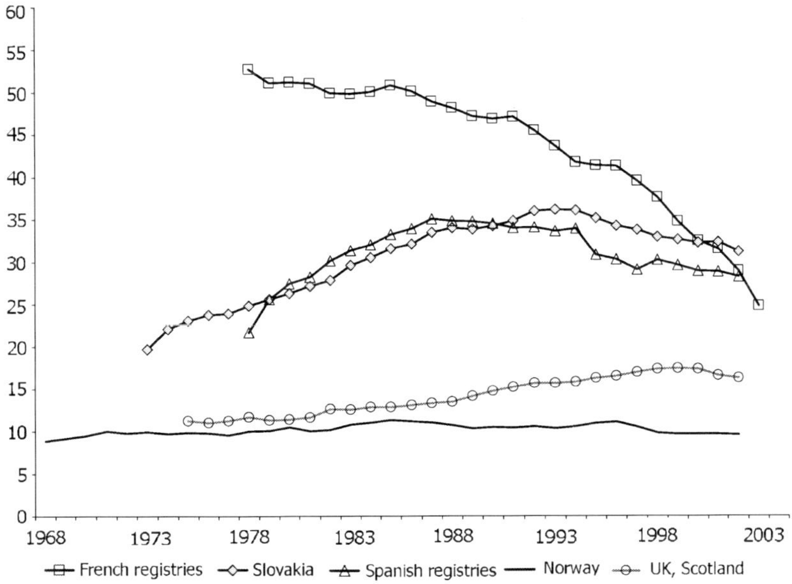

Fig. 14 Trends in age standardized incidence rates (ASR) of head and neck cancers in selected European regions, men. Rates have been smoothed using 3 years average

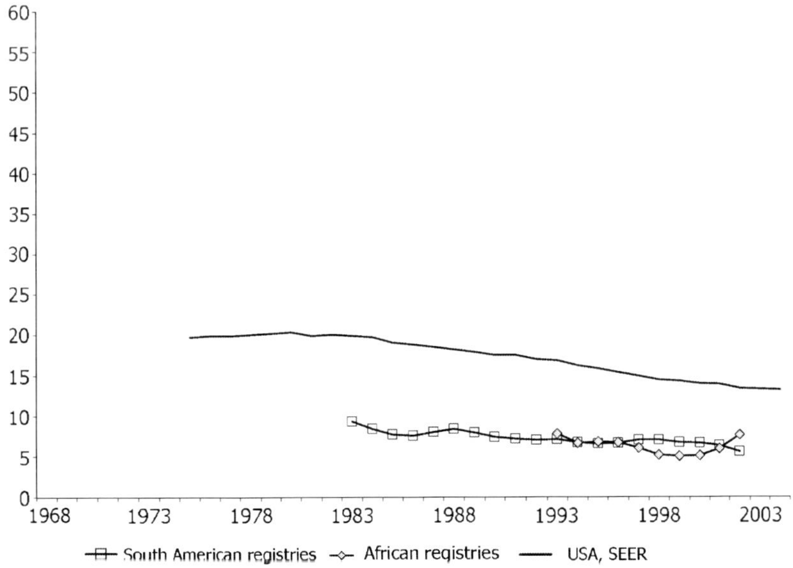

Fig. 15 Trends in age-standardized incidence rates (ASR) of head and neck cancers in selected regions of the Americas and Africa, men. Rates have been smoothed using 3 years average

The patterns for head and neck cancer mortality rates among men were largely consistent with the incidence rate trends. One notable increase was the mortality rate among Hungarian men (Fig. 16), as reported previously [11].

Figures 17–19 show the incidence trends among women in ASR of HNC in selected regions of the world. Among women, the incidence rates have also been declining in India and China. The HNC incidence rates in Australia, Japan, and Singapore have been fairly stable. In Europe, the HNC incidence rates among women appear largely stable, though there seems to be some indications of very small increases in Scotland, France, and Norway. In the Americas, the HNC incidence rates for women appear to be declining slowly. For Africa, a decline is suggested, though the data is available only for a 10-year period. Trends in mortality rates among women were largely consistent with those of incidence rates.

Histologic Distribution

The distribution of histologic subtypes of head and neck cancer for select countries is shown in Table 3. In Africa, Kaposi's sarcoma was the most common type of head and neck cancer, most likely due to the prevalence of HIV/AIDs [18]. In Europe and the United States [6, 12], over 90% of male head and neck cancer patients had squamous cell carcinomas, suggesting the importance of tobacco and

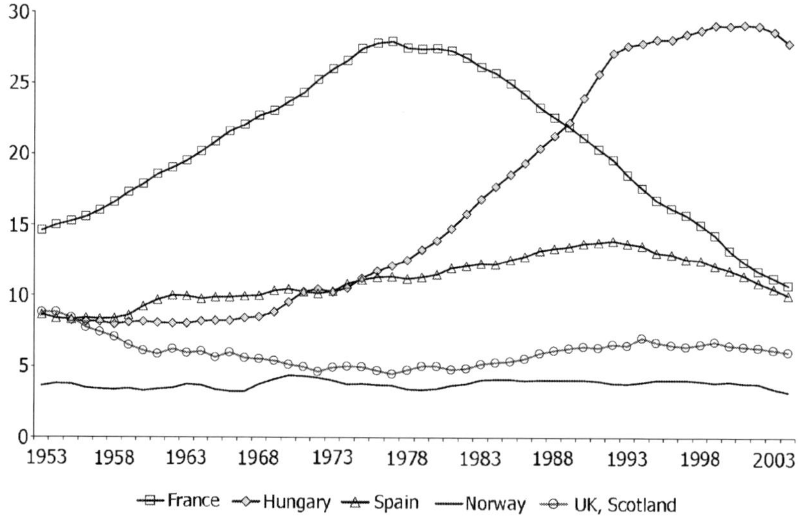

Fig. 16 Trends in age-standardized mortality rates (ASR) from head and neck cancers in selected European countries, men. Includes nasopharyngeal and salivary glands cancers. Rates have been smoothed using 3 years average

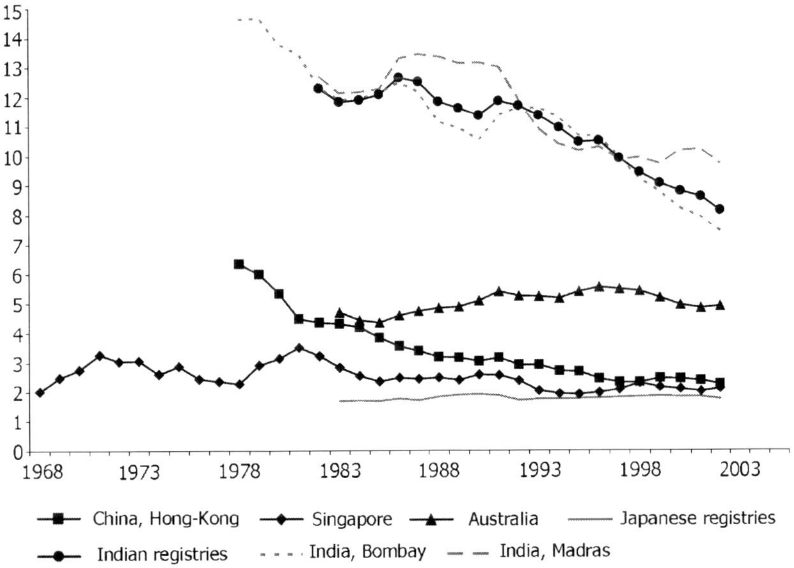

Fig. 17 Trends in age-standardized incidence rates (ASR) of head and neck cancers in selected Asia-Pacific regions, women. Rates have been smoothed using 3 years average

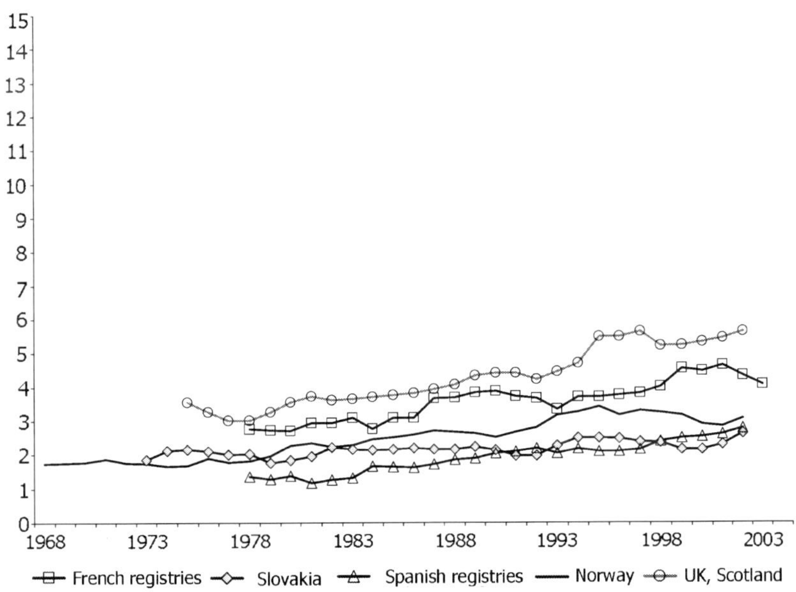

Fig. 18 Trends in age-standardized incidence rates (ASR) of head and neck cancers in selected European regions, women. Rates have been smoothed using 3 years average

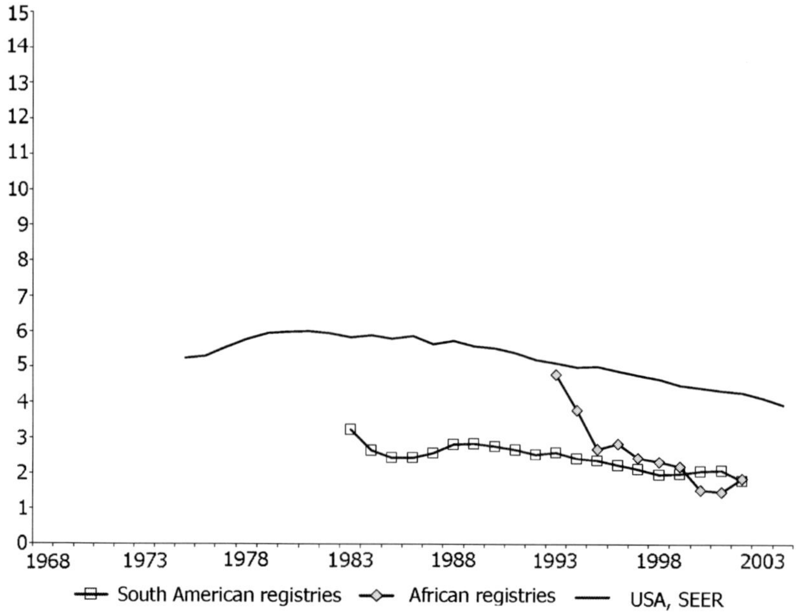

Fig. 19 Trends in age-standardized incidence rates (ASR) of head and neck cancers in selected regions of the Americas and Africa, women. Rates have been smoothed using 3 years average

Table 3 Histologic distribution of head and neck cancer in select countries

	Male	Female	Both sexes
Africa: Uganda, Kyadondo County and Zimbabwe, Harare			
Squamous cell carcinoma	24.5	9.8	18.6
Adenocarcinoma	0.5	1.0	0.7
Kaposi sarcoma	58.5	73.6	64.6
Lymphoma	4.5	5.4	4.8
Other and unspecified	11.9	10.3	11.3
India: Mumbai and Chennai			
Squamous cell carcinoma	79.5	77.6	79.1
Adenocarcinoma	1.0	1.8	1.2
Kaposi sarcoma	0.0	0.0	0.0
Lymphoma	0.1	0.2	0.1
Other and unspecified	19.4	20.4	19.7
USA, SEER			
Squamous cell carcinoma	91.6	85.8	90.0
Adenocarcinoma	1.0	3.2	1.6
Kaposi sarcoma	1.2	0.0	0.9
Lymphoma	1.9	3.8	2.4
Other and unspecified	4.3	7.1	5.1
France: Bas-Rhin, Calvados, Doubs, Isere, Somme and Tarn			
Squamous cell carcinoma	94.1	84.1	93.1
Adenocarcinoma	0.5	2.6	0.7
Kaposi sarcoma	0.1	0.0	0.1
Lymphoma	1.0	7.2	1.6
Other and unspecified	4.3	6.0	4.5

alcohol as risk factors. The majority of women in Europe and the United States also had squamous cell carcinomas, but the proportion was less than that for men. On the other hand, the proportion of adenocarcinomas in Europe and the United States was greater in women than men. Though adenocarcinomas are also related to tobacco and alcohol, these risk factors are thought to be more important for squamous cell carcinoma. The histologic distribution difference for women suggests that factors other than tobacco and alcohol are playing an important role for head and neck cancer etiology. In contrast, the proportion of squamous cell carcinomas in India was fairly similar among men and women. The proportion of other and unspecified histologic types was large in India, at approximately 20% for men and women.

Survival Experience

The 5-year relative survival rates reported from 21 countries in the European Cancer Registry-based Study of Survival and Care of Cancer Patients (EUROCARE-4) were 48.5 for oral cavity cancer, 39.8 for oropharyngeal cancer, 25.5 for hypopharyngeal cancer and 63.1 for laryngeal cancer during the period of 1995–1999 [7]. For the previous period (1990–1994), the 5-year relative survival rates were 44.4 for oral cavity cancer, 31.0 for oropharyngeal cancer, 24.2 for hypopharyngeal cancer and 60.6 for laryngeal cancer [7, 13]. Thus, compared to the previous period, the survival rates for oral cavity cancer, oropharyngeal and laryngeal cancer improved whereas survival among hypopharyngeal cancer patients remained approximately similar. The 5-year relative survival rate reported by the SEER program for the period 1996–2004 was 59.7% for oral cavity and pharyngeal cancers and 62.5% for larynx cancer [6].

Five year relative survival from a few selected low and medium resource countries [11] is shown in Table 4. Very low survival was observed in Thailand and India, whereas survival in Cuba and China were higher.

Table 4 5-year relative survival (%) by anatomical subsites in head and neck cancer in selected low and medium resource countries

	Chiang Mai, Thailand, 1983–1992	Khon Kaen, Thailand, 1985–1992	Chennai, India, 1984–1989	Cuba, 1988–1989	Shanghai, China, 1988–1991
Oral cavity	19.4	39.3	32.8	49.1	55.2
Oropharynx	23.3	26.7	20.9	33.7	55.8
Hypopharynx	21.4	na	17.5	–	24.8
Larynx	20.2	44.5	39.0	–	52.1

Sankaranarayanan R, Black RJ, Parkin DM (eds): Cancer Survival in Developing Countries. IARC Scientific Publications No. 145, International Agency for Research on Cancer, Lyon, 1998

Implication

More than 75% of HNC can be attributed to the use of tobacco and alcohol in various forms in Europe and the United States [14, 15]. In India, tobacco smoking and alcohol drinking are thought to contribute to about 35% of oral cavity cancers among men, while paan chewing accounted for 49% of oral cavity cancers among men and 87% of oral cavity cancers among women [16]. The trends in the incidence of these cancers are associated with patterns of tobacco and alcohol use.

The increase in the incidence of HNC in males observed in Central and Eastern Europe seem to be clearly related to the trends in prevalence of risk factors. Alcohol and cigarette consumption have substantially increased in Central and Eastern Europe in recent years. In France, the recent decline in incidence and mortality from oropharyngeal and laryngeal cancers are consistent with the declining trends in alcohol use. The decrease of incidence and mortality in India is likely related to some decreases in betel quid chewing and tobacco smoking, and possibly due to some improvement in nutrition, particularly in women. The descriptive epidemiology of HNC, though with some limitations, identifies regions of the world where primary prevention could be the most effective strategy to reduce the burden from this disease.

While primary prevention is an important strategy for long-term disease control, early detection and prompt treatment have the potential to improve the outcome in the short term. The role of screening in early detection and reducing mortality appear to be effective in developing countries [17], particularly in those countries where tongue and mouth cancers predominate.

Acknowledgments We would like to thank Mrs. Krittika Guinot for preparing select tables and figures.

References

1. Ferlay J, Bray F, Pisani P, Parkin DM (2004) GLOBOCAN 2002: cancer incidence, mortality and prevalence worldwide, version 2.0. IARC CancerBase No. 5. IARCPress, Lyon
2. Percy C, Van Holten V, Muir C (1990) International Classification of Diseases for Oncology, 2nd edn. World Health Organization, Geneva
3. Sun EC, Curtis R, Melbye M, Goedert JJ (1999) Salivary gland cancer in the United States. Cancer Epidemiol Biomarkers Prev 8:1095–100
4. Spano JP, Busson P, Atlan D, Bourhis J, Pignon JP, Esteban C, Armand JP (2003) Nasopharyngeal carcinomas: an update. Eur J Cancer 39(15):2121–35
5. Curado MP, Edwards B, Shin HR, Storm H, Ferlay J, Heanue M, Boyle P (2007) Cancer incidence in five continents. IARC Scientific Publications, No. 160, Lyon
6. Ries LAG, Melbert D, Krapcho M, Stinchcomb DG, Howlader N, Horner MJ, Mariotto A, Miller BA, Feuer EJ, Altekruse SF, Lewis DR, Clegg L et al. (2008) SEER cancer statistics review, 1975–2005, http://seer.cancer.gov/csr/1975_2005/, based on November 2007 SEER data submission, posted to the SEER web site. National Cancer Institute, Bethesda, MD

7. Karim-Kos HE, Vars E, Soerjomataram I, Lemmens V, Siesling S, Coebergh JW (2008) Recent trends of cancer in Europe: a combined approach of incidence, survival and mortality for 17 cancer sites since the 1990s. Eur J Cancer 44:1345–1389
8. Richards M (2007) EUROCARE-4 studies bring new data on cancer survival. Lancet Oncol 8(9):752–753
9. Sankaranarayanan R, Black RJ, Swaminathan R, Parkin DM (1998) An overview of Cancer Survival in developing countries. In Sankaranarayanan R, Black RJ, Parkin DM (eds) Cancer Survival in Developing Countries IARC Scientific Publications No 145. IARC, Lyon, pp. 135–173
10. WHO (1996) Mortality database. World Health Organization
11. Bray I, Brennan P, Boffetta P (2000) Projections of alcohol- and tobacco-related cancer mortality in Central Europe. Int J Cancer 87(1):122–128
12. Lambda SA, Ferlay J, Bray F, Parkin DM (2001) European Network of Cancer Registries. EUROCIM, version 4.0. European database V2.4 (2003), Lyon
13. Capocaccia R, Gatta G, Roazzi P, Carrani E, Santaquilani M, De Angelis R, Tavilla A (2003) The EUROCARE-3 database: methodology of data collection, standardisation, quality control and statistical analysis. Ann Oncol 14(suppl. 5):v14–v27
14. Blot WJ, McLaughlin JK, Winn DM, Austin DF, Greenberg RS, Preston-Martin S, Bernstein L, Schoenberg JB, Stemhagen A, Fraumeni JF Jr (1988) Smoking and drinking in relation to oral and pharyngeal cancer. Cancer Res 48(11):3282–3287
15. Negri E, La Vecchia C, Franceschi S, Tavani A (1993) Attributable risk for oral cancer in northern Italy. Cancer Epidemiol Biomarkers Prev 2(3):189–193
16. Balaram P, Sridhar H, Rajkumar T, Vaccarella S, Herrero R, Nandakumar A, Ravichandran K, Ramdas K, Sankaranarayanan R, Gajalakshmi V, Muñoz N, Franceschi S (2002) Oral cancer in southern India: the influence of smoking, drinking, paan-chewing and oral hygiene. Int J Cancer 98(3):440–445
17. Sankaranarayanan R, Ramadas K, Thomas G, Muwonge R, Thara S, Mathew B, Rajan B (2005) Effect of screening on oral cancer mortality in Kerala, India: a cluster-randomised controlled trial. Lancet 365(9475):1927–1933
18. Marimo C, Hille JJ (2006) The burden of oral malignancies in Zimbabwe 1988 to 1997: a population based study. Cent Afr J Med. 52(5–6):51–5

Risk Factors: Tobacco and Alcohol

Mia Hashibe

Tobacco and alcohol can be considered the two most important head and neck cancer risk factors since the majority of head and neck cancers are attributed to the two risk factors [1, 2]. Each is a head and neck cancer risk factor independent of the other factor [3]. An interaction between tobacco and alcohol on the risk of head and neck cancers was reported in the 1970s and is a paradigm of interaction between two environmental factors in human carcinogenesis [1, 2].

Tobacco

Tobacco use includes smoking of tobacco products such as cigarettes, cigars, and pipes, chewing smokeless tobacco products, and using snuff tobacco. Local smoking tobacco products such as bidi and chutta, hand rolled Indian cigarettes are important as well [2]. In regions including India and Taiwan, chewing areca nut and betel quid with or without tobacco is also the major risk factor for most head and neck cancers [4]. Additional types of tobacco use include water pipes in North Africa, the Mediterranean region, and parts of Asia; kreteks (clove flavored cigarettes) in Indonesia; and suipa, chilum, or hookli (clay pipes) in Southeast Asia.

An association between tobacco use and the risk of head and neck cancer was reported in the first IARC tobacco monograph in 1986 [5] and also in the update in 2004 [2]. Tobacco smoking is thought to confer a relative risk of approximately 4–5 for oral cavity, oropharyngeal, and hypopharyngeal cancers and 10 for laryngeal cancers [6].

While tobacco smoking is an established head and neck cancer risk factor, the association of several other related factors to head and neck cancer risk are not clear. Involuntary smoking (environmental tobacco smoke or passive smoking) is a

M. Hashibe (✉)
Division of Public Health
Department of Family & Preventive Medicine
University of Utah School of Medicine
Salt Lake City, Utah
e-mail: mia.hashibe@utah.edu

A.F. Olshan (ed.), *Epidemiology, Pathogenesis, and Prevention of Head and Neck Cancer*,
DOI 10.1007/978-1-4419-1472-9_4, © Springer Science+Business Media, LLC 2010

risk factor for lung cancer, but few studies have examined the relation to head and neck cancer. Marijuana use, which in some regions is smoked with tobacco and is also correlated with cigarette smoking behavior, has been investigated as a head and neck cancer risk factor.

Independent Effect

Alcohol drinking may act as a confounder in estimating the effect between tobacco smoking and head and neck cancer since it is a major risk factor for head and neck cancer, and there is an association between alcohol and tobacco use. Even when alcohol drinking is adjusted in the model, there is concern for residual confounding. Restricting to never-alcohol drinkers is ideal, yet it has been difficult to achieve in individual studies, because only a minority of head and neck cancer patients are never-drinkers. Previous studies had assessed this in small series that included <150 cases.

This issue was addressed as a priority in the International Head and Neck Cancer Epidemiology (INHANCE) consortium, a collaboration of researchers coordinating epidemiologic studies of head and neck cancer [3]. Individual level data were pooled across 14 case-control studies for a total of 1,598 head and neck cancer cases and 4,051 controls who were never-drinkers (Table 1). The odds ratio (OR) for ever tobacco smoking among never-drinkers was approximately twofold. Tobacco smoking is considered the use of cigarettes, cigars, and pipes. Dose-response relations were observed for the frequency, duration, and packyears of cigarette smoking among never-drinkers. The risk of laryngeal cancer was greater than the risk of oral cavity and pharyngeal cancer for cigarette smoking among never-drinkers.

Dose Response

The dose-response relation between tobacco use and the risk of head and neck cancer has been reported in epidemiologic studies from around the world. The IARC monograph on tobacco smoke reported that from 1987 to 2002, there were 3 cohort studies and 16 case-control studies on oral cavity cancer, 3 cohort studies and 12 case-control studies on pharyngeal cancer, and 5 cohort studies and 27 case-control studies on laryngeal cancer [2]. The studies were from various regions of the world including North America, Europe, Asia, and South America. Most of the studies reported dose-response relations with the risk of these cancers and frequency (cigarettes per day), duration (years), and cumulative consumption of cigarettes (packyears or lifetime consumption).

Since the increasing risk observed for increased cigarettes per day is not independent of the total exposure smoking (i.e., subjects who smoke greater number

Table 1 Tobacco smoking and the risk of head and neck cancer, results from INHANCE Consortium pooled analyses

Reference, cases/controls	Exposure	ORs
Never-alcohol drinkers	Ever cigarette smoking[a]	2.13 (1.52, 2.98)
Hashibe [3]	*Frequency*[a]	
1,598 cases, 4,051 controls from 14 case-control studies (INHANCE)	Never-smokers	1.00 (referent)
	1–10 cigarettes per day	1.82 (1.28–2.59)
	11–20 cigarettes per day	2.36 (1.60–3.47)
	21–30 cigarettes per day	3.58 (2.09–6.16)
	31–40 cigarettes per day	4.46 (2.54–7.83)
	>40 cigarettes per day	2.69 (1.21–5.98)
		P trend<0.001
	Duration[a]	
	Never-smokers	1.00 (referent)
	1–10 years	1.45 (1.04–2.03)
	11–20 years	1.10 (0.75–1.61)
	21–30 years	1.79 (1.20–2.67)
	31–40 years	3.61 (2.26–5.75)
	>40 years	4.83 (3.18–7.33)
		P trend<0.001
Age at start of tobacco smoking[b]	Never-tobacco users	1.00 (referent)
Chang [42]	≥30	2.36 (1.85–3.00)
14,633 cases and 19,501 controls from 20 studies (INHANCE)	25–29	2.40 (1.74–3.31)
	20–24	2.42 (1.74–3.38)
	15–19	2.35 (1.67–3.31)
	10–14	2.03 (1.35–3.07)
	1–9	2.22 (1.39–3.53)
	P trend	<0.001
Cessation of tobacco use[c]	Current smokers	1.00 (referent)
Marron [39]	>1–4 years	0.70 (0.61, 0.81)
12,040 cases, 16,884 controls from 17 case-control studies (INHANCE)	5–9 years	0.48 (0.40, 0.58)
	10–19 years	0.34 (0.28, 0.40)
	20+ years	0.23 (0.18, 0.31)
	Never-smokers	0.23 (0.16, 0.34)
	P trend	<0.01

[a]Adjusted for age, sex, race/ethnicity, education level, study center, years of cigar smoking, and years of pipe smoking
[b]Adjusted for sex, race/ethnicity, education, study center, frequency of alcohol drinking, tobacco pack-years, and duration of chew tobacco and snuff
[c]Cessation from cigarette, cigars or pipes. Adjusted for age, sex, race/ethnicity, study center, education level, tobacco pack-years, and drinking frequency

of cigarettes per day are exposed to greater cumulative exposure (packyears) even at a fixed duration of smoking), and vice-versa, consideration of total exposure and exposure rate can help separate out the effects. Lubin et al. [7] compared the risk for total exposure at higher frequency for shorter durations and the total exposure at lower frequency for longer durations with data from the INHANCE consortium. There was a "reduced potency" effect, where at a fixed level of packyears and for subjects smoking more than 15 cigarettes per day, smoking at higher frequency for shorter duration involved less risk than smoking at lower frequency for a longer duration. Furthermore, the results suggested that the greater risk observed with laryngeal cancer may be due to more sensitivity to the frequency exposure.

Age at Start of Tobacco Smoking

Age at starting tobacco smoking appears to be inversely correlated with the risk of head and neck cancers, when the frequency or duration of tobacco smoked is not adjusted for [8–10]; this may be because individuals who started smoking early also tended to smoke for a longer duration or possibly more frequently. On the other hand, the results from studies on age at start and head and neck cancer risk that adjusted on tobacco habits have not been consistent. A study from Cuba reported that the risk of oral cavity and oro-pharynx cancer was higher among people who started to smoke <17 years old compared to those who started to smoke later [11]. A study from Italy found a similar association with laryngeal cancer before adjustment for the duration of smoking [12]. Other studies from France [13], and India [14] reported no risk differences for the larynx, hypopharynx, and oral cavity cancers due to different age of starting tobacco habits. Reports from population-based case-control studies were also inconsistent. Some studies (without adjustment for frequency or duration of tobacco habits) reported that younger age at start of smoking was associated with higher head and neck cancer risk [15, 16], while others observed the association only among men [17, 18] or among African-Americans [19].

In a pooled analysis in the INHANCE Consortium of 20 case-control studies [20], the risk of head and neck cancer was fairly similar regardless of the age at which cigarette smoking was started with adjustment on tobacco packyears (Table 1). When tobacco packyears was not adjusted for, individuals who started smoking at a younger age had a greater risk of head and neck cancer relative to individuals who started at an older age; these results were probably due to the greater cumulative exposure that the individuals who started at a young age experienced.

Cessation of Tobacco Smoking

Most epidemiologic studies of head and neck cancer have shown a consistent reduction in risk with the cessation of tobacco smoking habits. The IARC monograph summarized that there were 1 cohort and 8 case-control studies that had reported a lower risk for former smokers compared to current smokers [2]. Longer time since quitting smoking is also associated with greater reduced risk, as reported in 7 case-control studies. The reduction in risk to a level similar to that of never-smokers may take approximately 10–20 years.

Pooled analysis in the INHANCE Consortium showed results similar to these previous studies (Table 1). Risk reduction was observed fairly immediately, after quitting tobacco smoking for 1–4 years, especially for people who smoked 10 or more cigarettes per day. The risk being reduced to a level that was comparable to that of never-smokers was observed in individuals who had quit for 20 or more years.

Types of Tobacco

Tobacco is smoked in the form of cigarettes, cigars, or pipe. By far, the most common form of tobacco smoking is cigarettes. Types of cigarette and the risk of head and neck cancer have been examined in a few studies. Black tobacco resulted in a higher relative risk than blond tobacco; and hand rolled cigarettes were associated with higher head and neck cancer risk than manufactured cigarettes [2].

While there is no question that smoking other types of tobacco such as cigars and pipes confer increased head and neck cancer risk, differences in the risk by tobacco use have been difficult to quantify since there are very few individuals who only smoke cigars or pipe. A few studies have attempted to examine this [2], but did not observe differences. Similarly, analysis in the INHANCE Consortium did not result in differences in risk for individuals who smoked only cigarettes or only cigars or only pipes (Table 2).

Smoking local tobacco products such as bidi and chutta in Southeast Asia are also important risk factors for head and neck cancer. A meta-analysis of 10 studies of oral cancer showed that the risk increased because bidi smoking was approximately fourfold [21] (Table 2). Similarly, a large-scale study that differentiated between individuals who smoked cigarettes only, bidi only, cigarette and bidi, and other types of tobacco products showed that the risk of hypopharyngeal and laryngeal cancers were increased [22] (Table 2). The point estimates suggested that bidi smoking may result in higher relative risks compared to cigarette smoking.

In addition to smoking tobacco, tobacco can also be chewed. In Southeast Asia, various types of local products are chewed with or without tobacco (betel quid, areca nut, khaini, zarda, pan, gutkha, mawa) [23]. A large-scale case-control study in India reported that chewing tobacco resulted in an increased risk of oral cavity cancers regardless of whether the chewing product included tobacco or not [24]. The IARC monograph concluded that betel quid without tobacco is carcinogenic for the oral cavity and that betel quid with tobacco is carcinogenic for the oral cavity, pharynx, and esophagus [4].

Table 2 Types of tobacco and the risk of head and neck cancer

Reference, cases/controls	Exposure	ORs	
Cigars and pipes		*Head and neck cancer*	
Layman et al. (43) 13,373 cases and 18,158 controls from 19 case-control studies (INHANCE)	Never-tobacco user[a]	1.00 (referent)	
	Predominantly cigarette (66.6-99%)	3.10 (2.13–4.50)	
	Cigarette only (100%)	4.07 (3.13–5.29)	
	Predominantly cigar (66.6-99%)	4.71 (2.42–9.17)	
	Cigar only (100%)	3.70 (1.96–6.98)	
	Predominantly pipe (66.6-99%)	3.32 (1.61–6.81)	
	Pipe only (100%)	2.55 (1.60–4.07)	
India			
Rahman [21]	Bidi smoking	*Oral cavity cancer* 4.0 (2.7, 4.4)	
4,778 cases and 6,271 controls from 10 studies			
Sapkota [22]	Smoking tobacco products	*Hypopharyngeal cancer*	*Larynx cancer*
512 hypopharyngeal, 511 laryngeal cancer cases and 718 controls	Never	1.00	1.00
	Cigarette	3.82 (2.32–6.29)	5.06 (2.50–10.26)
	Bidi	6.80 (4.64–9.97)	9.61 (5.65–16.35)
	Cigarette and bidi	4.74 (2.42–9.29)	9.52 (4.15–21.85)
	Other	4.21 (1.69–10.47)	5.85 (1.85–18.50)
Znaor [24]	Chewing product	*Oral cavity cancer*	*Pharyngeal cancer*
1,563 oral, 636 pharyngeal cases, 1,711 controls (male only)	Without tobacco	2.19 (1.63–2.95)	1.37 (0.89–2.10)
	With tobacco	5.05 (4.26–5.97)	1.83 (1.43–2.33)
In Europe and North America			
Boffetta [25]	Smokeless tobacco	*Oral cavity cancer*	
13 studies		1.8 (1.1, 2.9)	

[a]Adjusted on age (continuous), sex, race, educational level, centers, alcohol consumption in ml per day

Snuff, which is fine-cut or powered tobacco that is inhaled or sniffed through the nose [25], is an important risk factor for head and neck cancer. Snuff ranges in moistness from dry to moist; moist snuff is also called snus. Snus use is prevalent in the American and European regions, while dry snuff use is observed in African, Eastern Mediterranean, European, and South East Asia regions [23]. Smokeless tobacco in the US and Northern Europe, including snuff, tobacco chewing, and snus, is thought to confer an increased oral cavity cancer risk of approximately 1.8 (95%CI = 1.1, 2.9) [25]. Boffetta et al. estimated that the proportion of male oral cancer cases attributable to smokeless tobacco use ranged from 1.6% in Canada and 6.6% in the US, to 52.5% in India and 68.2% in Sudan [25]. The proportion of female oral cancer cases attributable to smokeless tobacco was estimated to be about 13.6% in Sudan and 51.6% in India [25].

Involuntary Smoking

Very few studies have been published on the possible association between involuntary tobacco smoking and the risk of head and neck cancers (Table 3). Zhang et al. reported an increased risk of head and neck cancer for regular exposure at home and at work, with a dose-response observed for the degree of exposure [26]. Though the odds ratios were adjusted for packyears of cigarette smoking, it is difficult to rule out residual confounding by cigarette smoking. Lee et al. investigated involuntary smoking and the risk of head and neck cancer in a pooled analysis of 5 case-control studies from the United States, Latin America, and Central Europe in the INHANCE Consortium [27]. The odds ratio for ever exposure was suggestive of an increased risk of laryngeal cancer. Dose response trends were observed with duration of exposure at home, duration of exposure at work, and the risk of laryngeal cancer. Lee et al. also investigated involuntary smoking on upper aerodigestive tract cancers (oral cavity, pharynx, larynx, and esophagus) in a large-scale study in Western Europe [28]. Among 178 UADT cancer cases and 702 controls who were never-tobacco users, an increased risk of UADT cancer of approximately 1.6 was observed for ever exposure to involuntary smoking at home or work (Table 3). Dose-response relations were apparent for the duration of exposure and the risk of UADT cancers. The risk was more apparent for oral cavity and oropharyngeal cancers, than for hypopharyngeal and laryngeal cancers.

Marijuana Use

Marijuana smoke contains several of the same carcinogens as the tar from tobacco, raising concerns that smoking of marijuana may be a risk factor for tobacco-related

Table 3 Epidemiologic studies on involuntary smoking and the risk of head and neck cancers

Reference	Study period	Cases	Controls	Exposure	OR[a]
Zhang [26][a]	1992–1994	155 head and neck, nasopharyngeal and esophageal cancers	166	Regularly exposed at both home and work	2.4 (95% CI 0.9–6.8)
				Dose-response: Degree of exposure (never, light, heavy)	*P* for trend = 0.0249
Lee [27][b]	1992–2006	542 head and neck cancer, never-tobacco users (146 oral cavity, 224 pharynx, 71 larynx; INHANCE)	2,197	Ever exposed	Head and neck cancer: 1.07 (0.85, 1.34) Oral cavity cancer: 0.93 (0.61, 1.41) Pharyngeal cancer 1.30 (0.31, 5.34) Laryngeal cancer: 1.71 (0.98, 3.00)
				Dose response:	
				duration at home	pharyngeal cancer: *p* for trend=0.02
				duration at home	laryngeal cancer: *p* for trend=0.02
				duration at work	laryngeal cancer: *p* for trend=0.07
Lee [28]	2002–2005	178 UADT cancer cases, never-tobacco users (111 oral cavity and oropharynx, 34 larynx and hypopharynx, 24 esophagus)	702	Ever exposed at home or work	UADT cancer: 1.59 (1.04–2.46)
				Duration of exposure at home or work	Oral cavity & oropharyngeal cancer: 1.78 (1.03–3.08) Hypopharyngeal and laryngeal cancer: 2.05 (0.81–5.22)
				Never	UADT cancer 1.00
				1–15 years	1.31 (0.75–2.28)
				>15 years	1.78 (1.13–2.80)
				P for trend	0.011

[a]adjusted for age, race, education, heavy alcohol use, marjiuana use, and packyears of cigarette smoking

[b]Pooled analysis of 6 case-control studies, not including the Zhang et al. study. Adjusted on age, sex, race, education, study center, alcohol drinking drinkyears

Table 4 Epidemiologic studies on marijuana use and the risk of head and neck cancers

Reference	Study period	Cases	Controls	Exposure	OR[a]
Zhang [29]	1992–1994	173 Head and neck, esophagus, salivary gland, nasal cavity cancers	176	Ever use	2.6 (1.1, 6.6)
Rosenblatt [30]	1985–1995	407 Oral cavity cancer	615	Ever use	0.9 (0.6, 1.3)
Llewellyn [32]	1990–1997	116 Oral cavity, oropharynx cancers, ≤45 years	207	Cannabis smoker	1.0 (0.5, 2.2)
Llewellyn [15]	1999–2001	53 Oral cavity, oropharynx cancers, ≤45 years	91	Cannabis smoker	0.3 (0.1, 1.8)
Hashibe [31]	1999–2004	303 oral cavity, 100 pharynx, 90 larynx cancers	1,040	50 joint year[b]	Oral cavity: 1.1 (0.80, 1.5) Pharynx: 0.75 (0.37, 1.5) Larynx: 0.93 (0.50, 1.7)
Aldington [33]	2001–2005	75 Head and neck, salivary gland, nasal cavity cancers, ≤55 years	319	Ever use	1.0 (0.5, 2.3)
Gillison [34]	2000–2006	92 HPV-16 positive, 148 HPV-16 negative head and neck, paranasal sinus cancers	184,296 respectively	Smoke marijuana monthly for ≥1 year	HPV-16 positive: 4.7 (1.3, 17) HPV-16 negative: 2.0 (0.62, 6.5)
Berthiller [35]	1985–2006	4,029 head and neck cancer, pooled analysis of 5 case-control studies (INHANCE)	5,015	Ever use	Overall: 0.88 (0.67, 1.16) Never-tobacco users: 0.93 (0.63, 1.37) Never-alcohol drinkers: 1.27 (0.77, 2.12)

[a]All odds ratios presented were adjusted for cigarette smoking

[b]Treating cumulative marijuana use as a continuous variable; the estimated OR is for a difference of 50 joint-years

cancers. Several epidemiologic studies have examined the possible association between marijuana use and head and neck cancer risk (Table 4).

Zhang et al. [29] first reported that marijuana use may increase risk of head and neck cancers in a hospital-based case-control study in the United States, with dose-response relations for both frequency ($p=0.0214$) and duration of use ($p = 0.0134$). The association was stronger in patients who were ≤55 years [29]. However, in population-based case-control studies from the US, Rosenblatt et al. reported no association with oral cavity cancer [30] and Hashibe et al. reported no association with oral cavity, pharynx, or larynx cancers [31]. Similarly, two small studies on subjects ≤45 years in the UK [15, 32] and a small study on subjects ≤55 years in New Zealand reported no associations [33]. A hospital-based case-control study reported that marijuana use was a risk factor for head and neck cancer patients who were HPV-16 positive but not for head and neck cancer patients who were HPV-16 negative [34]. Dose-response relations for both frequency ($p=0.007$), duration ($p=0.011$), and cumulative ($p=0.003$) use were reported for the HPV-16 positive head and neck cancer patients [34].

In a pooled analysis of 5 case-control studies from North America and South America including the two population-based studies mentioned above [30, 31], ever marijuana use was not correlated with the risk of head and neck cancer (Table 4) [35]. Results were stratified by tobacco and alcohol use, to address the potential residual confounding that may occur for marijuana estimates adjusted on tobacco and alcohol. No associations were observed among never-tobacco users or never-alcohol drinkers.

In summary, of the 7 case-control studies and 1 pooled analysis study on the association of marijuana use and head and neck cancer risk, only 2 of the case-control studies reported associations with dose-response relations. The 2 studies suggested that marijuana use is a risk factor for specific subgroups, such as patients ≤55 years or patients who have HPV-16 positive tumors. However, it is still far from established whether marijuana use is a risk factor for head and neck cancer overall or for select subgroups. It is possible that marijuana use, even with long-term or heavy use is not a strong risk head and neck cancer risk factor and will be difficult to detect in epidemiologic studies.

Alcohol

Alcohol consumption includes drinking of beverages containing ethanol such as wine, liquor, beer, and other local alcohol products. Relative to other alcohol related cancers, the risk conferred by alcohol drinking is strong for head and neck cancers [36]. Consuming 50 g of alcohol per day is thought to increase the risk of oral cavity and pharyngeal cancers by approximately threefold and the risk of laryngeal cancer by twofold relative to nondrinkers [37].

Independent Effect

The effect of alcohol drinking among never-smokers was examined by the INHANCE Consortium. Individual level data on never-tobacco users was pooled for 1,072 cases and 5,775 controls from 14 case-control studies (Table 5). Though ever-drinking in general was not associated with head and neck cancer risk, drinking at least three drinks a day was associated with a twofold increase in head and neck cancer risk.

Table 5 Alcohol drinking and the risk of head and neck cancer, results from INHANCE Consortium pooled analyses

Reference		ORs
Never-tobacco users[a]	Drinking ≥3 drinks/day	2.04 (1.29, 3.21)
Hashibe [3]	vs. never drinking	
1,072 cases, 5,775 controls from 14 studies (INHANCE)	*Frequency*	
	Never-drinkers	1.00 (referent)
	<1 drinks/day	1.04 (0.79–1.38)
	1–2 drinks/day	1.30 (0.94–1.80)
	3–4 drinks/day	1.82 (1.10–2.99)
	≥5 drinks/day	2.81 (1.49–5.27)
	P trend	0.001
	Duration	
	Never-drinkers	1.00 (referent)
	1–10	1.56 (1.11–2.19)
	11–20	1.22 (0.87–1.71)
	21–30	1.27 (0.87–1.87)
	31–40	1.17 (0.84–1.62)
	>40 years	1.05 (0.65–1.68)
	P trend	0.319
Age at start of alcohol drinking[b]	Never-alcohol drinkers	1.00 (referent)
Chang [42]	≥28	1.45 (1.10–1.89)
11,769 cases and 15,074 controls from 16 studies (INHANCE)	23–27	1.59 (1.06–2.40)
	18–22	1.53 (1.17–2.00)
	1–17	1.23 (0.88–1.71)
	P trend	0.91
Cessation of alcohol drinking[c]	Current drinkers	1.00 (referent)
Marron [39]	>1–4 years	0.99 (0.69, 1.43)
9,167 cases and 12,593 controls from 13 studies (INHANCE)	5–9 years	0.90 (0.62, 1.30)
	10–19 years	0.94 (0.75, 1.18)
	20+ years	0.60 (0.40, 0.89)
	Never-drinkers	0.74 (0.51, 1.06)
	P trend	0.05

[a]Adjusted for age, sex, race/ethnicity, education level, and study center
[b]Age at starting drinking wine, liquor or beer. Adjusted for sex, race/ethnicity, education, study center, tobacco-years and frequency of alcohol drinking
[c]Cessation of wine, beer or liquor. Adjusted for age, sex, race/ethnicity, study center, education level, tobacco pack-years, and drinking frequency

A dose-response relationship was observed between head and neck cancer risk and the frequency of alcohol consumption (drinks per day; p for trend=0.001), but not with the duration of alcohol drinking (years; p for trend=0.319). The risk associated with higher frequency of alcohol drinking was most pronounced for pharyngeal cancers and laryngeal cancer, compared to oral cavity cancer.

Dose Response

Between 1988 and 2007, the IARC monograph on alcohol reported that there were 5 cohort studies on oral cavity and pharyngeal cancers, 8 case-control studies on oral cavity cancer, 9 case-control studies on pharyngeal cancer, 19 case-control studies on oral cavity/pharyngeal cancers combined, and approximately 18 case-control studies on laryngeal cancer [37]. Most studies adjusted on tobacco smoking and consistently showed dose-response relations between alcohol drinking frequency and the risk of head and neck cancers. These results were observed across geographic regions including Europe, Asia, North America, and Latin America. The IARC monograph reported that there was little information on the duration of alcohol drinking and the risk of laryngeal cancer. The INHANCE Consortium results showed that there was no dose response relation between duration of alcohol drinking and the risk of head and neck cancers (Table 5); these results were consistent for the risk of oral cavity, pharyngeal, and laryngeal cancers separately.

Lubin et al. examined total exposure and exposure rate (frequency/intensity) for alcohol drinking and the risk of head and neck cancers based on the INHANCE Consortium pooled data [7]. The analysis suggested that for individuals who drink less than 10 drinks per day, at fixed cumulative alcohol levels, exposure to higher drinks per day over a shorter duration was more harmful than exposure to fewer drinks per day over a longer duration. Above 10 drinks per day, the data were sparse and interpretation was difficult. Greater risks of oral cavity and pharyngeal cancer compared to laryngeal cancer due to alcohol drinking were confirmed; these risk differences were attributed to drink-years (cumulative alcohol consumption) rather than the frequency of alcohol drinking.

Age at Start of Alcohol Drinking

Very few studies reported on the association between age at start of drinking alcoholic beverages and the risk of head and neck cancer. Two studies which did not control for smoking or drinking habits reported that there was no clear trends for age at starting drinking with oral cavity and pharyngeal cancer [16, 17]. One study which controlled for tobacco smoking habits also did not show any oral cavity cancer risk differences by various ages of starting drinking [38]. With further adjustment for alcohol drinking habits, age at starting drinking was still not suggested to be associated with the risk of oral and pharyngeal cancer [11, 14]. Age at start of drinking specific types of alcohol was seldom explored because of small sample sizes.

In the INHANCE pooled analysis [20], similar to the results on age at starting tobacco smoking, the risk of head and neck cancer was fairly similar regardless of the age at starting alcohol drinking (Table 5). There was a suggestion that earlier age at starting liquor drinking increased the risk of head and neck cancer more than starting at a later age. However, the confidence intervals were fairly wide and the difference was not statistically significant.

Cessation of Alcohol Drinking

In contrast to the studies on cessation of tobacco smoking, there are fewer published studies reporting on the effects of stopping alcohol drinking on the risk of head and neck cancers. In the INHANCE pooled analysis, a clear beneficial effect against head and neck cancer risk was demonstrated when individuals quit alcohol drinking [39]. The risk reduction due to alcohol cessation was not observed immediately in contrast to the benefit observed for tobacco cessation after 1–4 years. However, after 20 years of quitting, the risk was similar to that of never-drinkers.

Types of Alcohol

Previous studies have explored differences in head and neck cancer risk due to different alcoholic beverage types such as wine, liquor, and beer [37]. The overall consensus was that the most common type of alcoholic beverage type in a specific region conferred the greatest risk. More specifically, highest risks were observed for beer in North America, wine in Europe, and hard liquors in Latin America [37].

Since most drinkers will consume different types of alcoholic beverage types, it is difficult to separate any risk differences. A recent INHANCE Consortium analysis was able to examine alcoholic beverage types among individuals who reportedly drank only one type of alcoholic beverage [40]. Overall head and neck cancer risks were fairly consistent among individuals who drank only beer, liquor, or wine (Table 6); the head and neck cancer risk was approximately twofold for drinking 16–30 drinks per week for wine, liquor, or beer. For heavier drinking (>30 drinks per week), the odds ratios for head and neck cancer risk were approximately 4 for liquor, 5 for beer, and 6 for wine; though the point estimates were different, the confidence intervals were overlapped suggesting no significant differences. When stratified by region (Table 7), the head and neck cancer risk estimates for liquor and beer appeared to be slightly higher in the North American studies, whereas for wine the risk estimates were higher for Europe and Latin America.

Table 6 Types of alcoholic beverages and the risk of head and neck cancer in the INHANCE consortium

	Cases	Controls	OR (95%CI) for drinks/week[a]				
			≤5	6–15	16–30	>30	*P* trend
Beer only	1,963	4,417	1.6 (1.3, 2.1)	1.9 (1.4, 2.7)	2.2 (1.3, 3.5)	5.4 (3.1, 9.2)	<0.0001
Liquor only	4,605	3,962	1.6 (1.0, 2.6)	1.5 (1.0, 2.4)	2.3 (1.4, 4.0)	3.6 (2.2, 5.8)	<0.0001
Wine only	2,117	5,862	1.1 (0.8, 1.6)	1.2 (0.8, 1.9)	1.9 (0.9, 3.9)	6.3 (2.2, 18.6)	<0.0001

[a]OR adjusted for age, sex, race/ethnicity, study center, education level, pack-years of smoking, years of cigar smoking, years of pipe smoking. Modified from Purdue et al. [40]

Tobacco and Alcohol

When considering the combination of tobacco and alcohol, the countries with the highest prevalences of these habits are not necessarily the countries with the highest incidence of head and neck cancer in men or women (Figs. 1 and 2). For women, the countries with the highest incidence rates such as Bangladesh, Sri Lanka, and India do not have high smoking or heavy alcohol prevalences. The importance of chewing tobacco, betel quid (with or without tobacco), and other local products that contain tobacco as risk factors for head and neck cancer become apparent (Fig. 3). For men, the head and neck cancer incidence rates are high in countries such as Hungary, Bangladesh, France, and Sri Lanka; while Hungary and France have fairly high heavy alcohol prevalence and smoking prevalence, Sri Lanka and Bangladesh have low prevalence of heavy alcohol intake. Though these figures assess tobacco, alcohol, and head and neck cancer in an ecologic manner, the complexity in the role of other head and neck cancer risk factors is evident.

In terms of the interaction between tobacco and alcohol and the risk of head and neck cancers, numerous epidemiologic studies have examined interactions, but many reports assessed interactions only descriptively, without applying formal statistical testing [2]. Some studies tested for the presence of interactions on the additive scale while others tested on the multiplicative scale, and different categories were used for tobacco use and alcohol use. These results were therefore difficult to compare across studies.

In the INHANCE Consortium analysis, multiplicative interaction parameters and population attributable risks were estimated for tobacco and alcohol drinking [41]. A greater than multiplicative joint effect between ever tobacco and alcohol use was observed for head and neck cancer risk ($\psi = 2.15$, 95%CI = 1.53–3.04). The head and neck cancer risk for individuals who drank 3 or more drinks per day and smoked more than 20 cigarettes per day was approximately 14 (Fig. 3). The population attributable risk (PAR) for tobacco or alcohol was 72% (95%CI = 61–79%) for head and neck cancer, of which 4% was due to alcohol alone, 33% was due tobacco alone, and 35% was due to tobacco and alcohol combined (Fig. 4). The total PAR differed

Table 7 Alcoholic beverage type and the risk of head and neck cancer in the INHANCE consortium, by geographic region

	Number of standard drinks/week					
	Beer-only drinker		Liquor-only drinker		Wine-only drinker	
	≤15	>15	≤15	>15	≤15	>15
Region	$N_{Case}/N_{Control}$ OR (95% CI)	$N_{Case}/N_{Control}$ OR (95% CI)	$N_{Case}/N_{Control}$ OR (95% CI)	$N_{Case}/N_{Control}$ OR (95% CI)	$N_{Case}/N_{Control}$ OR (95% CI)	$N_{Case}/N_{Control}$ OR (95% CI)
North America	*292/382*	*314/143*	*101/171*	*123/69*	*70/236*	*12/9*
	2.0 (1.5, 2.6)	4.1 (2.2, 7.6)	1.9 (0.8, 4.4)	3.2 (1.5, 6.6)	1.1 (0.7, 1.8)	2.8 (0.5, 15.5)
Latin America	*104/211*	*67/88*	*34/24*	*61/36*	*39/48*	*50/15*
	1.5 (0.7, 3.2)	2.1 (0.8, 5.7)	2.1 (0.4, 9.6)	2.6 (0.6, 11.1)	1.1 (0.6, 1.9)	3.7 (1.7, 7.8)
Europe	*42/116*	*32/34*	*141/198*	*32/19*	*170/890*	*661/1,212*
	1.4 (0.6, 3.2)	3.5 (1.2, 10.4)	1.2 (0.6, 2.5)	1.7 (0.4, 6.9)	1.5 (0.6, 3.4)	4.0 (1.4, 11.2)

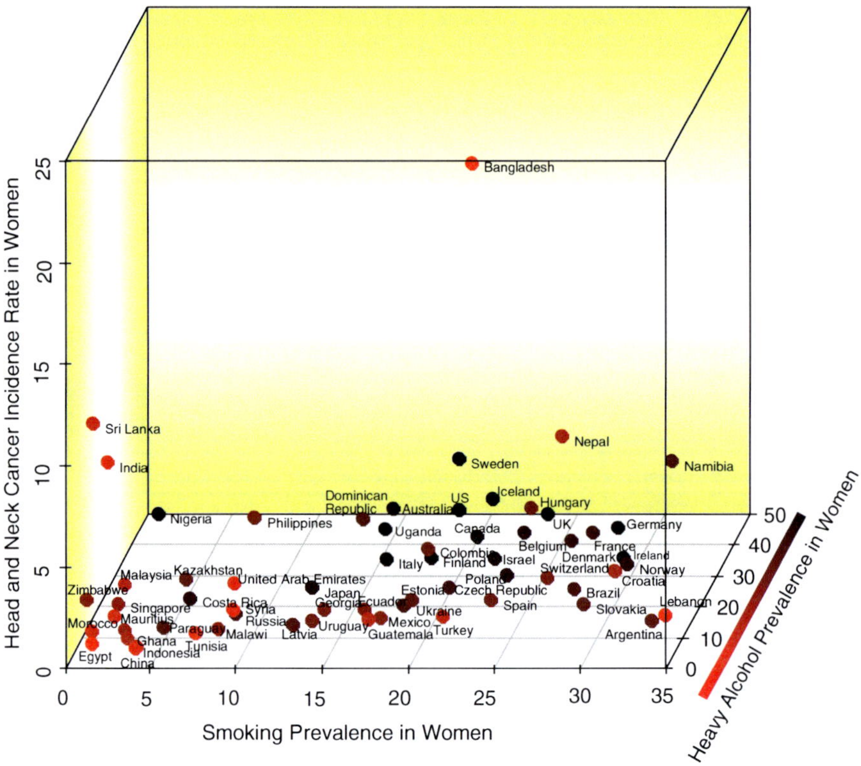

Fig. 1 Prevalence of smoking (%), heavy alcohol drinking (%), and head and neck cancer incidence rates (age-standardized, per 100,000) in women by country (sources: WHO Tobacco Atlas 2002, WHO Global Information System on Alcohol and Health 2007, GLOBOCAN 2002)

by subsite (64% for oral cavity cancer, 72% for pharyngeal cancer, 89% for laryngeal cancer), by sex (74% for men, 57% for women), by age (33% for cases<45 years, 73% for cases>60 years), and by region (84% in Europe, 51% in North America, 83% in Latin America). The importance of tobacco and alcohol thus appears to differ substantially by subsite, by sex, and by geographic region (Fig. 4).

Summary

Tobacco and alcohol are clearly important risk factors for head and neck cancers. A substantial amount of research effort has been applied, mainly in the form of case-control studies in clarifying the dose-response relations across geographic regions. Analytical methods to combine data from these numerous case-control studies, such as pooled- and meta-analyses have been beneficial in further addressing various research questions on tobacco and alcohol. Though the research area has

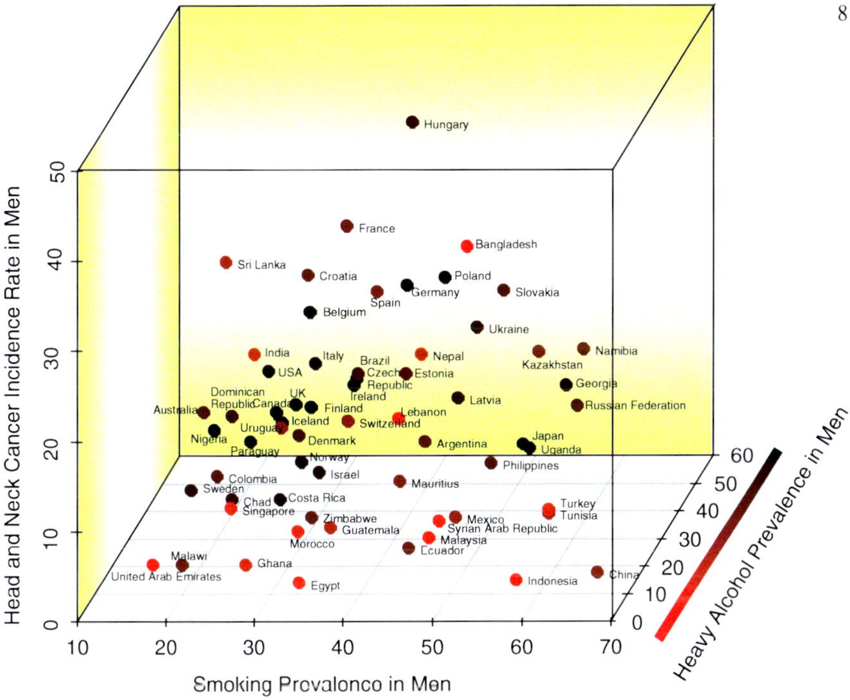

Fig. 2 Prevalence of smoking (%), heavy alcohol drinking (%), and head and neck cancer incidence rates (age-standardized, per 100,000) in men by country (sources: WHO Tobacco Atlas 2002, WHO Global Information System on Alcohol and Health 2007, GLOBOCAN 2002)

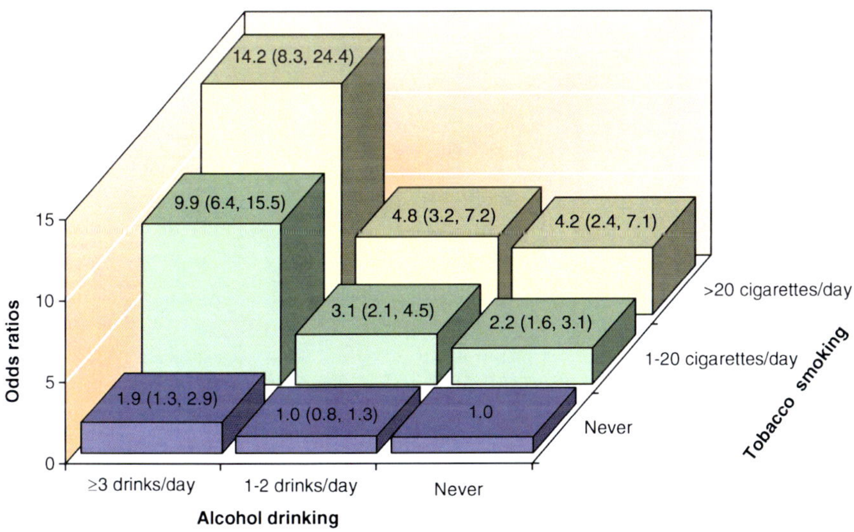

Fig. 3 Interaction between tobacco and alcohol on the risk of head and neck cancers, based on pooled data of 18 case-control studies (11,211 cases and 16,152 controls) from Western countries in the INHANCE consortium. Tobacco smoking combined cigarette, cigar and pipe use in cigarette equivalents

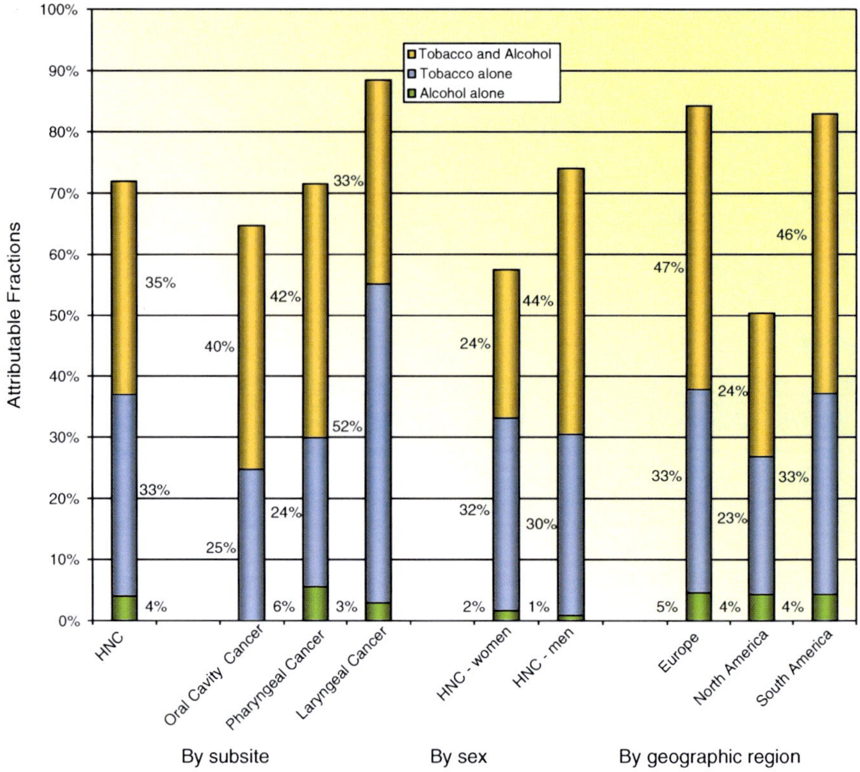

Fig. 4 Attributable fractions due to tobacco and alcohol for head and neck cancers, based on pooled data of 18 case-control studies (11,211 cases and 16,152 controls) from Western countries in the INHANCE consortium. Tobacco smoking combined cigarette, cigar and pipe use in cigarette equivalents

seen substantial collaborative efforts in this regard, the next step in intensifying collaborations may be to synchronize the next phase of epidemiologic studies on head and neck cancer around the globe, for an even larger scale study. In regions such as Africa and East Asia (particularly China), there is a lack of epidemiologic large-scale studies on head and neck cancer. Harmonizing the epidemiologic methods across the next generation of case-control studies will strengthen the data pooling capacity and may exponentiate the number of research questions that can be addressed not only for tobacco and alcohol but other important head and neck cancer research areas such as HPV infection.

References

1. (1988) Alcohol drinking. IARC Working Group, Lyon, 13–20 October 1987. IARC Monogr Eval Carcinog Risks Hum 44:1–378
2. (2004) Tobacco smoke and involuntary smoking. IARC Monogr Eval Carcinog Risks Hum 83:1–1438

3. Hashibe M, Brennan P, Benhamou S, Castellsague X, Chen C, Curado MP, Dal ML, Daudt AW, Fabianova E, Fernandez L, Wunsch-Filho V, Franceschi S et al (2007) Alcohol drinking in never users of tobacco, cigarette smoking in never drinkers, and the risk of head and neck cancer: pooled analysis in the International Head and Neck Cancer Epidemiology Consortium. J Natl Cancer Inst 99(10):777–789
4. (2004) Betel-quid and areca-nut chewing and some related nitrosamines. IARC Monogr Eval Carcinog Risks Hum 85
5. (1986) Tobacco smoking. IARC Monogr Eval Carcinog Risks Hum 38
6. Vineis P, Alavanja M, Buffler P, Fontham E, Franceschi S, Gao YT, Gupta PC, Hackshaw A, Matos E, Samet J, Sitas F, Smith J et al (2004) Tobacco and cancer: recent epidemiological evidence. J Natl Cancer Inst 96(2):99–106
7. Lubin JH, Purdue M, Kelsey K, Zhang ZF, Winn D, Wei Q, Talamini R, Szeszenia-Dabrowska N, Sturgis EM, Smith E, Shangina O, Schwartz SM, et al (2009) Total exposure and exposure rate effects for alcohol and smoking and risk of head and neck cancer: a pooled analysis of case-control studies. Am J Epidemiol 170(8):937–947
8. Barra S, Baron AE, Franceschi S, Talamini R, La Vecchia C (1991) Cancer and non-cancer controls in studies on the effect of tobacco and alcohol consumption. Int J Epidemiol 20(4):845–851
9. Franceschi S, Talamini R, Barra S, Baron AE, Negri E, Bidoli E, Serraino D, La Vecchia C (1990) Smoking and drinking in relation to cancers of the oral cavity, pharynx, larynx, and esophagus in northern Italy. Cancer Res 50(20):6502–6507
10. Choi SY, Kahyo H (1991) Effect of cigarette smoking and alcohol consumption in the aetiology of cancer of the oral cavity, pharynx and larynx. Int J Epidemiol 20(4):878–885
11. Garrote LF, Herrero R, Reyes RM, Vaccarella S, Anta JL, Ferbeye L, Munoz N, Franceschi S (2001) Risk factors for cancer of the oral cavity and oro-pharynx in Cuba. Br J Cancer 85(1):46–54
12. Talamini R, Bosetti C, La Vecchia C, Dal Maso L, Levi F, Bidoli E, Negri E, Pasche C, Vaccarella S, Barzan L, Franceschi S (2002) Combined effect of tobacco and alcohol on laryngeal cancer risk: a case-control study. Cancer Causes Control 13(10):957–964
13. Menvielle G, Luce D, Goldberg P, Bugel I, Leclerc A (2004) Smoking, alcohol drinking and cancer risk for various sites of the larynx and hypopharynx. A case-control study in France. Eur J Cancer Prev 13(3):165–172
14. Balaram P, Sridhar H, Rajkumar T, Vaccarella S, Herrero R, Nandakumar A, Ravichandran K, Ramdas K, Sankaranarayanan R, Gajalakshmi V, Munoz N, Franceschi S (2002) Oral cancer in southern India: the influence of smoking, drinking, paan-chewing and oral hygiene. Int J Cancer 98(3):440–445
15. Llewellyn CD, Johnson NW, Warnakulasuriya KA (2004) Risk factors for oral cancer in newly diagnosed patients aged 45 years and younger: a case-control study in Southern England. J Oral Pathol Med 33(9):525–532
16. Merletti F, Boffetta P, Ciccone G, Mashberg A, Terracini B (1989) Role of tobacco and alcoholic beverages in the etiology of cancer of the oral cavity/oropharynx in Torino, Italy. Cancer Res 49(17):4919–4924
17. Blot WJ, McLaughlin JK, Winn DM, Austin DF, Greenberg RS, Preston-Martin S, Bernstein L, Schoenberg JB, Stemhagen A, Fraumeni JF Jr (1988) Smoking and drinking in relation to oral and pharyngeal cancer. Cancer Res 48(11):3282–3287
18. Lewin F, Norell SE, Johansson H, Gustavsson P, Wennerberg J, Biorklund A, Rutqvist LE (1998) Smoking tobacco, oral snuff, and alcohol in the etiology of squamous cell carcinoma of the head and neck: a population-based case-referent study in Sweden. Cancer 82(7): 1367–1375
19. Day GL, Blot WJ, Austin DF, Bernstein L, Greenberg RS, Preston-Martin S, Schoenberg JB, Winn DM, McLaughlin JK, Fraumeni JF Jr (1993) Racial differences in risk of oral and pharyngeal cancer: alcohol, tobacco, and other determinants. J Natl Cancer Inst 85(6):465–473
20. Bosetti C, Gallus S, Peto R, Negri E, Talamini R, Tavani A, Franceschi S, La VC (2008) Tobacco smoking, smoking cessation, and cumulative risk of upper aerodigestive tract cancers. Am J Epidemiol 167(4):468–473

21. Rahman M, Sakamoto J, Fukui T (2003) Bidi smoking and oral cancer: a meta-analysis. Int J Cancer 106(4):600–604
22. Sapkota A, Gajalakshmi V, Jetly DH, Roychowdhury S, Dikshit RP, Brennan P, Hashibe M, Boffetta P (2007) Smokeless tobacco and increased risk of hypopharyngeal and laryngeal cancers: a multicentric case-control study from India. Int J Cancer 121(8):1793–1798
23. (2007) Smokeless tobacco and some tobacco-specific N-nitrosamines. IARC Monogr Eval Carcinog Risks Hum 89
24. Znaor A, Brennan P, Gajalakshmi V, Mathew A, Shanta V, Varghese C, Boffetta P (2003) Independent and combined effects of tobacco smoking, chewing and alcohol drinking on the risk of oral, pharyngeal and esophageal cancers in Indian men. Int J Cancer 105(5):681–686
25. Boffetta P, Hecht S, Gray N, Gupta P, Straif K (2008) Smokeless tobacco and cancer. Lancet Oncol 9(7):667–675
26. Zhang ZF, Morgenstern H, Spitz MR, Tashkin DP, Yu GP, Hsu TC, Schantz SP (2000) Environmental tobacco smoking, mutagen sensitivity, and head and neck squamous cell carcinoma. Cancer Epidemiol Biomarkers Prev 9(10):1043–1049
27. Lee YC, Boffetta P, Sturgis EM, Wei Q, Zhang ZF, Muscat J, Lazarus P, Matos E, Hayes RB, Winn DM, Zaridze D, Wunsch-Filho V et al (2008) Involuntary smoking and head and neck cancer risk: pooled analysis in the INHANCE consortium. Cancer Epidemiol Biomarkers Prev 17(8):1974–1981
28. Lee YC, Marron M, Benhamou S, Bouchardy C, Ahrens W, Pohlabeln H, Lagiou P, Trichopoulos D, Agudo A, Castellsague X, Bencko V, Holcatova I, Kjaerheim K, Merletti F, Richiardi L, Macfarlane GJ, Macfarlane TV, Talamini R, Barzan L, Canova C, Simonato L, Conway DI, McKinney PA, Lowry RJ, Sneddon L, Znaor A, Healy CM, McCartan BE, Brennan P, Hashibe M. Active and involuntary tobacco smoking and upper aerodigestive tract cancer risks in a multicenter case-control study. Cancer Epidemiol Biomarkers Prev. 2009 Dec;18(12):3353–61
29. Zhang ZF, Morgenstern H, Spitz MR, Tashkin DP, Yu GP, Marshall JR, Hsu TC, Schantz SP (1999) Marijuana use and increased risk of squamous cell carcinoma of the head and neck. Cancer Epidemiol Biomarkers Prev 8(12):1071–1078
30. Rosenblatt KA, Daling JR, Chen C, Sherman KJ, Schwartz SM (2004) Marijuana use and risk of oral squamous cell carcinoma. Cancer Res 64(11):4049–4054
31. Hashibe M, Morgenstern H, Cui Y, Tashkin DP, Zhang ZF, Cozen W, Mack TM, Greenland S (2006) Marijuana use and the risk of lung and upper aerodigestive tract cancers: results of a population-based case-control study. Cancer Epidemiol Biomarkers Prev 15(10):1829–1834
32. Llewellyn CD, Linklater K, Bell J, Johnson NW, Warnakulasuriya S (2004) An analysis of risk factors for oral cancer in young people: a case-control study. Oral Oncol 40(3):304–313
33. Aldington S, Harwood M, Cox B, Weatherall M, Beckert L, Hansell A, Pritchard A, Robinson G, Beasley R (2008) Cannabis use and cancer of the head and neck: case-control study. Otolaryngol Head Neck Surg 138(3):374–380
34. Gillison ML, D'Souza G, Westra W, Sugar E, Xiao W, Begum S, Viscidi R (2008) Distinct risk factor profiles for human papillomavirus type 16-positive and human papillomavirus type 16-negative head and neck cancers. J Natl Cancer Inst 100(6):407–420
35. Berthiller J, Lee YC, Boffetta P, Wei Q, Sturgis EM, Greenland S, Morgenstern H, Zhang ZF, Lazarus P, Muscat J, Chen C, Schwartz SM, et al (2009) Marijuana smoking and the risk of head and neck cancer: pooled analysis in the INHANCE consortium. Cancer Epidemiol Biomarkers Prev 18(5):1544–1551
36. Bagnardi V, Blangiardo M, La Vecchia C, Corrao G (2001) A meta-analysis of alcohol drinking and cancer risk. Br J Cancer 85(11):1700–1705
37. (2008) Consumption of alcoholic beverages and ethyl carbamate (urethane). IARC Monogr Eval Carcinog Risks Hum 96, in press
38. Lissowska J, Pilarska A, Pilarski P, Samolczyk-Wanyura D, Piekarczyk J, Bardin-Mikollajczak A, Zatonski W, Herrero R, Munoz N, Franceschi S (2003) Smoking, alcohol, diet, dentition and sexual practices in the epidemiology of oral cancer in Poland. Eur J Cancer Prev 12(1):25–33
39. Marron M, Boffetta P, Zhang ZF, Zaridze D, Wünsch-Filho V, Winn DM, Wei Q, Talamini R, Szeszenia-Dabrowska N, Sturgis EM, Smith E, Schwartz SM, Rudnai P, Purdue MP, Olshan

AF, Eluf-Neto J, Muscat J, Morgenstern H, Menezes A, McClean M, Matos E, Mates IN, Lissowska J, Levi F, Lazarus P, Vecchia CL, Koifman S, Kelsey K, Herrero R, Hayes RB, Franceschi S, Fernandez L, Fabianova E, Daudt AW, Maso LD, Curado MP, Cadoni G, Chen C, Castellsague X, Boccia S, Benhamou S, Ferro G, Berthiller J, Brennan P, Møller H, Hashibe M. Cessation of alcohol drinking, tobacco smoking and the reversal of head and neck cancer risk. Int J Epidemiol. 2009 Oct 5. [Epub ahead of print]
40. Purdue M et al (2009) Type of alcoholic beverage and risk of head and neck cancer – a pooled analysis within the INHANCE consortium. Am J Epidemiol 169(2):132–142
41. Hashibe M, Brennan P, Chuang SC, Boccia S, Castellsague X, Chen C, Curado MP, Dal Maso L, Daudt AW, Fabianova E, Fernandez L, Wünsch-Filho V, et al (2009) Interaction between tobacco and alcohol use and the risk of head and neck cancer: pooled analysis in the International Head and Neck Cancer Epidemiology Consortium. Cancer Epidemiol Biomarkers Prev 18(2):541–550
42. Chang SC, Zhang ZF, Eluf-Neto J, Schwartz SM, Matos E, Purdue M, Wei Q, Herrero R, Smith EM, Kelsey K, Koifman S, Sturgis EM et al (2008) Age at start of using tobacco and drinking alcohol on the risk of head and neck Cancer: pooled analysis in the International Head and Neck Cancer Epidemiology Consortium
43. Layman AB, Hashibe M, Chuang SC, Zhang ZF, Zatonski W, Winn DM, Wei QY, Talamini R, Szeszenia-Dabrowska N, Sturgis EM, Smith E, Shangina O et al. Smoking and Smokeless Tobacco Products and Risk of Head and Neck Cancers: Pooled Analysis in the International Head and Neck Cancer Epidemiology Consortium. (submitted)

Human Papillomavirus and Head and Neck Cancer

Anil Chaturvedi and Maura L. Gillison

Human Papillomaviruses

Human papillomaviruses (HPV) have been implicated in the pathogenesis of several cancers of the anogenital tract, including cervical, vulvar, vaginal, and anal cancers in women and penile and anal cancers among men. In 2007, the World Health Organization stated for the first time that there was sufficient molecular and epidemiological evidence to conclude that HPVs are also etiologic for a nonanogenital malignancy, specifically oral cancers [1]. HPV infection is necessary for the development of cervical carcinoma, where HPV genomic DNA is identified in virtually all cancers (>99%) [2]. By contrast, for all other HPV-associated malignancies inclusive of oral cancers, only a subset of cancers at that anatomic site is attributable to HPV [3, 4]. Taken together, an estimated 561,000 men and women worldwide were diagnosed with cancers attributable to HPV infection in 2002 [5], accounting for approximately 5.2% of the global cancer burden [6]. According to the Centers for Disease Control, approximately 20,000 cancers in the United States were attributable to HPV infection each year during the period from 1998 through 2003 [4, 7]. HPV infection is therefore a major cause of morbidity and mortality from cancers worldwide.

HPV infection of the genital tract and skin is extraordinarily common among healthy individuals. Although large epidemiological surveys have documented the prevalence rates for cervical HPV infection well among women, considerably less data are available for genital infection among men and nongenital HPV infection among men or women. Therefore, the summary estimates for HPV prevalence based largely on genital surveys in women alone likely underestimate exposure in the world population. Natural history studies of genital HPV infection indicate that HPV is acquired largely through sexual contact [8]. Approximately 10% of women worldwide have a prevalent cervical HPV infection [9], but prevalence varies substantially by age and geographic region [10]. In the US, CDC data from 2003 to 2004 indicated that 26.8% of women between the ages of 14 and 59 had a prevalent

A. Chaturvedi and M.L. Gillison (✉)
e-mail: Maura.Gillison@osumc.edu

A.F. Olshan (ed.), *Epidemiology, Pathogenesis, and Prevention of Head and Neck Cancer*, DOI 10.1007/978-1-4419-1472-9_5, © Springer Science+Business Media, LLC 2010 genital HPV infection [11]. Although significantly less data on HPV infection in men are available, genital HPV infection is at least as common among men as among women [12, 13]. Initial studies of small sample size indicate that cutaneous HPVs can be detected in the skin of the majority (~96%) of asymptomatic individuals with repeated testing [14] and that early transmission may occur within families [15]. DNA sequence analyses of HPVs isolated from different world populations have indicated that HPVs have evolved in concert with humans: HPV sequence divergence corresponds with human migratory patterns over several thousand years [16, 17]. Thus, HPV has evolved as human migration occurred, and infections of the skin and genital tract are extraordinarily common and the consequence of human to human contact, with the majority of individuals likely having been exposed.

Biology and Viral Transformation

Human papillomaviruses (HPV) are members of the Papillomaviridae family of double stranded, circular DNA viruses that have a specific tropism for human cutaneous (beta-papillomaviruses) or mucosal (alpha-papillomaviruses) epithelia. HPVs specifically infect the basal cell layer of the human epithelium and can either induce benign hyperproliferations of the epithelium (e.g. papillomas or warts) and/or promote the development of a premalignant or malignant lesion. Following infection, HPV exists as a circular episome within the host cell nucleus and is maintained at a low copy number. As basal cells divide, some daughter cells persist in the basal layers, while other daughter cells move toward the upper layers of the epithelium and begin to differentiate. It is during this differentiation process that HPV utilizes the host cell DNA machinery for viral replication and produces viral capsid proteins and virions that are contained within shed, terminally differentiated, surface epithelial cells [18].

Studies of the genomic organization of papillomaviruses reveal a well-conserved general organization. The episomal genome is of ~8,000 base pairs and encodes eight proteins. The early (E) genes encode proteins involved in viral DNA replication, maintenance of the viral episome, regulation of viral and host-cell gene expression, and host-cell proliferation. The two late (L) genes L1 and L2 encode the major and minor structural proteins of the viral protein capsid, respectively. The viral genome also contains the long control region (LCR), which includes the viral origin of replication and transcriptional regulatory regions.

The E1 and E2 genes are DNA binding proteins that form a complex at the viral origin of replication to recruit cellular polymerases necessary for viral replication and are also important for maintenance of the viral episome during cell division [19]. The E1 gene is also an ATP-dependent helicase that unwinds DNA during viral replication [20], whereas the E2 protein functions as a transcription factor that negatively regulates viral E6 and E7 expression [21]. The E4 protein is expressed primarily in differentiated epithelial cells and arrests cells in the G2 phase of the cell cycle, modulates late viral genome expression and viral replication, and may interact with the cellular cytokeratin network [22]. The E5 protein is an integral membrane protein that promotes cellular transformation via the EGFR pathway [23], including via phosphorylation and inhibition of degradation of the receptor [24]. It also functions to downregulate MHC class I expression on the infected cell, perhaps aiding in evasion of the host immune response [25].

The transforming potential of oncogenic HPV types is attributed to the viral E6 and E7 proteins that are capable of inactivating two human tumor suppressor proteins, p53 and pRb, respectively [26]. The E6 protein combines with a cellular protein E6-AP to form an ubiquitin ligase that targets p53 for degradation via the proteosome [27]. Another major function of E6 important for immortalization is activation of the catalytic subunit of telomerase, hTERT [28].The E7 protein binds the tumor suppressor pRb and blocks its binding to the E2F transcription factor, leading to constitutive activation of S phase genes [29]. In HPV-associated malignant transformation, viral DNA may be integrated into the host cell genome, and deletion of large portions of the viral genome may occur. The E2 gene is frequently disrupted during viral integration, one of several mechanisms that result in deregulated expression of the viral E6 and E7 oncoproteins [30], thereby promoting tumorigenesis. E6 and E7 are necessary for viral transformation and stimulate cellular proliferation, delay cellular differentiation, increase the frequency of spontaneous and mutagen-induced mutations, and induce chromosomal instability (i.e. gene amplification, polyploidy, and aneuploidy) in transfected cell lines [26].

Epidemiologic Classification as Oncogenic Types

Genomic sequences of HPVs were initially isolated from benign warts [31] and from cervical cancer specimens in the early 1980s by Harold zur Hausen, a discovery which earned him the Nobel Prize in 2008 [32, 33]. The classification schema for HPVs has since recognized over 120 different HPV types based on DNA sequence [34]. The HPV types first isolated from cervical cancers (HPV16 and 18) were initially classified as oncogenic or high-risk types based on cellular transformation assays that demonstrated the ability of these HPV types to immortalize human keratinocytes in vitro, whereas HPVs isolated from benign genital warts (referred to as low-risk, e.g. 6 and 11) were incapable [35, 36]. The viral E6 and E7 regions of HPV types 16 and 18 were demonstrated to be essential for cellular immortalization [37], and the ability of E6 [38] and E7 [39] proteins from these high-risk, but not low-risk, types to degrade cellular tumor suppressor proteins p53 and pRb correlated with this immortalization function.

More recently, HPV types have been classified as high-risk or low-risk based largely upon strong epidemiological associations observed in case–control studies of cervical cancer [40, 41]. Fifteen different HPV types were classified as high-risk, and an additional three as probably high-risk, based upon at least a fivefold increase in odds of cervical cancer in a pooled, case–control study of ~1,900 women with cervical cancer [40]. High-risk (and probably high-risk) types include most of the members of the phylogenetically related A7 (HPV18, 39, 45, 59, 68) and A9

(HPV16, 31, 33, 35, 52, 58) species, as well as some members of the A6 (HPV 53, 56, 66), A5 (HPV 26, 51 and 82), and A11 (HPV73) species within the genera alpha-papillomaviruses. "Low-risk" HPV types, e.g. HPV6 and 11, are associated with benign hyperproliferations of the infected epithelium, such as genital warts and upper airway papillomas.

Molecular Evidence for a Causal Role of HPV in Head and Neck Squamous Cell Carcinomas (HNSCCs)

Extensive research leading to the observation that HPV infection is a necessary cause of cervical cancer has provided a valuable molecular framework to evaluate the causal role of HPV infection in other cancers [3, 4]. This framework includes the detection of HPV genome in tumors, and more importantly, characteristics of specificity of HPV to tumor cell nuclei as well as HPV genome functionality (as evidenced by viral integration, high viral copy number, and expression of the E6 and E7 oncogenes) [3, 4]. Several studies have reported the detection of HPV DNA in tumors of the oropharynx, oral cavity, and the larynx [1, 42, 43]. A systematic review of worldwide published literature by Kreimer et al. [44] reported that HPV DNA was detected in 35.6% of oropharynx cancers, 24.0% of larynx cancers, and 23.5% of oral cavity cancers. Notably, HPV16 infection, which accounts for approximately 50% of all cervical cancers, constituted a vast majority of HPV-positive head and neck cancers – 86.7% of oropharynx cancers, 69.2% of larynx cancers, and 68.2% of oral cavity cancers [44]. It is, however, important to note that these prevalence estimates are predominantly based on the detection of HPV DNA in tumors by PCR-based methods. Given the high sensitivity, lack of specificity to tumor cells, and the susceptibility to contamination of PCR methods, these prevalence estimates may overestimate the true prevalence of HPV in tumors. On the other hand, degradation of archival tumor specimens may have contributed to the underestimation of HPV prevalence in tumors [44].

A summary of the molecular evidence for a causal role of HPV across constituent head and neck cancer subsites – oral cavity, oropharynx, and the larynx – is presented in Table 1. Cancers of the nasopharynx, paranasal sinuses, and salivary gland are excluded owing to a lack of evidence for a role for HPV in the literature. Molecular evidence for a causal role of HPV infection is the strongest for oropharynx cancers, including those arising from the base of tongue, lingual and palatine tonsil, Waldeyer's ring, and overlapping lesions of the pharynx [42]. Several studies have shown the presence of HPV DNA in oropharynx tumors [1, 42, 43], as well as specificity of the HPV genome to the tumor cell nuclei and frequent integration into the human genome [45–49], high viral copy numbers comparable to levels observed in cervical cancers [49–52], high-level expression of E6 and E7 oncogenes [48, 53, 54], and evidence of antibodies to E6 and E7 antigens [55–57]. On the other hand, beyond PCR detection of HPV DNA, additional evidence for a causal role of HPV in cancers of the oral cavity and larynx has been weak and inconsistent [4]. Thus,

Table 1 Molecular evidence for the association of HPV infection with head and neck cancers

	Oral cavity	Oropharynx	Larynx
Detection of HPV genome	+	++	+
Integrated HPV genome in tumor nuclei	+/–	++	+/–
High viral load/copy number	+/–	++	+/–
Expression of E6 and E7 oncogenes	+/–	++	+/–
Antibodies to E6 and E7 proteins	+/–	++	+/–

++ Strong evidence from multiple studies
+ Moderate evidence
+/– Weak evidence with inconsistent results across studies

molecular evidence indicates that HPV is a well-established cause of a high proportion of oropharynx cancers. A small proportion of oral cavity and larynx cancers, if any, could potentially be etiologically related to HPV infection.

Accruing evidence indicates that HPV-positive HNSCC is a distinct entity at the molecular level when compared to HPV-negative HNSCC [42]. Consistent with functional inactivation of p53 by HPV E6 protein, HPV-positive HNSCCs are characterized by a low frequency of inactivating TP53 mutations when compared to HPV-negative HNSCCs (0–10% versus 50–75%) [45, 53, 58, 59]. HPV-positive HNSCCs are also characterized by low frequency of chromosomal loss at 3p, 9p, and 17p loci [53]. Genomic alterations at 3p, 9p, and 17p are believed to be the early events in HNSCC carcinogenesis [53]. Therefore, the low frequency of alterations at these loci in HPV-positive cancers points to an etiologic role for HPV in tumor initiation [53]. On the other hand, because molecular progression models for HNSCCs are predominantly based on studies of oral cavity cancers, low frequency of these alterations in HPV-positive tumors may also reflect differences between oropharynx vs. oral cavity cancers. The presence of HPV DNA in tumors correlates with increased expression of p16 and decreased expression of epidermal growth factor receptor (EGFR) [42, 60–62]. Additionally, recent studies indicate that HPV-positive HNSCCs are characterized by a distinct gene expression profile, including overexpression of cell cycle regulators such as p18 and underexpression of immune response genes (IL-10 and IL-13) [63, 64].

Epidemiologic Evidence for a Causal Role of HPV in HNSCCs

HPV Exposure Measures

Analytic epidemiologic studies investigating the association of HPV infection with HNSCC have utilized different measures of HPV exposure. Serology-based exposure measures utilize the detection of antibodies to HPV L1 proteins [65]. Antibodies to HPV L1 are type-specific and have the advantage of measuring cumulative life-time exposure to HPV [65]. The utility of type-specific L1 antibodies is, however, hampered by the lack of anatomic site-specificity. Additionally, a considerable proportion of women (~30%) with cervical HPV16 infection fail to mount a detectable L1 antibody response, thus reducing assay sensitivity [65]. The presence of antibodies to HPV E6 and E7 antigens is strongly indicative of the presence of an HPV-related cancer [55]. However, similar to L1 antibodies, measurement of E6/E7 antibodies has low sensitivity given that only 60–70% of HPV16-positive cervical cancer patients show evidence of detectable HPV16 E6/E7 antibodies [66]. Studies of DNA-based HPV exposure assessment have utilized detection of type-specific HPV genomes or a broad-spectrum of mucosal HPV genotypes through PCR. While DNA-based exposure assessment is more sensitive than serology-based methods, the presence of HPV DNA is a transient measure of exposure, particularly among control subjects. Previous studies have found variable correlations across the different HPV exposure measures [67–71]. Herrero et al. [67] reported that presence of HPV in exfoliated oral cells correlated poorly with HPV detection in tumor biopsies (Kappa = 0.059). In contrast, Gillison et al. [70] reported that subjects with real-time PCR detection of HPV16 infection in oral rinse samples were 53-fold more likely to have HPV16 DNA-positive oropharyngeal cancers than those without evidence of HPV16 in oral rinses. Recent studies have also found high correlation between serologic measures of HPV exposure (L1 antibodies) and the presence of HPV16 in tumor tissues [50, 71]. For example, Kreimer et al. [50] reported that tumor HPV16-positive HNSCC cases were more likely to also have evidence of antibodies to HPV L1, E6, and E7 (Odds ratios of 14.6, 57.6, and 25.6, respectively) when compared to HPV16-negative cases.

Evidence from Case–Control and Cohort Studies

Several case–control studies have evaluated the association of HPV infection with oral cavity and oropharynx cancers using both serologic and DNA-based methods. HPV16 L1 seropositivity is associated with high increase in the risk of oropharynx cancer (odds ratios ranging from 3 to 180), but low increase in the risk of oral cavity cancers (odds ratios ranging from 2 to 3) (Table 2) [67, 68, 70–76]. A few serology-based case–control studies have associated the presence of HPV16 L1 antibodies with increased risk of larynx cancers, with two to threefold odds ratio [71, 72]. Furthermore, Smith et al. [77] reported that supraglottic were tenfold more likely than glottic laryngeal cancers to be HPV-associated. Nonetheless, given the anatomic proximity, it is likely that base of tongue cancers could have been misclassified as supraglottic larynx cancers. Consistent with antibodies to HPV16, E6/E7 being markers for the presence of HPV-related cancer, the odds of HPV16 E6/E7 antibody positivity are 50–400 fold higher among individuals with oropharyngeal cancer compared with control subjects (Table 3) [67, 71, 74, 75].

The low sensitivity of HPV16 L1 serology assays may have underestimated the true association between HPV16 and cancer risk. Indeed, studies that have utilized

Table 2 Selected case–control and cohort studies for the association of HPV 16 L1 antibodies with head and neck cancer

Author, year	#cases/#controls	All HNSCCs OR (95% CI)	Oral cavity OR (95% CI)	Oropharynx OR (95% CI)	Larynx OR (95% CI)	Adjustment factors
Schwartz, 1998 [68]	259/446	2.3 (1.6–3.3)	1.1 (0.5–2.5)	3.9 (2.0–7.8)	–	a, b, d, and f
Mork, 2001 [72]	292/1568	2.1 (1.4–3.2)	2.8 (1.2–6.6) [Tongue]	14.4 (3.6–58.2)	2.1 (1.4–3.2)	e
Dahlstrom, 2003 [73]	120/120	6.6 (3.0–14.9)	–	59.5 (5.7–620.2)	–	a, b, c, d, and f
Herrero, 2003 [67]	1610/1732	–	1.5 (1.1–2.1)	3.5 (2.1–5.9)	–	a, b, d, f, g, and k
Smith, 2007 [74]	204/326	1.7 (1.1–2.5)	1.2 (0.7–2.0)	3.5 (1.9–6.5)	–	a, d, f
Furniss, 2007 [71]	486/550	4.0 (2.8–5.7)	1.4 (0.9–2.4)	6.0 (4.9–8.7)	2.7 (1.5–5.1)	a, b, c, d, f, and h
D'Souza, 2007 [75]	100/200	–	–	32.2 (14.6–71.3)	–	a, b, d, f, i, and j
Pintos, 2008 [76]	72/129	7.4 (2.8–27.2)	3.8 (0.9–17.5)	182 (7–4753)	–	a, b, d, f, h
Gillison. 2008 [70]	92/184(HPV 16+ tumors)	–	–	18.3 (6.8–49)		a, b, d, f, i, and j

a age, *b* sex, *c* race, *d* smoking, *e* smoking by cotinine measurements; *f* alcohol; *g* chewing tobacco; *h* education; *i* oral health status; *j* family history of head and neck cancers.

Table 3 Selected case–control studies for the association of HPV 16 E6/E7 antibodies with head and neck cancer

Author, year	#cases/ #controls	All HNSCCs OR (95% CI)	Oral cavity OR (95% CI)	Oropharynx OR (95% CI)	Adjustment factors
Herrero, 2003 [67]	1670/1732	–	2.9 (1.7–4.8)	9.2 (4.8–17.7)	a, b, d, f, g, and k
Smith, 2007 [74]	204/326	15.0 (4.2–53.4)	4.7 (0.5–45.3)	384.0 (49.3–)	a, d, f
D'Souza, 2007 [75]	100/200	–	–	58.4 (24.2–138.3)	a, b, d, f, i, and j

a age, *b* sex, *c* race, *d* smoking, *e* smoking by cotinine measurements; *f* alcohol; *g* chewing tobacco; *h* education; *i* oral health status; *j* family history of head and neck cancers.

DNA-based oral HPV detection have generally found stronger associations (Table 4). The presence of oral HPV infection is associated with 10–200 fold increased risk of oropharyngeal cancer and two to fourfold increased risk of oral cavity cancers [67–70, 75, 76, 78, 79]. Importantly, a majority of these studies have incorporated adjustment for a range of confounders, including the important HNSCC risk factors – tobacco and alcohol use.

Increased risk of oropharyngeal cancer is predominantly observed for high-risk HPV infections, particularly HPV16 [68–70, 76, 79]. Infection with low-risk HPV types is not associated with increased risk of either oropharynx or oral cavity cancers [68–70, 76, 79]. Additionally, serologic studies of HPV types18, 31, 33, or 35 (L1 antibodies) have reported weak and inconsistent associations with oropharyngeal cancer, which is consistent with <10% of oropharyngeal cancers being attributable to non-HPV16 high-risk types [70, 72, 74].

Only one study has evaluated the HPV-HNSCC association prospectively [72]. This study reported that HPV16 L1 seropositivity was associated with a 14-fold increased risk of oropharynx cancer and a twofold increased risk of oral cavity or larynx cancer [72]. The increased HNSCC risk was observed more than 15 years prior to cancer diagnosis, indicating that HPV exposure precedes cancer development by many years [72]. No prospective study has evaluated the association of oral HPV infection with HNSCC.

Given the predominantly sexual transmission of HPV infection [80], association of sexual behaviors with HNSCC risk represents another important line of evidence in support of an HPV etiology [75]. Associations of sexual behaviors with HNSCC risk have been inconsistent in several studies [68, 69, 81], perhaps as a result of the lack of stratification of HNSCCs by anatomic site [75]. In a recent case–control study of oropharynx cancers, D'Souza et al. [75] reported that markers of high-risk sexual behavior such as number of lifetime vaginal sex partners, number of lifetime oral sex partners, and early age at sexual debut were associated with four to eightfold increased risk of oropharyngeal cancer after adjustment for tobacco and alcohol use. Notably, these associations failed to retain statistical significance when models incorporated adjustment for HPV16 seropositivity, indicating that the sexual behavior associations were mediated through increased HPV exposure [75].

Table 4 Selected case–control studies for the association of oral HPV infection with head and neck cancer

Author, year	#cases/ #controls	Sampling method	HPV PCR–genotyping	HPV types	All HNSCCs OR (95% CI)	Oral cavity OR (95% CI)	Oropharynx OR (95% CI)	Adjustment factors
Schwartz, 1998 [68]	284/477	Tap water rinse and cytobrush	MY09/11 – Southern blot	16, 18, 31, 33, 35	1.3 (0.6–2.9)	–	–	a, b, d, f
				6, 11	0.5 (0.2–1.4)			
Strome, 2002 [78]	52/48 Tonsil cancers	Tumor and normal tissues	MY09/11 – Sequencing	Any HPV	–	–	18.2 (4.6–73.1)	a, b
Herrero, 2003 [67]	1670/1732	Saline oral rinse and cytobrush	GP5+/6+ – EIA and Southern blot	Any HPV	–	0.6 (0.3–1.1)	1.0 (0.4–2.5)	a, b, d, f, g, k
Smith, 2004 [69]	201/333	Saline oral rinse	MY09/11 – Sequencing	High-risk	2.6 (1.5–4.2)	–	–	a, b, d, f
				Low-risk	0.8 (0.4–1.7)			
Hansson, 2005 [79]	131/320	Saline oral rinse and swabs of tonsillar fossa	MY09/11 and GP5+/6+ nested PCR – Sequencing	High-risk	63 (14–230)	24 (3.2–180)	230 (44–1,200)	a, b, d, f
				Low-risk	1.4 (0.5–4.3)	2.4 (0.5–11.0)	0.8 (0.1–6.9)	
Pintos, 2008 [76]	72/129	Saline oral rinse and cytobrush	PGMY09/11 – Line blot	High-risk	4.8 (1.2–19.4)	2.1 (0.4–13.0)	19.3 (2.3–159)	a, b, d, f, h
				Low-risk	0.2 (0.0–4.4)	0.3 (0.0–5.5)	NR	
D'Souza, 2007 [75]	100/200	Saline oral rinse and cytobrush	PGMY09/11 – Line blot	Any HPV	–	–	12.3 (5.4–26.4)	a, b, d, f, i, j
				HPV16	–	–	14.6 (6.3–36.6)	
Gillison, 2008 [70]	92/184	Oral rinse and cytobrush	HPV16 Real-time PCR	HPV16	–	–	53 (8.5–333)	a, b, d, f, i, j

a age, *b* sex, *c* race, *d* smoking, *e* smoking by cotinine measurements, *f* alcohol, *g* chewing tobacco, *h* education, *i* oral health status, *j* family history of head and neck cancers

In summary, epidemiologic evidence for an etiologic role of HPV seems the strongest and most consistent for cancers of the oropharynx and weak and inconsistent for cancers of the oral cavity and larynx. Although some studies have found significant associations between markers of HPV exposure and risk of oral cavity and laryngeal cancers, it is likely that misclassification of the primary tumor site may have contributed to a large part of the increased risk. Misclassification of oropharyngeal cancers as oral cancers is particularly likely given that oral cancers are relatively more common in most populations [5]. Likewise, misclassification of base of tongue cancers as larynx cancers may have contributed to positive associations for larynx cancers.

Interaction of HPV with Other HNSCC Risk Factors

Numerous case-series have reported that the proportion of HPV-positive HNSCCs is significantly higher among never smokers and never drinkers [45, 82–85]. Nonetheless, evidence from case–control studies regarding the statistical interaction of HPV with smoking and alcohol use has been equivocal (Table 5). Pertaining to interaction with cigarette smoking, previous studies have reported the lack of any additive or multiplicative interactions (i.e., the joint effect of HPV and smoking is similar to the predicted sum/product of individuals effects) [68, 69, 73, 75], super-additive interactions (i.e., joint effect of HPV and smoking higher than the predicted sum of individual effects) [68], as well as significant negative interactions (i.e., joint effect of HPV and smoking significantly less than the product of individual effects) [86]. Likewise, previous studies have reported the lack of additive or multiplicative interactions between HPV and alcohol use [67, 68, 75], the presence of super-additive interactions [69], and significant negative interactions [86]. Several study design and methodological aspects in previous studies may have contributed to the inconsistent results. For example, studies reporting significant negative interactions between HPV and tobacco/alcohol have predominantly utilized serologic assessments of HPV16 [67, 86]. The low sensitivity of HPV serology assays and recent observations that smokers are less likely to develop HPV antibodies affect the validity of these interactions [87]. Further, lack of stratification of HNSCCs by anatomic site may also have contributed to inconsistent results.

Several case-series and case–control studies have shown that HPV-positive HNSCCs are more common among younger individuals, men, and among whites [42, 75]. These associations with age, sex, and race may, in part, arise from differences in sexual behaviors and consequent differences in risk of oral HPV exposure. Recently, HPV16 seropositivity was reported to modify the association between fruit consumption and head and neck cancer [88]. Whereas odds of cancer decreased with high fruit consumption among HPV-seronegative subjects, the opposite was true for seropositive subjects. However, in a case–case comparison, the odds of HPV-DNA positive versus HPV-negative cancer was not related to fruit consumption

Table 5 Selected studies addressing the statistical interaction of HPV infection with smoking and alcohol

Reference	# cases/ controls	Method of HPV exposure	Assessment of interactions	Interaction with smoking	Interaction with alcohol
Schwartz, 1998 [68]	259/446	HPV16 L1 serology	Synergy index (additive)	Super-additive	Not significant
Herrero, 2003 [67]	1670/1732	HPV16 L1, E6, and E7 serology	Multiplicative	L1: Not significant for oral cavity or oropharynx cancers E6/E7: Significantly less than predicted by individual effects. Consistent with risk additivity	Not reported
Dahlstorm, 2003 [73]	120/120	HPV16 L1 serology	Multiplicative	Not significant	Not reported
Smith, 2004 [69]	201/333	HPV DNA in exfoliated cells	Synergy index (additive) Multiplicative	Not significant on additive or multiplicative scales	Super-additive. Not significant on multiplicative scale.
Applebaum, 2007 [86]	485/549	HPV16 L1 serology	Multiplicative	Significantly less than predicted by individual effects	Significantly less than predicted by individual effects
D' Souza, 2007 [75]	100/200	HPV16 L1 serology HPV DNA in oral rinse	Synergy index (additive)	Not significant	Not significant

as would be expected, consistent with an alternate explanation that diet may affect seroconvertion among HPV16-exposed individuals. No previous study has investigated the statistical interaction of HPV with other known HNSCC risk factors such as host genetic susceptibility, or a family history of HNSCC.

An alternative strategy for evaluating statistical interactions of HPV with other risk factors is to compare risk factor profiles for HPV-positive and HPV-negative HNSCCs, as recently reported by Gillison et al. [70]. Distinct risk factor profiles were observed for HPV-positive and HPV-negative HNSCCs in this study. HPV-positive HNSCCs were unrelated to tobacco or alcohol use or markers of poor oral hygiene, but were significantly associated with oral sex behaviors. In contrast, HPV-negative HNSCCs were significantly associated with tobacco and alcohol use and markers of poor oral hygiene, but were unrelated to sexual behaviors. This study also reported a novel interaction between marijuana use (duration and intensity) and HPV infection, with significantly increased risks among individuals with joint exposures. Conceivably, the carcinogenic and immunosuppressive effects of marijuana may act in concert with HPV infection [70].

The absence of overt statistical interactions between HPV and the dominant HNSCC risk factors – tobacco/alcohol use – indicates that HPV infection and tobacco/alcohol target similar pathways in HNSCC carcinogenesis [53, 70]. Indeed, HPV-positive and HPV-negative HNSCCs share common oncogenic pathways – disruption of host tumor suppressor genes p53 and pRb either via genotoxic damage from tobacco and/or alcohol use or via functional inactivation by HPV oncoproteins [53, 70].

In summary, although HPV attributable proportions are relatively higher among never smokers and never drinkers, current evidence indicates that HPV-positive HNSCCs occur among both individuals with or without exposure to tobacco or alcohol.

Epidemiologic Assessment of Causality for HPV in Oropharyngeal Cancer

The association of HPV with oropharynx cancers fulfills all of the modern criteria for causality (Table 6) [89]. Studies conducted in multiple populations have shown that HPV exposed individuals have a more than tenfold increased risk of oropharyngeal cancer than unexposed (strength and consistency of association) [67–70, 75, 76, 78, 79]. The HPV association seems specific for oropharyngeal cancers across HNSCC subsites (specificity) [67–70, 75, 76, 78, 79]. HPV exposure precedes the development of oropharyngeal cancer (temporality) [72]. Although increasing oropharyngeal cancer risk with increasing HPV antibody titers [71] suggests a dose-response effect (biologic gradient of increasing risk with increasing degree of exposure), there is little evidence that antibody titers to HPV antigens are indicative of increased exposure. Molecular mechanisms of HPV-induced cervical,

Table 6 Epidemiologic assessment of causality for HPV in oropharyngeal cancer

Criterion	Evidence	Strength of evidence
Strength	Measures of HPV exposure (serological or DNA-based) have been associated with > tenfold increased risk of oropharyngeal cancer in retrospective and prospective studies.	++
Consistency	HPV infection has been consistently associated with increased oropharyngeal cancer risk in studies conducted across different geographic locations/populations.	++
Specificity	Across head and neck cancer anatomic subsites, the association of HPV seems specific for cancers arising in the oropharynx, including the base of tongue, lingual and palatine tonsil, and other parts of the oropharynx.	++
Temporality	Only one cohort study has evaluated the association of HPV with prospective oropharyngeal cancer risk. HPV infection (measured by antibodies to HPV16 L1) precedes oropharyngeal cancer development by more than 15 years.	+
Biologic gradient	Risk of oropharyngeal cancer increased significantly with increasing HPV16 L1 antibody titers indicating a dose-response effect.	+/−
Plausibility	E6 and E7 proteins of HPV bind to and inactivate tumor suppressor proteins p53 and pRB, respectively, leading to malignant transformation of infected cells.	++
Coherence	HPV-positive oropharyngeal cancers have evidence of integrated, high copy number HPV genomes in tumor cells as well as expression of E6 and E7 gene products. Consistent with HPVs being predominantly transmitted sexually, markers of sexual activity, including oral sex and number of lifetime oral sex partners have also been associated with increased oropharyngeal cancer risk in several studies.	++
Experiment	Downregulation of E6 and E7 oncoproteins in HPV-positive cell lines resulted in increased apoptosis and reversal of malignant phenotype (as evidenced by increase in p53 and pRB levels).	+
Analogy	HPV-induced oropharyngeal carcinogenesis is analogous to HPV-induced cervical, anal, penile, vaginal, and vulvar carcinogenesis.	++

++ Strong evidence from multiple studies
+ Moderate evidence in single or few studies
+/− Weak evidence

anal, penile, vaginal, and vulvar carcinogenesis lend support for plausibility and analogy [3]. Additionally, reversal of malignant phenotype through inhibition of HPV E6 and E7 gene expression provides experimental evidence [90]. Finally, associations with markers of high-risk sexual behavior are coherent within the sexual transmission framework of mucosal HPV infections [80].

Epidemiology of Oral HPV Infections

In contrast to the knowledge regarding the epidemiology of anogenital HPV infections, little is currently known regarding the transmission, epidemiology, and natural history of oral HPV infections. Cross-sectional studies have utilized multiple sampling strategies to assess the prevalence of oral HPV infection, including exfoliated oral cells, buccal swabs, saliva, tissue scrapings, and oral rinse samples, and have reported varying prevalence estimates (Table 7). Prevalence of oral HPV infection has varied widely across different populations, from 2.4% among pregnant women [91] to 33% among HIV-infected individuals [92]. Similar to the high prevalence of HPV16 in HNSCCs [44], HPV16 is the most prevalent oral HPV type in the general population, with prevalence estimates of at least 1%. A few studies that have assessed predictors of oral HPV infections show that: (1) oral HPV prevalence is associated with sexual behaviors, including practicing oral sex, number of lifetime oral sex partners, and number of lifetime sexual partners [91–93], thus underscoring sexual transmission of HPV to the oral mucosa; (2) nonsexual transmission of HPV to the oral cavity through auto-inoculation or salivary transmission is also plausible [91, 94]; (3) oral HPV prevalence is significantly higher among HIV-infected men and women [92, 93]. Among HIV-infected individuals, oral HPV prevalence increases with increasing immunosuppression (low CD4 T-cell counts and high HIV-1 viral loads) [92, 93, 95]. However, prevalence is significantly higher among individuals receiving highly-active antiretroviral therapies (HAART) [92, 95], perhaps as a result of confounding by indication; (4) oral HPV prevalence is higher among individuals with a history of genital warts or sexually transmitted diseases [93]; (5) oral HPV prevalence does not decrease with increasing age [69, 92, 93]; (6) men have a higher prevalence of oral HPV than women [91, 93, 95]; and (7) oral HPV prevalence is higher among whites than other races [95]. Although reasons for gender/racial differences in oral HPV prevalence are unclear, differences in sexual behaviors may explain these observations.

Several observations indicate that the epidemiology of oral HPV infection is distinct from the epidemiology of cervical HPV [92, 96]. Across different populations, prevalence of oral HPV infection is lower than prevalence of cervical HPV infection [92]. The HPV genotype distribution in the oral cavity is also significantly different from that in the cervix [96]. Studies that have assessed dual infection patterns at the oral cavity and the cervix have shown that women with cervical HPV infection were more likely to have a concomitant oral HPV infection; nonetheless, type-specific concordance was poor [96]. In contrast to decreasing prevalence of cervical HPV infections with increasing age [97], prevalence of oral HPV infection is reportedly stable or increases with increasing age [69, 92, 93]. Although distinct from the cervix, the pattern of age-specific prevalence of oral HPV infection appears similar to that of anal and penile HPV infections [98, 99]. A distinct hormonal milieu in the cervix may, in part, contribute to differences in age-specific prevalence of oral versus cervical HPV infection [98, 100]. Differences in immune responses between the oral cavity and the genital tract may also contribute to age-specific differences.

Table 7 Selected studies of the prevalence and predictors of oral HPV infections

Reference	# subjects	Population	Sampling method	HPV PCR and genotyping method	HPV prevalence	Common genotypes	Predictors
Kreimer, 2004 [93]	586	396 HIV-infected 190 HIV-uninfected women. Baltimore, USA	Saline oral rinse	PCR: PGMY09/11 Genotyping: Linear probe array (Roche, 37 types)	25.3% in HIV-infected 7.6% in HIV-uninfected	16, 89, and 84	*HIV-infected:* Number of recent oral sex partners, low CD4 count, presence of oral mucosal abnormalities, and HSV-2 seropositivity *HIV-uninfected:* Older age, men, and HSV-2 seropositivity
Canadas, 2004 [133]	187	Female sex workers. Spain	Buccal cells	PCR: MY09/11 Genotyping: Dot blot	7.9%	6 and 16	Not reported
Smith, 2004 [69]	625	557 pregnant women and 68 men. Iowa, USA	Saline oral rinse	PCR: MY09/11 Genotyping: Sequencing	2.4% among women 5.9% among men	16	*Women:* Older age, multi- parity *Men:* Number of female sex partners
Cameron, 2005 [95]	98	HIV-infected subjects. New Orleans, USA	Saliva	PCR: PGMY09/11 Genotyping: Line blot assay (Roche, 27 types)	35%	16, 55, and 83	Higher prevalence among whites, intravenous drug users, and subjects on HAART regimens
Fakhry, 2006 [96]	221	143 HIV-infected and 78 HIV-uninfected women in the Women's Interagency HIV Cohort Study (WIHS). Multi-center, USA	Saline oral rinse	PCR: PGMY09/11 Genotyping: Linear probe array (Roche, 37 types)	25.2% in HIV-infected 9% in HIV-uninfected	72, 62, and 89	Not reported

(continued)

Table 7 (continued)

Reference	# subjects	Population	Sampling method	HPV PCR and genotyping method	HPV prevalence	Common genotypes	Predictors
Rintala, 2006 [101]	462	331 pregnant women and 131 male partners. Turku, Finland	Oral mucosal cells	PCR: MY09/11 and GP5+/6+ nested PCR Genotyping: DNA hybridization	16% in women 18% in men	Not reported	–Not associated with sexual behavior. –faster clearance among men –oral HPV persistence associated with persistence in the partner
Sacramento, 2006 [134]	50	Non-malignant surgey patients. Sao Jose, Brazil	Oropharyngeal tissue scrapings	PCR : MY09/11 Genotyping : Dot blot (19 types)	5.2% overall 1.7% in tonsil 1.7% in soft palate 1.2% in base of tongue 0.6% in pharynx	16, 52, and 61	Not reported
D'souza, 2007 [92]	182	123 HIV-infected and 59 HIV-uninfected women in the Women's Interagency HIV Cohort Study (WIHS). Multi-center, USA	Saline oral rinse	PCR: PGMY09/11 Genotyping: Linear probe array (Roche, 37 types)	33% in HIV-infected 15.3% in HIV-uninfected	72, 16, and 83	*Predictors of persistence:* Older age, current smoking, HAART regimens, time on HAART therapy, low CD4 counts, and higher HIV-1 viral loads
Marais, 2008 [135]	105	33 HIV-infected and 72 HIV-uninfected women referred for colposcopy Cape Town, South Africa	Exfoliated buccal cells	PCR: PGMY09/11 Genotyping: Linear probe array (Roche, 37 types)	33% in HIV-infected 23.6% in HIV-uninfected	33, 13, and 72 among HIV-infected 11, 28, and 33 among HIV-uninfected	Not reported

Furthermore, infection prevalence being a function of both incidence and persistence (duration), differences in age-specific prevalence may arise from distinct incidence and persistence patterns for oral and cervical HPV infections.

Very few studies have assessed the natural history of oral HPV infections. In a short-term natural history study of oral HPV infections among HIV-infected and HIV-uninfected women, D'Souza et al. [92] reported oral HPV incidence rates of 3.3 per 100 person-months among HIV-infected women and 1.7 per 100 person-months among HIV-uninfected women. Although oral HPV incidence rates were significantly lower than cervical HPV incidence (10.7 and 10.4 per 100 person-months among HIV-infected and HIV-uninfected women, respectively), six-month persistence was similar for oral and cervical HPV infections. Significant predictors of 6-month oral HPV persistence included older age, current smoking, and use of HAART regimens. In a prospective Finnish family study of pregnant women and male partners, Rintala et al. [101] assessed the natural history of oral HPV infections, defined as any HPV infection irrespective of genotype, over 24 months of follow-up. Incidence of oral HPV was similar among women and men. However, oral HPV persistence was significantly higher among women. Although individual factors such as oral sex behaviors were not associated with persistence, persistent oral HPV infection in the spouse was highly predictive of HPV persistence within an individual [101].

Clinical Features of HPV-Positive Head and Neck Cancers

In addition to differences in molecular and epidemiologic features, HPV-positive oropharynx cancers have distinct clinical characteristics [42, 45, 60, 102]. HPV-positive oropharyngeal cancers are diagnosed at a more advanced TNM stage than HPV-negative cancers: HPV-positive tumors tend to be diagnosed at a lower tumor size, with lymph node positivity, and presence of metastases [42, 59, 62, 103]. Histologically, HPV-positive oropharyngeal cancers are poorly differentiated and are characterized by a basaloid pathology [45]. Several retrospective studies have shown that HPV-positive oropharynx cancers have improved prognosis than HPV-negative oropharyngeal cancers. Despite the advanced stage at diagnosis, patients with HPV-positive oropharyngeal cancers have better response to induction chemotherapy [103, 104], and better overall, disease-specific, and disease-free survival rates [45, 59, 61, 62, 84, 103–107], with a 20–80% reduction in the hazard of death (Table 8).

While the clinical benefit may in part arise from epidemiologic features of patients with HPV-positive cancers such as younger age at diagnosis and low prevalence of smoking/alcohol use, previous studies have shown that the survival benefit is independent of important prognostic factors – age, tumor stage, treatment modality, smoking, and alcohol use. Nonetheless, the majority of previous studies have been small and retrospective in nature, thus precluding adequate adjustment for a range of potential confounders. In the first prospective evaluation, Fakhry et al.

Table 8 Selected studies comparing prognosis for HPV-positive oropharyngeal cancers versus HPV-negative oropharyngeal cancers

Reference	# of oropharyngeal cancers (% HPV positive)	Treatments	Follow-up time	Overall survival/ disease-specific survival HPV+ vs. HPV- HR (95% CI)	Disease-free survival HPV+ vs. HPV- HR (95% CI)	Adjustment factors	Effect modifiers
Gillison, 2000 [45]	60 (57.0)	Surgery Radiation Surgery+ radiation Chemoradiation	5 years	0.26 (0.07–0.98)	–	None	None
Lindel, 2001 [84]	99 (14.0)	Radiation Radiation+ chemotherapy	6 years	0.35 (0.13–0.98)	0.50 (0.20–1.26)	None	None
Dahlgren, 2004 [105]	25 (40.0)	Radiation Surgery	5 years	Disease-specific (KM estimates): HPV+: 60% HPV–: 20% $p=0.036$	–	Tumor stage	None
Licitra, 2006 [59]	90 (19.0)	Surgery Surgery+radiation	5 years	KM estimates HPV+/TP53 wt: 79% HPV–/TP53 wt or HPV–/+ and TP53 mut: 46% $p=0.001$	HPV+/TP53 wt: 21% HPV-/TP53 wt or HPV–/+ and TP53 mut: 53% $p=0.037$	Treatment, age, and tumor stage	TP53 mutations Survival for HPV+/ TP53 wt > HPV+/– and TP53 mut
Weinberger, 2006 [62]	107 (61.0)	Radiation and chemotherapy	5 years	Overall survival: HPV+/p16–: 0.80 (0.40–1.8) HPV+/p16+: 0.19 (0.10–0.70)	HPV+/p16–: 0.74 (0.40–1.6) HPV+/p16+: 0.20 (0.10–0.60)	Tumor type, treatment, TNM stage, histologic grade	p16 expression Survival for HPV+/ p16+ > HPV+/p16–

Reimers, 2007 [106]	106 (28.0%)	Surgery Surgery–radiation/ chemoradiation Cemoradiation	5 years	0.42 (0.10–1.76)	0.34 (0.06–1.85)	p16, EGFR, tumor stage	None
Worden, 2008 [103]	42 (64.3%)	Chemoradiation Surgery/radiation	4 years	0.81 (0.70–0.94)	0.77 (0.63–0.93)	age, KPS score, T class, N class, smoking	HPV viral load High viral load associated with improved treatment response, overall survival, and disease-free survival
Hafkamp, 2008 [107]	81 (41.0%)	Surgery Radiation Chemotherapy Combinations of S+R+C	5 years	0.43 (0.22–0.90)	HPV+: 73% HPV–: 48% $p=0.038$	Smoking Alcohol T classification	Smoking HPV+ non-smokers > HPV+ smokers
Fakhry, 2008 [104]	62 (62%)	Radiation	5 years	0.39 (0.15–1.05)	0.38 (0.12–1.15)	ECOG performance status	None

[104] recently reported the association of tumor HPV status with prognosis among patients with oropharynx or larynx cancer in the Eastern Cooperative Oncology Group trial. Patients with HPV-positive tumors had a significantly better response to induction chemotherapy (82 vs. 55%) and chemoradiation (84 vs. 57%). Over a follow-up of ~3 years, patients with HPV-positive oropharyngeal cancers had a 61% reduction in the hazard of death and a 62% reduction in the hazard of progression when compared to those with HPV-negative tumors [104].

The survival benefit for HPV-positive cancers is believed to arise from enhanced tumor sensitivity to the effects of chemoradiation [60]. However, studies have shown better survival for HPV-positive patients treated by surgery alone [59], indicating that the improved prognosis may not be treatment-specific. Prognosis for patients with HPV-positive oropharyngeal cancers has also been shown to be modified by factors such as presence of TP53 mutations, p16 overexpression, and smoking. It is, however, important to note that a majority of these observations arise from studies with small sample sizes. Tumor TP53 mutations are observed in approximately 50% of patients with oropharyngeal cancers and the presence of mutations is associated with worse prognosis [108]. Licitra et al. [59] reported that patients with HPV+/TP53 wild-type oropharyngeal cancers had significantly higher 5-year survival when compared to those with HPV-positive or – negative tumors with TP53 mutations. Similarly, in an analysis that included both oral cavity and oropharyngeal cancers, Smith et al. [109] reported that patients with HPV-positive tumors with overexpression of p53 had significantly higher tumor recurrence compared to those with HPV-positive tumors without p53 overexpression. Weinberger et al. [62] reported that in a series of 78 oropharyngeal cancers, 61% of tumors were HPV-positive, but only 38% of HPV-positive tumors had evidence of p16 expression. Patients with HPV-positive/p16-positive tumors had significantly better 5-year overall and disease-free survival when compared to patients with HPV-positive/p16-negative tumors, suggesting that the survival benefit of HPV-positive tumors is mediated through p16 expression [62]. In contrast, most previous studies have observed a high correlation between p16 expression and tumor HPV positivity [61, 104, 106, 107], which has precluded an assessment of the independent effect of p16 or the effect modification between p16 and HPV [104]. Finally, nonsmokers with HPV-positive tonsil cancers have been shown to have significantly higher disease-specific survival compared to smokers with HPV-positive cancers [107].

Although several theories have been proposed, the precise mechanisms involved in the enhanced treatment response and improved survival of HPV-positive oropharyngeal cancers are currently unclear. These theories include: (1) Low rates of genomic damage in HPV-positive tumors, (2) The absence of field cancerization in HPV-induced cancers, and (3) The presence of immune responses to HPV antigens [59, 102, 104]. As noted in Sect. 2, HPV-positive oropharyngeal cancers are characterized by a low frequency of TP53 mutations and low rates of loss of heterozygosity and microsatellite instability at chromosomal loci 3p, 9p, and 17p [45, 53, 58]. As a result, HPV-positive tumors have intact apoptotic responses, which are believed to enhance response to chemoradiation [59, 60, 104]. Tobacco/alcohol cause genetic damage at multiple foci in the head and neck region (i.e., field cancerization). In contrast, tumors caused by HPV are believed to arise from limited foci of infection [47, 59], resulting in reduced incidence of second tumors [59]. Finally, immune responses to HPV antigens, particularly E6 and E7 oncoproteins [55–57], are also believed to aid in improved treatment responses and prognosis among patients with HPV-positive tumors [59, 104].

Burden of HPV-Related Head and Neck Cancers

The proportion of HNSCCs that are oropharyngeal in origin, and hence etiologically related to HPV infection, varies geographically and is relatively higher in developed than developing countries [5]. There is wide variability in the literature regarding the proportion of oropharynx cancers that is attributable to HPV infections, ranging from 12 to 63% [5, 44, 67, 104] (Table 9). Across these ranges, current data indicate that between 6,000 to 33,000 oropharynx cancers worldwide and 800 to 4,600 cancers in the US are potentially caused by HPV infection (Table 9). These estimates show that the burden of HPV-associated head and neck cancer is considerable. Moreover, recent studies in the US and Scandinavian countries show that the burden of HPV-associated head and neck cancers may have increased substantially over the past couple of decades [110–116]. In the US, incidence rates for HPV-related head and neck cancer subsites (base of tongue, tonsil, and pharynx) increased substantially during 1973–2004. In contrast, incidence of HPV-unrelated head and neck cancers decreased during the same period [110]. This increase for HPV-related head and neck cancers was predominantly observed among young individuals and white males [110]. It is likely that changes in sexual behaviors during the 1960s might have led to increased oral HPV exposure, and as a result, an increase in the proportion of HPV-positive oropharyngeal cancers. Indeed, a recent study from Sweden reported an approximately threefold increase in the proportion of HPV-positive tonsil cancers from the 1970s to the 2000s [116].

Table 9 Estimated annual burden of HPV-associated oropharynx cancers in the United States and worldwide

	HPV attributable proportions	US: 7,360 oropharynx cases annually[a]	Worldwide: 52,100 oropharynx cases annually[b]
		Number of HPV-attributable cases	
International case–control study. Herrero, 2003 [67]	18.3%	1,325	9,378
Parkin and Bray, 2006 [5]	12%	883	6,252
Systematic review. Kreimer, 2005 [44]	35.6%	2,620	18,548
Contemporary US estimates. Fakhry, 2008 [104]	63%	4,637	32,823

[a]Estimate from Parkin and Bray [5]
[b]Estimate from Watson et al. [7]

Prospects for Prevention of HPV-Associated Head and Neck Cancers

Populations at High Risk of HPV-Associated Head and Neck Cancer

Populations at particularly increased risk of HPV-associated HNSCCs include immunosuppressed HIV-infected individuals [117], individuals with a history of genital warts or sexually transmitted diseases [68, 75], survivors of HPV-associated cancers [118], and partners of individuals with HPV-associated cancers [119]. The increased risk among these populations predominantly arises from increased exposure to oral HPV infection. For example, the two to fivefold increased risk of oropharyngeal cancer among persons with AIDS when compared to individuals in the general population is consistent with increased oral HPV prevalence and persistence among HIV-infected individuals [92]. Likewise, increased risk of tonsil/oropharynx cancers among cervical cancer survivors and among partners of women with cervical cancer may indicate increased oral HPV exposure.

Potential for Prevention of HPV-Associated Head and Neck Cancer Through Prophylactic HPV Vaccination

Current virus-like particle-based prophylactic HPV vaccines – Gardasil (targeting HPV types 16, 18, 6, and 11) and Cervarix (targeting HPV types 16 and 18) – have been shown to have 90–95% efficacy against persistent cervical HPV infection and related disease (cervical intraepithelial neoplasia2/3) among women naïve for vaccine-targeted HPV types [120–122]. The quadrivalent HPV vaccine is also 100% efficacious in preventing genital warts, vulvar intraepithelial neoplasia, and vaginal intraepithelial neoplasia caused by vaccine HPV types [121]. The mechanism of protection of these vaccines is believed to be through generation of type-specific neutralizing IgG antibodies [123], which prevent establishment of persistent HPV infection, and as a consequence, related diseases. The HPV vaccines are prophylactic and not therapeutic [124]. In that, vaccination is not efficacious in clearing established HPV infections or preexisting disease [124]. Finally, although efficacy among men has not yet been reported, the vaccine is safe and immunogenic among males [125].

Several observations point to the potential for HPV vaccines to prevent oral HPV infection and associated HNSCCs through prophylactic HPV vaccination [126]. Prevention of oral papillomas through VLP-based vaccination in animal models provides proof-of-principle [127]. Additionally, levels of IgG antibodies in oral mucosal transudates correlate with systemic IgG responses in unvaccinated individuals [128, 129]. These results indicate that vaccine-induced systemic IgG responses would correlate with correspondingly high local IgG antibodies in the oral cavity, as has been observed in the cervix [130].

A majority of HPV-associated HNSCCs (90–95%) are attributable to HPV16 [44], underscoring the potential for prevention of a high proportion of HPV-associated HNSCCs. In the US, HPV vaccination is currently recommended only among females aged 9–26 years [131]. Nonetheless, the high burden of HPV-associated HNSCCs among males argues for gender neutral HPV vaccination [126, 132].

Conclusions and Future Directions

Extensive epidemiologic and molecular evidence has established HPV infection as an etiologic agent for oropharyngeal cancers, including those arising from the base of tongue and tonsil. The etiologic role of HPV in other head and neck cancers such as oral cavity and larynx cancers is currently unclear. HPV-positive head and neck cancers represent a distinct disease at the molecular, epidemiologic, and clinical levels. Several features pertaining to HPV-associated head and neck cancers need further investigation, including the natural history of oral HPV infection and premalignant lesions, interaction of HPV with other HNSCC risk factors such as tobacco, alcohol, diet, genetic susceptibility, and family history, reasons underlying the improved prognosis for HPV-positive HNSCCs, and the efficacy of currently available prophylactic HPV vaccines in preventing oral HPV infections.

References

1. International Agency for Research on Cancer (2007) IARC Monographs on the Evaluation of Carcinogenic Risks to Humans. vol 90: Human Papillomaviruses
2. Walboomers JM, Jacobs MV, Manos MM, Bosch FX, Kummer JA, Shah KV et al (1999) Human papillomavirus is a necessary cause of invasive cervical cancer worldwide. J Pathol 189(1):12–9
3. Gillison ML, Shah KV (2003) Chapter 9: role of mucosal human papillomavirus in nongenital cancers. J Natl Cancer Inst Monogr (31):57–65
4. Gillison ML, Chaturvedi AK, Lowy DR (2008) HPV prophylactic vaccines and the potential prevention of noncervical cancers in both men and women. Cancer 113(10):3036–46
5. Parkin DM, Bray F (2006) Chapter 2: The burden of HPV-related cancers. Vaccine 24(Suppl 3): S11–S25
6. Parkin DM (2006) The global health burden of infection-associated cancers in the year 2002. Int J Cancer 118(12):3030–44
7. Watson M, Saraiya M, Ahmed F, Cardinez CJ, Reichman ME, Weir HK et al (2008) Using population-based cancer registry data to assess the burden of human papillomavirus-associated cancers in the United States: overview of methods. Cancer 113(10 Suppl):2841–54
8. Bosch FX, Burchell AN, Schiffman M, Giuliano AR, de Sanjose S, Bruni L et al (2008) Epidemiology and natural history of human papillomavirus infections and type-specific implications in cervical neoplasia. Vaccine 26(Suppl 10):K1–16

9. Clifford GM, Gallus S, Herrero R, Munoz N, Snijders PJ, Vaccarella S et al (2005) Worldwide distribution of human papillomavirus types in cytologically normal women in the International Agency for Research on Cancer HPV prevalence surveys: a pooled analysis. Lancet 366(9490):991–8
10. Franceschi S, Herrero R, Clifford GM, Snijders PJ, Arslan A, Anh PT et al (2006) Variations in the age-specific curves of human papillomavirus prevalence in women worldwide. Int J Cancer 119(11):2677–84
11. Dunne EF, Unger ER, Sternberg M, McQuillan G, Swan DC, Patel SS et al (2007) Prevalence of HPV infection among females in the United States. JAMA 297(8):813–9
12. Dunne EF, Nielson CM, Stone KM, Markowitz LE, Giuliano AR (2006) Prevalence of HPV infection among men: a systematic review of the literature. J Infect Dis 194(8):1044–57
13. Partridge JM, Hughes JP, Feng Q, Winer RL, Weaver BA, Xi LF et al (2007) Genital human papillomavirus infection in men: incidence and risk factors in a cohort of university students. J Infect Dis 196(8):1128–36
14. De Koning MN, Struijk L, Bavinck JN, Kleter B, Ter SJ, Quint WG et al (2007) Betapapillomaviruses frequently persist in the skin of healthy individuals. J Gen Virol 88(Pt 5):1489–95
15. Weissenborn SJ, De Koning MN, Wieland U, Quint WG, Pfister HJ (2009) Intrafamilial transmission and family-specific spectra of cutaneous betapapillomaviruses. J Virol 83(2):811–6
16. Ho L, Chan SY, Burk RD, Das BC, Fujinaga K, Icenogle JP et al (1993) The genetic drift of human papillomavirus type 16 is a means of reconstructing prehistoric viral spread and the movement of ancient human populations. J Virol 67(11):6413–23
17. Ong CK, Chan SY, Campo MS, Fujinaga K, Mavromara-Nazos P, Labropoulou V et al (1993) Evolution of human papillomavirus type 18: an ancient phylogenetic root in Africa and intratype diversity reflect coevolution with human ethnic groups. J Virol 67(11):6424–31
18. Stubenrauch F, Laimins LA (1999) Human papillomavirus life cycle: active and latent phases. Semin Cancer Biol 9(6):379–86
19. Wang XM, Jansen KU, McClements WL (2003) DNA replicative functions of highly-expressed, codon-optimized human papillomavirus proteins E1 and E2. J Virol Methods 108(1):83–90
20. Wilson VG, West M, Woytek K, Rangasamy D (2002) Papillomavirus E1 proteins: form, function, and features. Virus Genes 24(3):275–90
21. Soeda E, Ferran MC, Baker CC, McBride AA (2006) Repression of HPV16 early region transcription by the E2 protein. Virology 351(1):29–41
22. Wilson R, Ryan GB, Knight GL, Laimins LA, Roberts S (2007) The full-length E1E4 protein of human papillomavirus type 18 modulates differentiation-dependent viral DNA amplification and late gene expression. Virology 362(2):453–60
23. Genther Williams SM, Disbrow GL, Schlegel R, Lee D, Threadgill DW, Lambert PF (2005) Requirement of epidermal growth factor receptor for hyperplasia induced by E5, a high-risk human papillomavirus oncogene. Cancer Res 65(15):6534–42
24. Tsai TC, Chen SL (2003) The biochemical and biological functions of human papillomavirus type 16 E5 protein. Arch Virol 148(8):1445–53
25. Ashrafi GH, Brown DR, Fife KH, Campo MS (2006) Down-regulation of MHC class I is a property common to papillomavirus E5 proteins. Virus Res 120(1–2):208–11
26. Munger K, Howley PM (2002) Human papillomavirus immortalization and transformation functions. Virus Res 89(2):213–28
27. Mantovani F, Banks L (2001) The human papillomavirus E6 protein and its contribution to malignant progression. Oncogene 20(54):7874–87
28. Klingelhutz AJ, Foster SA, McDougall JK (1996) Telomerase activation by the E6 gene product of human papillomavirus type 16. Nature 380(6569):79–82
29. Munger K, Basile JR, Duensing S, Eichten A, Gonzalez SL, Grace M et al (2001) Biological activities and molecular targets of the human papillomavirus E7 oncoprotein. Oncogene 20(54):7888–98
30. Romanczuk H, Howley PM (1992) Disruption of either the E1 or the E2 regulatory gene of human papillomavirus type 16 increases viral immortalization capacity. Proc Natl Acad Sci U S A 89(7):3159–63

31. Gissmann L, zur Hausen H (1980) Partial characterization of viral DNA from human genital warts (Condylomata acuminata). Int J Cancer 25(5):605–9
32. zur Hausen H (2009) Papillomaviruses in the causation of human cancers – a brief historical account. Virology 384:260–265
33. Durst M, Gissmann L, Ikenberg H, zur Hausen H (1983) A papillomavirus DNA from a cervical carcinoma and its prevalence in cancer biopsy samples from different geographic regions. Proc Natl Acad Sci U S A 80(12):3812–5
34. de Villiers EM, Fauquet C, Broker TR, Bernard HU, zur Hausen H (2004) Classification of papillomaviruses. Virology 324(1):17–27
35. Schlegel R, Phelps WC, Zhang YL, Barbosa M (1988) Quantitative keratinocyte assay detects two biological activities of human papillomavirus DNA and identifies viral types associated with cervical carcinoma. EMBO J 7(10):3181–7
36. Storey A, Pim D, Murray A, Osborn K, Banks L, Crawford L (1988) Comparison of the in vitro transforming activities of human papillomavirus types. EMBO J 7(6):1815–20
37. Phelps WC, Yee CL, Munger K, Howley PM (1988) The human papillomavirus type 16 E7 gene encodes transactivation and transformation functions similar to those of adenovirus E1A. Cell 53(4):539–47
38. Hiller T, Poppelreuther S, Stubenrauch F, Iftner T (2006) Comparative analysis of 19 genital human papillomavirus types with regard to p53 degradation, immortalization, phylogeny, and epidemiologic risk classification. Cancer Epidemiol Biomarkers Prev 15(7):1262–7
39. Heck DV, Yee CL, Howley PM, Munger K (1992) Efficiency of binding the retinoblastoma protein correlates with the transforming capacity of the E7 oncoproteins of the human papillomaviruses. Proc Natl Acad Sci U S A 89(10):4442–6
40. Munoz N, Bosch FX, de Sanjose S, Herrero R, Castellsague X, Shah KV et al (2003) Epidemiologic classification of human papillomavirus types associated with cervical cancer. N Engl J Med 348(6):518–27
41. Munoz N, Castellsague X, de Gonzalez AB, Gissmann L (2006) Chapter 1: HPV in the etiology of human cancer. Vaccine 24(Suppl 3):S31–S310
42. Gillison ML (2004) Human papillomavirus-associated head and neck cancer is a distinct epidemiologic, clinical, and molecular entity. Semin Oncol 31(6):744–54
43. Syrjanen S (2005) Human papillomavirus (HPV) in head and neck cancer. J Clin Virol 32(Suppl 1):S59–S66
44. Kreimer AR, Clifford GM, Boyle P, Franceschi S (2005) Human papillomavirus types in head and neck squamous cell carcinomas worldwide: a systematic review. Cancer Epidemiol Biomarkers Prev 14(2):467–75
45. Gillison ML, Koch WM, Capone RB, Spafford M, Westra WH, Wu L et al (2000) Evidence for a causal association between human papillomavirus and a subset of head and neck cancers. J Natl Cancer Inst 92(9):709–20
46. Ragin CC, Reshmi SC, Gollin SM (2004) Mapping and analysis of HPV16 integration sites in a head and neck cancer cell line. Int J Cancer 110(5):701–9
47. Begum S, Cao D, Gillison M, Zahurak M, Westra WH (2005) Tissue distribution of human papillomavirus 16 DNA integration in patients with tonsillar carcinoma. Clin Cancer Res 11(16):5694–9
48. van Houten V, Snijders PJ, van den Brekel MW, Kummer JA, Meijer CJ, van Leeuwen B et al (2001) Biological evidence that human papillomaviruses are etiologically involved in a subgroup of head and neck squamous cell carcinomas. Int J Cancer 93(2):232–5
49. Koskinen WJ, Chen RW, Leivo I, Makitie A, Back L, Kontio R et al (2003) Prevalence and physical status of human papillomavirus in squamous cell carcinomas of the head and neck. Int J Cancer 107(3):401–6
50. Kreimer AR, Clifford GM, Snijders PJ, Castellsague X, Meijer CJ, Pawlita M et al (2005) HPV16 semiquantitative viral load and serologic biomarkers in oral and oropharyngeal squamous cell carcinomas. Int J Cancer 115(2):329–32
51. Mellin H, Dahlgren L, Munck-Wikland E, Lindholm J, Rabbani H, Kalantari M et al (2002) Human papillomavirus type 16 is episomal and a high viral load may be correlated to better prognosis in tonsillar cancer. Int J Cancer 102(2):152–8

52. Klussmann JP, Weissenborn SJ, Wieland U, Dries V, Kolligs J, Jungehuelsing M et al (2001) Prevalence, distribution, and viral load of human papillomavirus 16 DNA in tonsillar carcinomas. Cancer 92(11):2875–84
53. Braakhuis BJ, Snijders PJ, Keune WJ, Meijer CJ, Ruijter-Schippers HJ, Leemans CR et al (2004) Genetic patterns in head and neck cancers that contain or lack transcriptionally active human papillomavirus. J Natl Cancer Inst 96(13):998–1006
54. Balz V, Scheckenbach K, Gotte K, Bockmuhl U, Petersen I, Bier H (2003) Is the p53 inactivation frequency in squamous cell carcinomas of the head and neck underestimated? Analysis of p53 exons 2–11 and human papillomavirus 16/18 E6 transcripts in 123 unselected tumor specimens. Cancer Res 63(6):1188–91
55. Zumbach K, Hoffmann M, Kahn T, Bosch F, Gottschlich S, Gorogh T et al (2000) Antibodies against oncoproteins E6 and E7 of human papillomavirus types 16 and 18 in patients with head-and-neck squamous-cell carcinoma. Int J Cancer 85(6):815–8
56. Hoffmann TK, Arsov C, Schirlau K, Bas M, Friebe-Hoffmann U, Klussmann JP et al (2006) T cells specific for HPV16 E7 epitopes in patients with squamous cell carcinoma of the oropharynx. Int J Cancer 118(8):1984–91
57. Albers A, Abe K, Hunt J, Wang J, Lopez-Albaitero A, Schaefer C et al (2005) Antitumor activity of human papillomavirus type 16 E7-specific T cells against virally infected squamous cell carcinoma of the head and neck. Cancer Res 65(23):11146–55
58. Dai M, Clifford GM, le Calvez F, Castellsague X, Snijders PJ, Pawlita M et al (2004) Human papillomavirus type 16 and TP53 mutation in oral cancer: matched analysis of the IARC multicenter study. Cancer Res 64(2):468–71
59. Licitra L, Perrone F, Bossi P, Suardi S, Mariani L, Artusi R et al (2006) High-risk human papillomavirus affects prognosis in patients with surgically treated oropharyngeal squamous cell carcinoma. J Clin Oncol 24(36):5630–6
60. Fakhry C, Gillison ML (2006) Clinical implications of human papillomavirus in head and neck cancers. J Clin Oncol 24(17):2606–11
61. Kumar B, Cordell KG, Lee JS, Worden FP, Prince ME, Tran HH et al (2008) EGFR, p16, HPV Titer, Bcl-xL and p53, sex, and smoking as indicators of response to therapy and survival in oropharyngeal cancer. J Clin Oncol 26(19):3128–37
62. Weinberger PM, Yu Z, Haffty BG, Kowalski D, Harigopal M, Brandsma J et al (2006) Molecular classification identifies a subset of human papillomavirus–associated oropharyngeal cancers with favorable prognosis. J Clin Oncol 24(5):736–47
63. Slebos RJ, Yi Y, Ely K, Carter J, Evjen A, Zhang X et al (2006) Gene expression differences associated with human papillomavirus status in head and neck squamous cell carcinoma. Clin Cancer Res 12(3 Pt 1):701–9
64. Schlecht NF, Burk RD, Adrien L, Dunne A, Kawachi N, Sarta C et al (2007) Gene expression profiles in HPV-infected head and neck cancer. J Pathol 213(3):283–93
65. Carter JJ, Galloway DA (1997) Humoral immune response to human papillomavirus infection. Clin Dermatol 15(2):249–59
66. Meschede W, Zumbach K, Braspenning J, Scheffner M (1998) itez-Bribiesca L, Luande J et al. Antibodies against early proteins of human papillomaviruses as diagnostic markers for invasive cervical cancer. J Clin Microbiol 36(2):475–80
67. Herrero R, Castellsague X, Pawlita M, Lissowska J, Kee F, Balaram P et al (2003) Human papillomavirus and oral cancer: the International Agency for Research on Cancer multicenter study. J Natl Cancer Inst 95(23):1772–83
68. Schwartz SM, Daling JR, Doody DR, Wipf GC, Carter JJ, Madeleine MM et al (1998) Oral cancer risk in relation to sexual history and evidence of human papillomavirus infection. J Natl Cancer Inst 90(21):1626–36
69. Smith EM, Ritchie JM, Summersgill KF, Hoffman HT, Wang DH, Haugen TH et al (2004) Human papillomavirus in oral exfoliated cells and risk of head and neck cancer. J Natl Cancer Inst 96(6):449–55
70. Gillison ML, D'Souza G, Westra W, Sugar E, Xiao W, Begum S et al (2008) Distinct risk factor profiles for human papillomavirus type 16-positive and human papillomavirus type 16-negative head and neck cancers. J Natl Cancer Inst 100(6):407–20

71. Furniss CS, McClean MD, Smith JF, Bryan J, Nelson HH, Peters ES et al (2007) Human papillomavirus 16 and head and neck squamous cell carcinoma. Int J Cancer 120(11):2386–92
72. Mork J, Lie AK, Glattre E, Hallmans G, Jellum E, Koskela P et al (2001) Human papillomavirus infection as a risk factor for squamous-cell carcinoma of the head and neck. N Engl J Med 344(15):1125–31
73. Dahlstrom KR, Adler-Storthz K, Etzel CJ, Liu Z, Dillon L, El Naggar AK et al (2003) Human papillomavirus type 16 infection and squamous cell carcinoma of the head and neck in never-smokers: a matched pair analysis. Clin Cancer Res 9(7):2620–6
74. Smith EM, Ritchie JM, Pawlita M, Rubenstein LM, Haugen TH, Turek LP et al (2007) Human papillomavirus seropositivity and risks of head and neck cancer. Int J Cancer 120(4):825–32
75. D'Souza G, Kreimer AR, Viscidi R, Pawlita M, Fakhry C, Koch WM et al (2007) Case-control study of human papillomavirus and oropharyngeal cancer. N Engl J Med 356(19):1944–56
76. Pintos J, Black MJ, Sadeghi N, Ghadirian P, Zeitouni AG, Viscidi RP et al (2008) Human papillomavirus infection and oral cancer: a case-control study in Montreal, Canada. Oral Oncol 44(3):242–50
77. Smith EM, Summersgill KF, Allen J, Hoffman HT, McCulloch T, Turek LP et al (2000) Human papillomavirus and risk of laryngeal cancer. Ann Otol Rhinol Laryngol 109(11):1069–76
78. Strome SE, Savva A, Brissett AE, Gostout BS, Lewis J, Clayton AC et al (2002) Squamous cell carcinoma of the tonsils: a molecular analysis of HPV associations. Clin Cancer Res 8(4):1093–100
79. Hansson BG, Rosenquist K, Antonsson A, Wennerberg J, Schildt EB, Bladstrom A et al (2005) Strong association between infection with human papillomavirus and oral and oropharyngeal squamous cell carcinoma: a population-based case-control study in southern Sweden. Acta Otolaryngol 125(12):1337–44
80. Trottier H, Franco EL (2006) The epidemiology of genital human papillomavirus infection. Vaccine 24(Suppl 1):S1–15
81. Maden C, Beckmann AM, Thomas DB, McKnight B, Sherman KJ, Ashley RL et al (1992) Human papillomaviruses, herpes simplex viruses, and the risk of oral cancer in men. Am J Epidemiol 135(10):1093–102
82. Koch WM, Lango M, Sewell D, Zahurak M, Sidransky D (1999) Head and neck cancer in nonsmokers: a distinct clinical and molecular entity. Laryngoscope 109(10):1544–51
83. Ringstrom E, Peters E, Hasegawa M, Posner M, Liu M, Kelsey KT (2002) Human papillomavirus type 16 and squamous cell carcinoma of the head and neck. Clin Cancer Res 8(10):3187–92
84. Lindel K, Beer KT, Laissue J, Greiner RH, Aebersold DM (2001) Human papillomavirus positive squamous cell carcinoma of the oropharynx: a radiosensitive subgroup of head and neck carcinoma. Cancer 92(4):805–13
85. Haraf DJ, Nodzenski E, Brachman D, Mick R, Montag A, Graves D et al (1996) Human papilloma virus and p53 in head and neck cancer: clinical correlates and survival. Clin Cancer Res 2(4):755–62
86. Applebaum KM, Furniss CS, Zeka A, Posner MR, Smith JF, Bryan J et al (2007) Lack of association of alcohol and tobacco with HPV16-associated head and neck cancer. J Natl Cancer Inst 99(23):1801–10
87. Wiley DJ, Wiesmeier E, Masongsong E, Gylys KH, Koutsky LA, Ferris DG et al (2006) Smokers at higher risk for undetected antibody for oncogenic human papillomavirus type 16 infection. Cancer Epidemiol Biomarkers Prev 15(5):915–20
88. Meyer MS, Applebaum KM, Furniss CS, Peters ES, Luckett BG, Smith JF et al (2008) Human papillomavirus-16 modifies the association between fruit consumption and head and neck squamous cell carcinoma. Cancer Epidemiol Biomarkers Prev 17(12):3419–26
89. AB Hill (1965) The environment and disease: association or causation? Proc R Soc Med 58:295–300
90. Rampias T, Sasaki C, DiMaio D, Psyrri A (2007) Retrovirus-mediated delivery of short hairpin RNA targeting human papillomavirus (HPV) 16 E6 and E7 oncogenes and induction of apoptosis in oropharyngeal squamous cell cancer (OSCC) cell line. J Clin Oncol (Meeting Abstracts) 25(18 Suppl):6002

91. Smith EM, Ritchie JM, Yankowitz J, Swarnavel S, Wang D, Haugen TH et al (2004) Human papillomavirus prevalence and types in newborns and parents: concordance and modes of transmission. Sex Transm Dis 31(1):57–62
92. D'Souza G, Fakhry C, Sugar EA, Seaberg EC, Weber K, Minkoff HL et al (2007) Six-month natural history of oral versus cervical human papillomavirus infection. Int J Cancer 121:143–150
93. Kreimer AR, Alberg AJ, Daniel R, Gravitt PE, Viscidi R, Garrett ES et al (2004) Oral human papillomavirus infection in adults is associated with sexual behavior and HIV serostatus. J Infect Dis 189(4):686–98
94. Rintala MA, Grenman SE, Puranen MH, Isolauri E, Ekblad U, Kero PO et al (2005) Transmission of high-risk human papillomavirus (HPV) between parents and infant: a prospective study of HPV in families in Finland. J Clin Microbiol 43(1):376–81
95. Cameron JE, Mercante D, O'Brien M, Gaffga AM, Leigh JE, Fidel PL Jr et al (2005) The impact of highly active antiretroviral therapy and immunodeficiency on human papillomavirus infection of the oral cavity of human immunodeficiency virus-seropositive adults. Sex Transm Dis 32(11):703–9
96. Fakhry C, D'Souza G, Sugar E, Weber K, Goshu E, Minkoff H et al (2006) Relationship between prevalent oral and cervical human papillomavirus infections in human immunodeficiency virus-positive and -negative women. J Clin Microbiol 44(12):4479–85
97. Winer RL, Kiviat NB, Hughes JP, Adam DE, Lee SK, Kuypers JM et al (2005) Development and duration of human papillomavirus lesions, after initial infection. J Infect Dis 191(5):731–8
98. Chin-Hong PV, Vittinghoff E, Cranston RD, Buchbinder S, Cohen D, Colfax G et al (2004) Age-Specific prevalence of anal human papillomavirus infection in HIV-negative sexually active men who have sex with men: the EXPLORE study. J Infect Dis 190(12):2070–6
99. Giuliano AR, Lu B, Nielson CM, Flores R, Papenfuss MR, Lee JH et al (2008) Age-specific prevalence, incidence, and duration of human papillomavirus infections in a cohort of 290 US men. J Infect Dis 198(6):827–35
100. Chin-Hong PV, Vittinghoff E, Cranston RD, Browne L, Buchbinder S, Colfax G et al (2005) Age-related prevalence of anal cancer precursors in homosexual men: the EXPLORE study. J Natl Cancer Inst 97(12):896–905
101. Rintala M, Grenman S, Puranen M, Syrjanen S (2006) Natural history of oral papillomavirus infections in spouses: a prospective Finnish HPV Family Study. J Clin Virol 35(1):89–94
102. Schlecht NF, Burk RD, Palefsky JM, Minkoff H, Xue X, Massad LS et al (2005) Variants of human papillomaviruses 16 and 18 and their natural history in human immunodeficiency virus-positive women. J Gen Virol 86(Pt 10):2709–20
103. Worden FP, Kumar B, Lee JS, Wolf GT, Cordell KG, Taylor JM et al (2008) Chemoselection as a strategy for organ preservation in advanced oropharynx cancer: response and survival positively associated with HPV16 copy number. J Clin Oncol 26(19):3138–46
104. Fakhry C, Westra WH, Li S, Cmelak A, Ridge JA, Pinto H et al (2008) Improved survival of patients with human papillomavirus-positive head and neck squamous cell carcinoma in a prospective clinical trial. J Natl Cancer Inst 100(4):261–9
105. Dahlgren L, Dahlstrand HM, Lindquist D, Hogmo A, Bjornestal L, Lindholm J et al (2004) Human papillomavirus is more common in base of tongue than in mobile tongue cancer and is a favorable prognostic factor in base of tongue cancer patients. Int J Cancer 112(6):1015–9
106. Reimers N, Kasper HU, Weissenborn SJ, Stutzer H, Preuss SF, Hoffmann TK et al (2007) Combined analysis of HPV-DNA, p16 and EGFR expression to predict prognosis in oropharyngeal cancer. Int J Cancer 120(8):1731–8
107. Hafkamp HC, Manni JJ, Haesevoets A, Voogd AC, Schepers M, Bot FJ et al (2008) Marked differences in survival rate between smokers and nonsmokers with HPV 16-associated tonsillar carcinomas. Int J Cancer 122(12):2656–64
108. Poeta ML, Manola J, Goldwasser MA, Forastiere A, Benoit N, Califano JA et al (2007) TP53 mutations and survival in squamous-cell carcinoma of the head and neck. N Engl J Med 357(25):2552–61

109. Smith EM, Wang D, Rubenstein LM, Morris WA, Turek LP, Haugen TH (2008) Association between p53 and human papillomavirus in head and neck cancer survival. Cancer Epidemiol Biomarkers Prev 17(2):421–7
110. Chaturvedi AK, Engels EA, Anderson WF, Gillison ML (2008) Incidence trends for human papillomavirus-related and -unrelated oral squamous cell carcinomas in the United States. J Clin Oncol 26(4):612–9
111. Carvalho AL, Nishimoto IN, Califano JA, Kowalski LP (2005) Trends in incidence and prognosis for head and neck cancer in the United States: a site-specific analysis of the SEER database. Int J Cancer 114(5):806–16
112. Sturgis EM, Cinciripini PM (2007) Trends in head and neck cancer incidence in relation to smoking prevalence: an emerging epidemic of human papillomavirus-associated cancers? Cancer 110(7):1429–35
113. Frisch M, Hjalgrim H, Jaeger AB, Biggar RJ (2000) Changing patterns of tonsillar squamous cell carcinoma in the United States. Cancer Causes Control 11(6):489–95
114. Shiboski CH, Shiboski SC, Silverman S Jr (2000) Trends in oral cancer rates in the United States, 1973–1996. Community Dent Oral Epidemiol 28(4):249–56
115. Shiboski CH, Schmidt BL, Jordan RC (2005) Tongue and tonsil carcinoma: increasing trends in the U.S. population ages 20–44 years. Cancer 103(9):1843–9
116. Hammarstedt L, Lindquist D, Dahlstrand H, Romanitan M, Dahlgren LO, Joneberg J et al (2006) Human papillomavirus as a risk factor for the increase in incidence of tonsillar cancer. Int J Cancer 119(11):2620–3
117. Frisch M, Biggar RJ, Goedert JJ (2000) Human papillomavirus-associated cancers in patients with human immunodeficiency virus infection and acquired immunodeficiency syndrome. J Natl Cancer Inst 92(18):1500–10
118. Chaturvedi AK, Engels EA, Gilbert ES, Chen BE, Storm H, Lynch CF et al (2007) Second cancers among 104, 760 survivors of cervical cancer: evaluation of long-term risk. J Natl Cancer Inst 99(21):1634–43
119. Hemminki K, Dong C, Frisch M (2000) Tonsillar and other upper aerodigestive tract cancers among cervical cancer patients and their husbands. Eur J Cancer Prev 9(6):433–7
120. Paavonen J, Jenkins D, Bosch FX, Naud P, Salmeron J, Wheeler CM et al (2007) Efficacy of a prophylactic adjuvanted bivalent L1 virus-like-particle vaccine against infection with human papillomavirus types 16 and 18 in young women: an interim analysis of a phase III double-blind, randomised controlled trial. Lancet 369(9580): 2161–70
121. Garland SM, Hernandez-Avila M, Wheeler CM, Perez G, Harper DM, Leodolter S et al (2007) Quadrivalent vaccine against human papillomavirus to prevent anogenital diseases. N Engl J Med 356(19):1928–43
122. FUTURE II Study Group (2007) Quadrivalent vaccine against human papillomavirus to prevent high-grade cervical lesions. N Engl J Med 356(19):1915–27.
123. Schiller JT, Lowy DR (2006) Prospects for cervical cancer prevention by human papillomavirus vaccination. Cancer Res 66(21):10229–32
124. Hildesheim A, Herrero R, Wacholder S, Rodriguez AC, Solomon D, Bratti MC et al (2007) Effect of human papillomavirus 16/18 L1 viruslike particle vaccine among young women with preexisting infection: a randomized trial. JAMA 298(7):743–53
125. Petaja T, Keranen H, Karppa T, Kawa A, Lantela S, Siitari-Mattila M et al (2009) Immunogenicity and safety of human papillomavirus (HPV)-16/18 AS04-adjuvanted vaccine in healthy boys aged 10–18 years. J Adolesc Health 44(1):33–40
126. Gillison ML (2008) Human papillomavirus-related diseases: oropharynx cancers and potential implications for adolescent HPV vaccination GILLISON2008A. J Adolesc Health 43 (4 Suppl):S52–S60
127. Suzich JA, Ghim SJ, Palmer-Hill FJ, White WI, Tamura JK, Bell JA et al (1995) Systemic immunization with papillomavirus L1 protein completely prevents the development of viral mucosal papillomas. Proc Natl Acad Sci U S A 92(25):11553–7

128. Cameron JE, Snowhite IV, Chaturvedi AK, Hagensee ME (2003) Human papillomavirus-specific antibody status in oral fluids modestly reflects serum status in human immunodeficiency virus-positive individuals. Clin Diagn Lab Immunol 10(3):431–8
129. Buchinsky FJ, Carter JJ, Wipf GC, Hughes JP, Koutsky LA, Galloway DA (2006) Comparison of oral fluid and serum ELISAs in the determination of IgG response to natural human papillomavirus infection in university women. J Clin Virol 35(4):450–3
130. Kemp TJ, Garcia-Pineres A, Falk RT, Poncelet S, Dessy F, Giannini SL et al (2008) Evaluation of systemic and mucosal anti-HPV16 and anti-HPV18 antibody responses from vaccinated women. Vaccine 26(29–30):3608–16
131. Markowitz LE, Dunne EF, Saraiya M, Lawson HW, Chesson H, Unger ER (2007) Quadrivalent human papillomavirus vaccine: recommendations of the Advisory Committee on Immunization Practices (ACIP). MMWR Recomm Rep 56(RR-2):1–24
132. Giuliano AR, Salmon D (2008) The case for a gender-neutral (universal) human papillomavirus vaccination policy in the United States: Point. Cancer Epidemiol Biomarkers Prev 17(4):805–8
133. Canadas MP, Bosch FX, Junquera ML, Ejarque M, Font R, Ordonez E et al (2004) Concordance of prevalence of human papillomavirus DNA in anogenital and oral infections in a high-risk population. J Clin Microbiol 42(3):1330–2
134. do Sacramento PR, Babeto E, Colombo J, Cabral Ruback MJ, Bonilha JL, Fernandes AM et al (2006) The prevalence of human papillomavirus in the oropharynx in healthy individuals in a Brazilian population. J Med Virol 78(5):614–8
135. Marais DJ, Passmore JA, Denny L, Sampson C, Allan BR, Williamson AL (2008) Cervical and oral human papillomavirus types in HIV-1 positive and negative women with cervical disease in South Africa. J Med Virol 80(6):953–9

Dietary Factors

Ersilia Lucenteforte, Werner Garavello, Cristina Bosetti, and Carlo La Vecchia

Cancer of the Oral Cavity and Pharynx

Introduction

Besides tobacco and alcohol – the two major recognized risk factors for oral and pharyngeal cancer in most populations – diet and nutrition have been suggested to play an important role in the etiology of these neoplasms [1–4]. The epidemiological evidence on diet and oral and pharyngeal cancer comes mainly from case–control studies, and the few prospective studies that generally analyzed cancers of the head and neck combined. The main results of epidemiological studies on diet and the risk of cancers of the oral cavity are summarized below.

Food Groups

Several studies have analyzed the risk of oral and pharyngeal cancer in relation to consumption of various food groups, including vegetables and fruits; meat, fish, and eggs; cereals; milk and dairy products; coffee and other hot drinks.

E. Lucenteforte (✉), W. Garavello, C. Bosetti, and C.La. Vecchia
Istituto di Ricerche Farmacologiche "Mario Negri", via Giuseppe La Masa 19, 20156 Milan, Italy
e-mail: lucenteforte@marionegri.it

W. Garavello
Clinica Otorinolaringoiatrica, DNTB, Università Milano-Bicocca, via Donizetti 106, 20052 Monza, Italy

C.La. Vecchia
Istituto di Statistica Medica e Biometria, "G.A. Maccacaro", Università degli Studi di Milano, via Venezian 1, 20133 Milan, Italy

A.F. Olshan (ed.), *Epidemiology, Pathogenesis, and Prevention of Head and Neck Cancer,* DOI 10.1007/978-1-4419-1472-9_6, © Springer Science+Business Media, LLC 2010

Vegetables and Fruits

Vegetables and fruits are the food groups most consistently related to oral and pharyngeal cancer. At least three cohort studies [5–7] and about 30 case–control studies [8–44] investigated the role of vegetables and fruits on the risk of cancer of the oral cavity and pharynx. Three other cohort studies evaluated the association for all cancers of the upper aerodigestive tract combined [45–47].

A cohort study of 265,118 Japanese adults found a decreased risk of cancer of the oral cavity and pharynx in relation to high consumption of green and yellow vegetables [5]. The Iowa Women's Health Study (IWHS) on 34,651 postmenopausal women from the USA, including 53 women who developed oral and pharyngeal cancer, reported a relative risk (RR) of 0.69 for the highest level of yellow/orange vegetable consumption [6]. Another US prospective study on 490,802 participants of the National Institutes of Health-American Association of Retired Persons (NIH-AARP) Diet and Health cohort, including 319 cancers of the oral cavity and 142 cancers of the oro-hypopharynx, reported a significant inverse association between total fruit and vegetable consumption and the risk of cancer of the oral cavity (RR=0.61); however, no association was found for oro-hypopharynx (RR=0.90) [7]. Moreover, when vegetables and fruits were analyzed separately, a stronger inverse association was found for vegetables than for fruits, both for cancer of the oral cavity (RR=0.56 and RR=0.84, respectively) and oro-hypopharynx (RR=0.56 and RR=1.19, respectively).

About 30 studies reported inverse associations with oral and pharyngeal cancer risk for at least one category of vegetables and/or fruits [8–16, 18–24, 26–29, 31, 33–39, 41–43]. Most studies that examined the relation with total vegetables reported a protective association (Fig. 1) [9, 10, 13, 14, 16, 19, 20, 22, 25, 28, 35–37, 41–44]. Similarly, most case–control studies that investigated the association with total fruit reported an inverse relation [8, 10, 11, 13–17, 19, 20, 22, 23, 25, 28, 29, 32, 34–38, 41–44] (Fig. 2). After allowance for the two major risk factors for oral and pharyngeal cancer (tobacco and alcohol), the protective association for fruit and vegetable consumption remained significant.

The beneficial effect of fruits and vegetables on oral and pharyngeal cancer risk is more consistent for raw and green/leafy vegetables [8, 11–15, 17, 18, 21, 23, 24, 26, 29, 33, 34, 36–38, 41, 43, 44], tomatoes [14, 21, 28, 33, 35–37, 43, 44, 48], carrots [12, 14, 15, 17, 21, 29, 33, 36, 37, 43], and citrus fruit [11–14, 18, 21, 24, 26, 28, 29, 31, 33, 35–38, 40, 41, 44]. The evidence is more limited and less convincing for other specific vegetables or fruits (such as cruciferous vegetables or apples/pears).

Among cohort studies which analyzed the risk of upper aerodigestive tract cancers combined (Fig. 3), a cohort study of 7,995 Hawaiian–Japanese men including 92 incident cases reported that a frequent consumption of fruit was inversely associated to the risk (RR=0.65) [45]. In a prospective study of 10,960 Norwegian men including 71 cases, a significant inverse trend in risk was found for oranges (RR=0.5 for the highest level of consumption) [46]. Increasing consumption of apples, bananas, and preserved fruit gave nonsignificant decreased RRs. However, the sum-score of fruits showed no significant relation. Moreover, none of the

Study	Cases	RR	95% CI
Winn et al. 1984	227	0.70	0.47-1.04
Notani and Jayant 1987	278	0.42	0.25-0.71
Franco et al. 1989	232	0.70	0.37-1.31
La Vecchia et al. 1991	105	0.40	0.20-0.80
De Stefani et al. 1994	246	0.40	0.19-0.85
Levi et al. 1998	156	0.30	0.16-0.57
Franceschi et al. 1999	512	0.40	0.28-0.57
Garrote et al. 2001	200	0.78	0.40-1.52
Tavani et al. 2001	132	0.37	0.16-0.87
Marchioni et al. 2002	260	0.86	0.54-1.38
Lissowska et al. 2003	122	0.17	0.07-0.43
Rajkumar et al. 2003	591	0.44	0.28-0.69
Sanchez et al. 2003	375	0.54	0.34-0.86
De Stefani et al. 2005	230	0.60	0.33-1.10
Suzuki et al. 2006	193	0.57	0.36-0.91
Sapkota et al. 2008	378	0.80	0.54-1.19

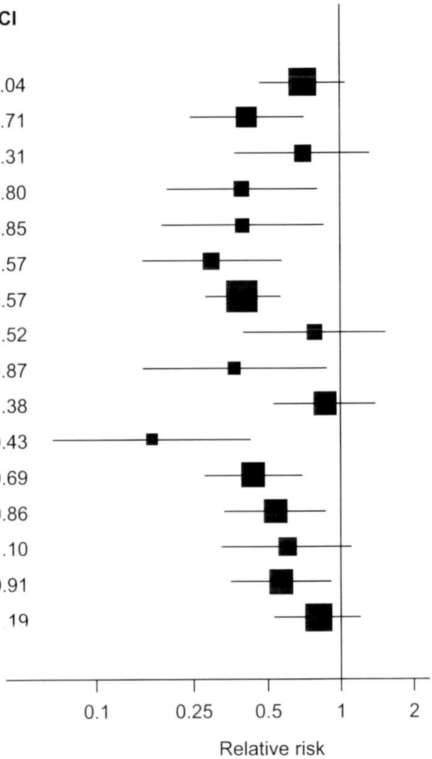

Fig. 1 Relative risks (RR) of oral and pharyngeal cancer and corresponding 95% confidence intervals (CI) for the highest level of vegetable consumption from selected case–control studies

vegetables analyzed showed any consistent relation with risk. The European Prospective Investigation into Cancer and Nutrition (EPIC) conducted in ten European countries on 345,904 subjects, including 352 cases, reported a significant inverse association with total vegetables and fruits combined (RR=0.60) and with total fruits (RR=0.60). No significant inverse association was, however, found for total vegetables (RR=0.80) [47].

Thus, epidemiological studies conducted in several countries provide consistent evidence for the fact that a diet characterized by high vegetable and fruit consumption has a beneficial effect on oral and pharyngeal cancer, with a reduction of risk of about 50-70%.

Meat, Fish, and Eggs

At least two cohort [45, 46] and 30 case–control studies [8, 9, 11–18, 21–26, 28, 30, 32–37, 40, 41, 43, 44, 49] analyzed the relation between meat and the risk of cancer of the oral cavity and pharynx.

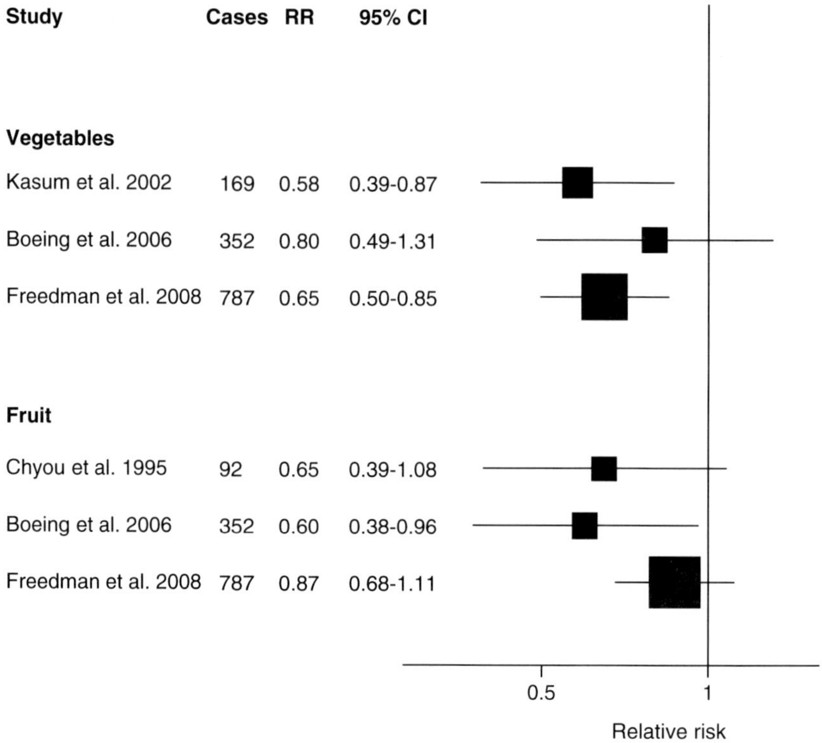

Fig. 2 Relative risks (RR) of oral and pharyngeal cancer and corresponding 95% confidence intervals (CI) for the highest level of fruit consumption from selected case–control studies

A cohort study on Hawaiian-Japanese found a non-significant inverse association with total meat, with a RR of 0.77 [45], while a Norwegian cohort study reported an increased risk of upper aerodigestive tract cancers for a high consumption of various types of meat, including beef (RR = 2.8), mutton (RR = 2.1), processed meat (RR = 1.6), pork (RR = 1.5), and bacon (RR = 2.2). However, a sum-score of meat consumption showed no significant relation [46].

An increased risk in relation to high meat consumption was also observed in various case–control studies [8, 11–14, 16, 18, 22, 24, 26, 28, 32–34, 36, 40, 41, 43], although inverse or no association between meat or meat products was reported in other studies [9, 15, 17, 21, 23, 25, 30, 35, 37, 44, 49].

A cohort study on Hawaiian-Japanese, found a non-significant positive association between consumption of fish upper aerodigestive tract cancers (RR = 1.37) [45]. In a cohort study from Norway, a non significant RR of 0.8 for the highest consumption of fresh/frozen fish was observed, while a sum-score of fish consumption did not significantly influence upper aerodigestive cancer risk [46]. Conversely, several case–control studies reported a decreased risk of cancers of

Study	Cases	RR	95% CI
Winn et al. 1984	227	0.60	0.42-0.85
Notani and Jayant 1987	278	1.12	0.67-1.88
La Vecchia et al. 1991	105	0.14	0.07-0.28
De Stefani et al. 1994	246	0.60	0.28-1.30
Levi et al. 1998	156	0.22	0.11-0.44
Franceschi et al. 1999	512	0.70	0.47-1.04
Garrote et al. 2001	200	0.43	0.21-0.89
Tavani et al. 2001	132	0.34	0.13-0.88
Marchioni et al. 2002	260	0.87	0.55-1.37
Lissowska et al. 2003	122	0.40	0.17-0.95
Rajkumar et al. 2003	591	0.55	0.38-0.80
Sanchez et al. 2003	375	0.52	0.34-0.79
De Stefani et al. 2005	230	0.70	0.39-1.26
Suzuki ot al. 2006	103	0.38	0.22-0.65
Sapkota et al. 2008	378	0.74	0.45-1.21

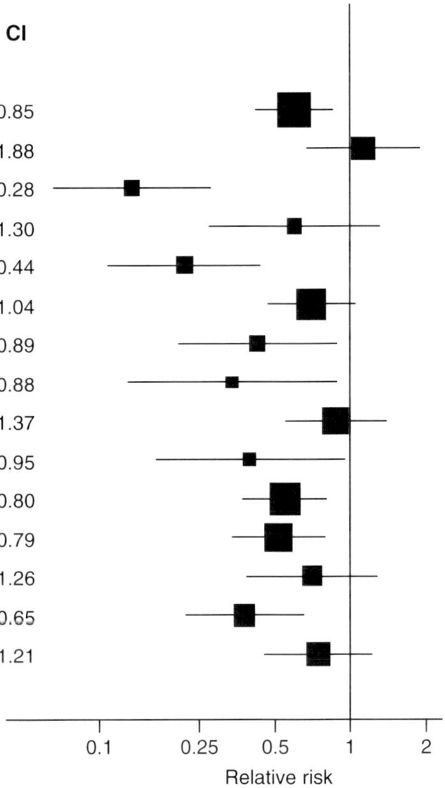

Fig. 3 Relative risks (RR) of upper aerodigestive tract cancers and corresponding 95% confidence intervals (CI) for the highest level of vegetable and fruit consumption from selected cohort studies

the oral cavity and pharynx for high consumption of fish [9, 11, 13, 15, 21, 24, 26, 29, 34–36, 44]. However, a few other case–control studies found a direct association [8, 18, 28, 43] or no association [14, 17, 23, 32, 37, 49] with oral and pharyngeal cancer risk.

The relation between eggs and oral and pharyngeal cancer risk was evaluated in various studies, which provided, however, conflicting results. A direct association was found in a cohort study on Japanese-Americans (RR = 1.33) [45], but no association (RR = 1.1) was observed in a cohort study from Norway [46]. Moreover, at least 10 case–control studies reported a direct association [9, 14, 15, 23–26, 28, 40, 41], while, a few other studies, reported an inverse [21, 35, 36], or no association [8, 17, 37].

The results on the association between protein-rich foods and oral and pharyngeal cancer risk are not consistent, although they suggest a detrimental effect of a diet rich in meat and eggs, and a more favorable one of a diet rich in fish.

Cereals

The role of cereals on the risk of cancer of the oral cavity and pharynx was investigated in at least three cohort [6, 45, 46] and 25 case–control studies [8, 9, 11, 13–15, 17, 20, 21, 24–26, 28, 30, 32, 34–37, 40, 41, 49–51].

In the IWHS cohort of postmenopausal women from the USA, a significant inverse association with oral and pharyngeal cancer was observed for the highest level of consumption of whole (RR = 0.47) and refined grains (RR = 0.70) [6]. In a Japanese–American cohort study, consumption of rice was positively associated with the risk of the upper aerodigestive tract cancers (RR = 1.43), while consumption of bread was inversely associated (RR = 0.80), although the dose-response relation was not statistically significant [45]. In a Norwegian prospective study, consumption of bread was significantly associated with a reduced risk of upper aerodigestive tract cancers (RR = 0.2 for the highest level of consumption) [46].

Various case–control studies reported an increased risk of oral and pharyngeal cancer with high consumption of cereals and cereal products [13, 14, 24, 25, 28, 40, 41, 50, 51]. Other studies, however, reported an inverse [8, 9, 20, 26, 30, 32, 34], or no association [11, 21, 35–37]. This may well reflect different consumption of cereal foods or different correlates of diets rich in cereals in various populations. An inverse association with whole-grains bread and wheat bread and pasta was found in various case–control studies [8, 14, 15, 17, 52].

The epidemiological evidence on cereal consumption and the risk of cancer of the oral cavity and pharynx is not completely consistent, but it suggests that cereals (mainly refined) may increase the risk of this neoplasm, while whole grain cereals may reduce it.

Milk and Dairy Products

At least one cohort study [45] and 25 case–control studies [8, 9, 11, 13–15, 17, 20–24, 26, 28, 30, 32, 34–37, 40, 41, 43] investigated the association between consumption of milk and dairy products and the risk of oral and pharyngeal cancer.

Results on milk have been mixed, with one cohort [45] and eight case–control studies [15, 20, 21, 24, 28, 35, 37, 40] reporting inverse associations with oral and pharyngeal cancer risk, other studies reporting no meaningful association [9, 14, 17, 22, 26, 36, 43], and others reporting a direct association [23, 44].

A direct relation between cheese consumption and the risk of oral and pharyngeal cancer was observed in a few studies [14, 24, 26, 28, 40, 44], although others observed a inverse one [15, 35–37, 43], or no association [17].

The relation between yoghurt consumption was considered in a few studies [28, 35–37, 43, 44], three of which reported a significant protective association [35, 37, 44], the remaining ones reported a direct non-significant association [28, 36], and another reported no association [43]. One study which evaluated buttermilk showed a protective association [9].

Finally, a few studies observed a direct association between dairy products in general and oral cavity and pharyngeal cancer risk [11, 13, 44], while a few others found an inverse one [25, 32, 34, 43] or no association [8, 30, 41].

The evidence regarding a diet high in milk and dairy products and the risk of oral cavity and pharynx is thus inconsistent, although it is possible now to exclude any strong association.

Tea, Coffee and Other Hot Drinks

In a cohort study on Hawaiian–Japanese people, coffee was directly associated to upper aerodigestive tract cancers, black tea was inversely related, and green tea was not associated to the risk [45]. A prospective study on Norwegian men reported inconsistent inverse associations between coffee consumption and oral and pharyngeal cancer risk [53]. A few case–control studies suggested a protective effect of tea [17, 23, 26, 40], as well as coffee [15, 17, 26] consumption on oral carcinogenesis, while other case–control studies found positive [12, 14, 21, 23, 54] or no associations [44].

Maté – a popular herbal infusion traditionally consumed in Argentina and some areas of Brazil – was positively related to the risk of oral and pharyngeal cancer [10, 12, 16, 25, 31, 40, 54]. This association was attributed to the fact that maté is generally consumed very hot through a metal straw, and can thus produce heat damage in the oral cavity.

Epidemiological studies on coffee and tea do not show any consistent association with the risk of cancer of the oral cavity and pharynx. There is some evidence of an excess risk for maté drinkers.

Nutrients and Other Food Components

Various studies investigated the role of vitamins and minerals on the risk of cancer of the oral cavity and pharynx. A limited number of studies investigated the role of other food components such as flavonoids, as well as of macronutrients (including mainly fats) and fibers.

Micronutrients

Various micronutrients and vitamins have been suggested to be responsible for the protective role of fruits and vegetables on oral/pharyngeal cancer.

The IWHS on 34,691 women and including 33 postmenopausal women with cancers of the mouth, pharynx, and esophagus found inverse associations for consumption of carotene (RR = 0.7) and vitamin C (RR = 0.7), but found no associations for vitamin E and retinol [55]. A cohort study on Japanese-American men found an inverse non-significant association with cancers of the upper aerodigestive tract, and consumption of calcium (RR = 0.67), and a positive one for sodium (RR = 1.26) [45].

At least eight case–control studies reported an inverse association between carotene (mainly β-carotene) intake and the risk of oral and pharyngeal cancer [11, 13, 19–21, 31, 42, 56], although another case–control study found a direct non significant association [18], and others found no consistent associations [32, 57, 58].

Inverse associations were also reported for intake of vitamin C [11, 13, 19–21, 32, 42, 56–60] and vitamin E [42, 56, 60, 61].

Case–control studies regarding other nutrients, such as vitamin A [21, 59, 60], folate [11, 62], iron [21, 32, 49, 56, 60], and calcium [21, 32, 49, 56] suggested a beneficial effect on oral and pharyngeal cancer of these nutrients, too.

No consistent relation has been reported for riboflavin [11, 21, 25, 32, 56, 63], retinol [11, 13, 20, 32, 56, 57, 59, 63], and thiamine [11, 21, 25, 32, 56, 60, 61, 63].

High dietary intake of carotene (mainly β-carotene), vitamin C and E have been suggested to decrease the risk of cancer of the oral cavity and pharynx, and the results regarding folate are suggestive of a possible beneficial effect. However, the evidence on the protective effect of carotenoids and other antioxidant vitamins comes mainly from dietary sources, not supplements, and it is difficult to disentangle the effect of these nutrients from that of fruits and vegetables, as well as other components found in plant foods.

Flavonoids

Flavonoids – a class of polyphenols found mainly in foods of vegetable origin, with antioxidant, antimutagenic, and antiproliferative properties – have also been suggested to be responsible for the beneficial effect of fruits and vegetables on oral and pharyngeal cancer. Two case–control studies conducted in Uruguay [58] and in Italy [64], reported RRs of 0.8 and 0.56, respectively for the highest level of intake of total flavonoids. In particular, the Italian study found a significant inverse association for flavanones (RR = 0.51) and flavonols (RR = 0.62) (Table 1), while for other classes of flavonoids (including isoflavones, anthocyanidins, flavan-3-ols, and flavones) the estimates were below unity, but not significant [64].

Fats

A reduced risk of oral cancer for a high intake of total fat was reported in a case–control study from China (RR = 0.56) [21], and in a cohort study on Hawaiian–Japanese (RR = 0.61) [45]. A positive association was reported in two other case–control studies from the United States [11, 63], and no association was found in two case–control studies, one conducted in Uruguay (RR = 1.0) [58] and the other conducted in Greece [32].

Table 1 Multivariate relative risk (RR) and 95% confidence intervals (CI) of oral and pharyngeal cancer and laryngeal cancer according to intake of selected flavonoids. Italy, 1991–2007 [64, 84]

	Quintile of intake, RR (95% CI)[a]				
Cancer, flavonoids	2	3	4	5	χ^2_{trend} (*p*-value)
Oral and pharyngeal					
Flavanones	0.90 (0.68–1.18)	0.70 (0.52–0.94)	0.61 (0.45–0.83)	0.51 (0.37–0.71)	22.03 (<0.001)
Flavonols	0.92 (0.66–1.28)	0.80 (0.57–1.12)	0.65 (0.46–0.92)	0.62 (0.43–0.89)	9.33 (0.002)
Total flavonoids	0.77 (0.56–1.06)	0.64 (0.46–0.89)	0.63 (0.45–0.87)	0.56 (0.40–0.78)	11.92 (0.001)
Laryngeal					
Flavan-3-ols	0.63 (0.40–1.01)	0.57 (0.35–0.91)	0.49 (0.31–0.77)	0.64 (0.41–0.99)	3.26 (0.071)
Flavanones	0.55 (0.38–0.81)	0.54 (0.37–0.80)	0.39 (0.26–0.59)	0.60 (0.41–0.89)	10.53 (0.001)
Flavonols	0.53 (0.34–0.82)	0.49 (0.31–0.75)	0.30 (0.19–0.48)	0.32 (0.20–0.52)	24.61 (<0.001)
Total flavonoids	0.62 (0.39–0.99)	0.56 (0.36–0.88)	0.57 (0.36–0.89)	0.60 (0.38–0.94)	3.55 (0.060)

[a]Reference category first quintile of intake

Table 2 Multivariate relative risks (RR) and corresponding 95% confidence intervals (CI) of oral and pharyngeal, and laryngeal cancer according to intake quintile of olive oil and other added fats [26, 74]

	Quintile of intake, RR (95% CI)[a]				
	2	3	4	5	χ^2_{trend}
Oral and pharyngeal cancer					
Olive oil	0.6 (0.4–0.9)	0.7 (0.5–1.1)	0.7 (0.5–1.1)	0.4 (0.3–0.7)	7.15[a]
Mixed seed oils	0.7 (0.5–1.1)	1.0 (0.7–1.4)	0.9 (0.6–1.3)	1.1 (0.7–1.7)	0.12
Butter	1.2 (0.8–1.8)	1.3 (0.8–1.9)	1.8 (1.2–2.7)	2.3 (1.6–3.5)	22.32[a]
Laryngeal cancer					
Olive oil	0.6 (0.4–0.9)	0.8 (0.5–1.2)	0.6 (0.4–1.0)	0.4 (0.3–0.7)	8.62[b]
Mixed seed oils	1.29 (0.8–2.1)	1.8 (1.1–2.9)	2.6 (1.6–4.1)	2.2 (1.3–3.5)	16.16[c]
Butter	1.4 (0.9–2.2)	1.0 (0.6–1.5)	1.4 (0.9–2.1)	0.9 (0.6–1.4)	0.33

Reference category first quintile of intake
[a] $p<0.01$
[b] $p<0.005$
[c] $p<0.0005$

Specific fatty acids were examined in three control–case studies. The study from the United States showed a direct association with saturated fatty acids (RR = 1.6/1.5 for men/women) [11]. In an Italian case–control study, the RR of oral and pharyngeal cancer was 1.4 for high intake of saturated fatty acids, and 0.8 for high intake of monounsaturated fatty acids deriving mainly from olive oil [65]. No association was found with polyunsaturated fatty acids in the same study. In contrast, in a case–control study conducted in Uruguay, an inverse association was observed for saturated fat and a direct one for polyunsaturated fat, while monounsaturated fat was not related to the risk of oral and pharyngeal cancer [58].

With respect to seasoning fats, two Italian case–control studies [14, 26] found a significant association with butter intake, but another one showed no association [15], while a case–control study from Brazil [40] observed an inverse nonsignificant association. Conversely, one study observed a significantly lower risk for high intake of olive oil and no association for mixed seed oils and margarine [26] (Table 2).

The evidence of a role of fat in the etiology of oral and pharyngeal cancer is thus inconclusive.

Fibers

A few studies from the USA [13, 63], China [21], Australia [20], Italy [66] and one study conducted in the USA, Italy and China [67] indicated that a diet high in fiber had a reduced risk of oral and pharyngeal cancer. Another US study reported a significant inverse association in men only [11].

With reference to the source of fiber, in a Chinese study, dietary fiber derived from vegetables and fruits was associated with a reduced risk of oral cancer, while fiber derived from other sources did not show any protective effect [21]. Fiber from vegetables, fruits, or grains have been shown to have a protective role on oral and pharyngeal cancer among an Italian population [66]. Legumes, which are a rich source of dietary fiber, have also been related to a reduced risk of oral cancer [25].

Thus, there is an indication that fiber may be inversely associated to the risk of oral and pharyngeal cancer, although the evidence is limited and inconclusive.

Cancer of The Larynx

Introduction

Besides tobacco and alcohol which are the two major risk factors for laryngeal cancer, diet has been suggested to be an important determinant of laryngeal cancer risk [1, 3, 68]. Epidemiological evidence on diet and laryngeal cancer is, however, more limited than that for oral and pharyngeal cancer, and derives mainly from case–control studies.

Food Groups and Hot Drinks

In this section, we will summarize the main findings with relation to vegetables and fruits; other foods; and hot drinks.

Vegetables and Fruits

At least three cohort studies [5–7] and at least 20 case–control studies, conducted in Europe [33, 43, 69–74], the USA [38], Brazil [31], Uruguay [25, 48, 75, 76], India [9, 77], China [78], and Japan [42], investigated the relation between vegetables and fruits and the risk of laryngeal cancer. Three other cohort studies – already mentioned in the previous section on oral cancer – analyzed the association with all upper aerodigestive tract cancers combined [45–47].

In a cohort study of Hawaiian–Japanese adults, a considerably lower RR of laryngeal cancer was observed for daily consumption of green/yellow vegetables [5]. The IWHS study including 21 cases of laryngeal cancer, reported RR of 0.80 for the highest consumption of yellow/orange vegetables [6]. The NIH-AARP cohort study including 279 laryngeal cancer cases reported a non-significant inverse association with total fruits and vegetables (RR=0.69), with similar results for fruits (RR=0.80) and vegetables (RR=0.77) [7].

Most case–control studies found a protective association for at least one category of vegetables and/or fruits [9, 31, 43, 48, 70–74, 76–78]. Moreover, most case–control studies that examined total vegetables as a broad category reported inverse associations with laryngeal cancer risk [9, 42, 43, 73–76] (Fig. 4). Similarly, most case–control studies that evaluated the role of total fruit consumption found a

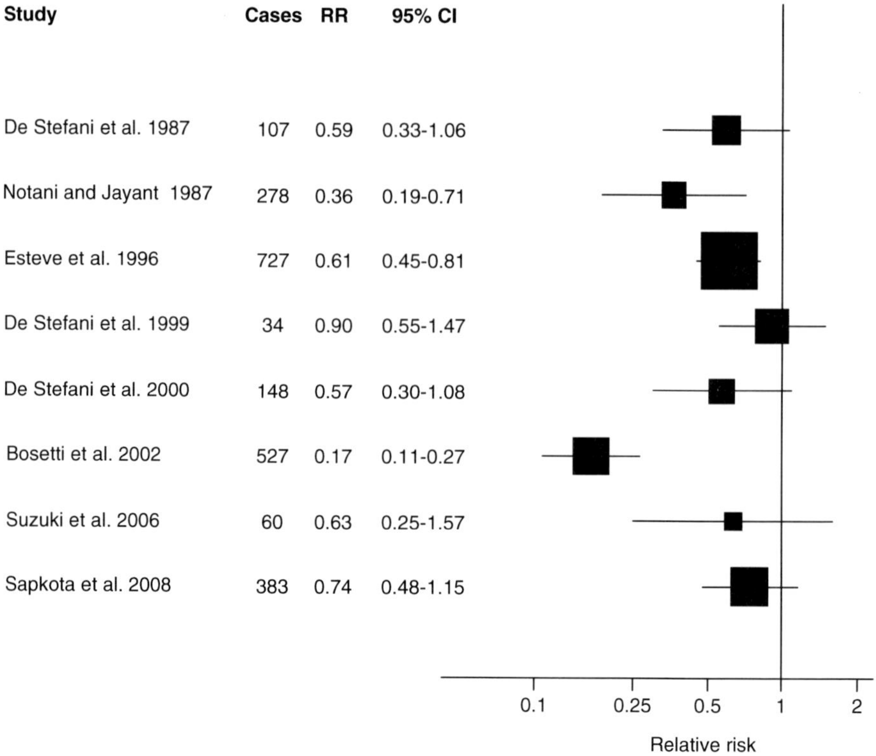

Fig. 4 Relative risks (RR) of laryngeal cancer and corresponding 95% confidence intervals (CI) for the highest level of vegetables consumption from selected case–control studies

protective effect [9, 25, 38, 42, 43, 69, 71, 73–78] (Fig. 5). Few data are available on particular types of fruits or vegetables, although consistent protective effects were observed for high intake of green/leafy vegetables and citrus fruits [25, 31, 33, 38, 43, 69, 71, 73, 74, 76–78]. In most case–control studies, which allowed for tobacco and alcohol consumption, the protective association for fruits and vegetables remained significant after adjustment for these two major risk factors for laryngeal cancer.

Epidemiological studies thus suggest that a diet high in vegetables and fruits reduces the risk of laryngeal cancer, although the evidence comes mainly from case–control studies.

Other Foods and Beverages

Case–control studies conducted in various countries suggested that meat consumption is generally not associated with the risk of laryngeal cancer [9, 25, 49, 71, 72, 77]. A increased risk has been reported for specific types of meats (such as fresh,

Study	Cases	RR	95% CI
De Stefani et al. 1987	107	0.77	0.42-1.42
Notani and Jayant 1987	80	0.50	0.25-1.01
Esteve et al. 1996	727	0.72	0.55-0.95
De Stefani et al. 1999	34	0.80	0.50-1.29
De Stefani et al. 2000	148	0.38	0.20-0.72
Bosetti et al. 2002	527	0.52	0.35-0.77
Suzuki et al. 2006	60	0.55	0.23-1.32
Sapkota et al. 2008	383	0.65	0.41-1.03

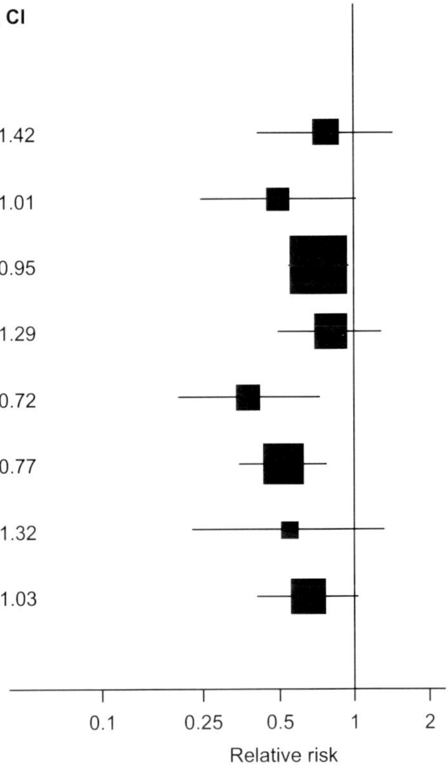

Fig. 5 Relative risks (RR) of laryngeal cancer and corresponding 95% confidence intervals (CI) for the highest level of fruit consumption from selected case–control studies

red, processed meat, and liver), although the evidence is quite limited [33, 43, 73, 74, 78, 79].

In contrast to meat, high fish consumption has been associated with a decreased risk of laryngeal cancer in a few studies [9, 49, 71–73, 78]. Two studies, however, found no [43] or a positive association [74].

An increased risk of laryngeal cancer was reported for high consumption of eggs in few studies [9, 25, 71, 74, 77].

With reference to milk and dairy products, an inverse relation with laryngeal cancer risk was reported in two case–control studies [43, 71] and in a prospective study [69], although no or positive association was found in three other case–control studies [9, 72, 74, 77]. Moreover, a significant inverse association was found for buttermilk [9].

Evidence on tea and coffee consumption and laryngeal cancer risk is limited, but does not suggest the existence of any meaningful association [54, 71, 72, 74]. As for oral cancer, however, a few studies suggested that hot maté drinking may increase the risk of this neoplasm [25, 31, 54, 75].

Nutrients and Other Food Components

Only a few studies collected dietary histories detailed enough to examine the potential relationship of laryngeal cancer with a wide variety of micro and macronutrients.

Micronutrients

Carotenoid intake was inversely related to the risk of laryngeal cancer in a few studies [31, 42, 73, 78, 80–82]. Similarly, vitamin C was suggested to have a protective effect on laryngeal cancer [42, 58, 73, 78, 82, 83], although the evidence is not consistent [81]. Conversely, retinol was associated with an increased risk in a few investigations [80–82], even if two studies found no association [73, 83].

With reference to minerals, intake of iron and zinc was associated with a reduced risk of laryngeal cancer in one case–control study, although there was no significant difference in the concentration of iron and zinc measured in nails between cases and controls [49]. Another case–control study observed a direct association with consumption of zinc, no association with iron, and a significant inverse one with potassium [82]. Moreover, a case–control study observed a direct association with iron [58]. Dietary intake of various minerals and laryngeal cancer risk (including iron, zinc, sodium, potassium, calcium, and phosphorus) was also evaluated in a multicentric European study, which found no significant association with any of the micronutrients examined [73].

Flavonoids

Two case–control studies conducted in Uruguay and Italy examined the relation between flavonoid intake and the risk of laryngeal cancer, and found significant inverse relations with total flavonoids (RR = 0.6 for both studies) [58, 84]. In particular, in the case–control study from Italy [84] the association was more consistent for two classes of flavonoids, i.e., flavanones (RR = 0.60) and flavonols (RR = 0.32) (Table 1). Thus, these studies suggest that flavonoids may at least in part account for the consistent inverse association observed between fruits, especially citrus fruits, and vegetable consumption and laryngeal cancer.

Macronutrients

A positive association with elevated consumption of fats has been reported in a few studies [58, 79, 81], although there is some indication of a more favorable effect of mono- and polyunsaturated fats, deriving mainly from olive oil on laryngeal carcinogenesis as compared to saturated fats [73, 74, 85] (Table 2).

The evidence of an association with other macronutrients, such as cholesterol [58, 85], proteins [58, 73, 81, 85], and carbohydrates [58, 73, 85] is limited and not consistent.

Conclusions

Epidemiological studies conducted in various populations consistently reported a protective effect of high consumption of vegetables and fruit on the risk of cancers of the oral cavity, pharynx, and larynx. The evidence, however, comes mainly from case–control studies.

Vegetables and fruits are rich in carotenoids, vitamins C and E, as well as flavonoids, with antioxidant and antitumor effects which may help prevent head and neck cancer [86–88]. Antioxidant nutrients and other food components have indeed shown protective effects on the risk of these neoplasms. However, the relations with single nutrients are less consistent than those for vegetables and fruits, and, it is difficult to disentangle the role of each single component. The protective effect of plant foods may indeed result from a combination of several nutrients, with complementary and overlapping mechanisms of action. It is also possible that more frequent consumption of fruits and vegetables is a non-specific indicator of a more affluent and better-planned diet [89, 90]. Moreover, although in most studies the inverse association for vegetables and fruit remained significant even after adjusting for the two major recognized risk factors for oral, pharyngeal, and laryngeal cancer (i.e., tobacco and alcohol), it is possible that at least part of the protective effect of fruits and vegetables may be explained by residual confounding. Smokers for instance have been reported to consume fewer vegetables than non smokers [91], and heavy alcohol drinkers tend to modify their diet, reducing the intake of other more beneficial foods and consequently of essential nutrients [92, 93].

Oral and pharyngeal cancer risk has been associated – although not consistently – to high intake of cereals. Compared with refined grains, whole grains are rich in soluble and insoluble fibers, which have been inversely related to the risk of oral and pharyngeal cancer. Furthermore, whole grain cereals share many micronutrients and other components with vegetables and fruits, including antioxidant nutrients and polyphenols [56, 71, 94]. Moreover, refined cereals and sugars have a higher rate of absorption than do whole-grain cereals, causing glycemic overload and compensatory increases in blood insulin level, and consequently insulin-like growth factor I (IGF-I), an important mitogenic stimulant of tumor cell growth in vitro [95, 96]. Glycemic index and load – indicators of the rate of absorption of carbohydrates and hence a measure of insulin demand – have indeed been directly associated to the risk of head and neck cancers [97].

Meat consumption has been related to an increased risk of oral and pharyngeal cancer in some studies, and some types of meat have also been associated with an increased risk of laryngeal cancer. Not all epidemiological studies, however, consistently support this association [98]. This effect may be attributable to their content of fats and cholesterol, but other nutrients or substances may be responsible for the increased risk, including heterocyclic amines, resulting from cooking, found to be associated with the risk of several neoplasms [99].

Fish, on the other hand, has been suggested to have a beneficial role on both oral and laryngeal cancers, possibly on account of its high content of polyunsaturated n-3 fatty acids, which have a chemopreventive role on various other neoplasms [100].

The evidence on the role of milk and dairy products, as well as coffee and tea on the risk of cancers of the head and neck is limited, particularly for laryngeal cancer.

In conclusion, consumption of vegetables and fruits appears to have the most consistent protective effect on the risk of head and neck cancers. In a network of studies from Italy, about 20–25% of cancers of the head and neck were attributed to low vegetable and fruit consumption, and the population attributable risk rose to 85–95% when tobacco and alcohol consumption were also considered [101].

References

1. World Cancer Research Fund/American Institute for Cancer Research (1997) Food, nutrition and the prevention of cancer: a global prospective. American Institute for Cancer Research, Washington, DC
2. Mayne ST, Morse DE, Winn DM (2006) Cancers of the oral cavity and pharynx. In: Schottenfeld D, Fraumeni JF Jr (eds) Cancer epidemiology and prevention, 3rd edn. Oxford University Press, New York, pp 674–696
3. World Cancer Research Fund/American Institute for Cancer Research (2007) Food, nutrition, physical activity, and the prevention of cancer: a global prospective. American Institute for Cancer Research, Washington, DC
4. Lucenteforte E, Garavello W, Bosetti C, La Vecchia C (2008) Dietary factors and oral and pharyngeal cancer risk. Oral Oncol 45:461–467
5. Hirayama T (1985) A large scale cohort study on cancer risks by diet-with special reference to the risk reducing effects of green-yellow vegetable consumption. Princess Takamatsu Symp 16:41–53
6. Kasum CM, Jacobs DR Jr, Nicodemus K, Folsom AR (2002) Dietary risk factors for upper aerodigestive tract cancers. Int J Cancer 99:267–272
7. Freedman ND, Park Y, Subar AF et al (2008) Fruit and vegetable intake and head and neck cancer risk in a large United States prospective cohort study. Int J Cancer 122:2330–2336
8. Winn DM, Ziegler RG, Pickle LW, Gridley G, Blot WJ, Hoover RN (1984) Diet in the etiology of oral and pharyngeal cancer among women from the southern United States. Cancer Res 44:1216–1222
9. Notani PN, Jayant K (1987) Role of diet in upper aerodigestive tract cancers. Nutr Cancer 10:103–113
10. De Stefani E, Correa P, Oreggia F et al (1988) Black tobacco, wine and mate in oropharyngeal cancer. A case–control study from Uruguay. Rev Epidemiol Sante Publique 36:389–394
11. McLaughlin JK, Gridley G, Block G et al (1988) Dietary factors in oral and pharyngeal cancer. J Natl Cancer Inst 80:1237–1243
12. Franco EL, Kowalski LP, Oliveira BV et al (1989) Risk factors for oral cancer in Brazil: a case–control study. Int J Cancer 43:992–1000
13. Gridley G, McLaughlin JK, Block G et al (1990) Diet and oral and pharyngeal cancer among blacks. Nutr Cancer 14 :219–225
14. Franceschi S, Bidoli E, Baron AE et al (1991) Nutrition and cancer of the oral cavity and pharynx in north-east Italy. Int J Cancer 47:20–25
15. La Vecchia C, Negri E, D'Avanzo B, Boyle P, Franceschi S (1991) Dietary indicators of oral and pharyngeal cancer. Int J Epidemiol 20:39–44
16. Oreggia F, De Stefani E, Correa P, Fierro L (1991) Risk factors for cancer of the tongue in Uruguay. Cancer 67:180–183
17. Franceschi S, Barra S, La Vecchia C, Bidoli E, Negri E, Talamini R (1992) Risk factors for cancer of the tongue and the mouth. A case–control study from northern Italy. Cancer 70:2227–2233

18. Zheng W, Blot WJ, Shu XO et al (1992) Risk factors for oral and pharyngeal cancer in Shanghai, with emphasis on diet. Cancer Epidemiol Biomarkers Prev 1:441–448
19. Day GL, Blot WJ, Austin DF et al (1993) Racial differences in risk of oral and pharyngeal cancer: alcohol, tobacco, and other determinants. J Natl Cancer Inst 85:465–473
20. Kune GA, Kune S, Field B et al (1993) Oral and pharyngeal cancer, diet, smoking, alcohol, and serum vitamin A and beta-carotene levels: a case–control study in men. Nutr Cancer 20:61–70
21. Zheng T, Boyle P, Willett WC et al (1993) A case–control study of oral cancer in Beijing, People's Republic of China. Associations with nutrient intakes, foods and food groups. Eur J Cancer B Oral Oncol 29B:45–55
22. De Stefani E, Oreggia F, Ronco A, Fierro L, Rivero S (1994) Salted meat consumption as a risk factor for cancer of the oral cavity and pharynx: a case–control study from Uruguay. Cancer Epidemiol Biomarkers Prev 3:381–385
23. Takezaki T, Hirose K, Inoue M et al (1996) Tobacco, alcohol and dietary factors associated with the risk of oral cancer among Japanese. Jpn J Cancer Res 87:555–562
24. Levi F, Pasche C, La Vecchia C, Lucchini F, Franceschi S, Monnier P (1998) Food groups and risk of oral and pharyngeal cancer. Int J Cancer 77:705–709
25. De Stefani E, Deneo-Pellegrini H, Mendilaharsu M, Ronco A (1999) Diet and risk of cancer of the upper aerodigestive tract–I. Foods. Oral Oncol 35:17–21
26. Franceschi S, Favero A, Conti E et al (1999) Food groups, oils and butter, and cancer of the oral cavity and pharynx. Br J Cancer 80:614–620
27. Brown LM, Gridley G, Diehl SR et al (2001) Family cancer history and susceptibility to oral carcinoma in Puerto Rico. Cancer 92:2102–2108
28. Fernandez Garrote L, Herrero R, Ortiz Reyes RM et al (2001) Risk factors for cancer of the oral cavity and oro-pharynx in Cuba. Br J Cancer 85:46–54
29. Tavani A, Gallus S, La Vecchia C et al (2001) Diet and risk of oral and pharyngeal cancer. An Italian case–control study. Eur J Cancer Prev 10:191–195
30. Marchioni DL, Fisberg RM, do Rosario M, Latorre DO, Wunsch V (2002) Diet and cancer of oral cavity and pharynx: a case–control study in Sao Paulo, Brazil. IARC Sci Publ 156:559–561
31. Nishimoto IN, Pintos J, Schlecht NF et al (2002) Assessment of control selection bias in a hospital-based case–control study of upper aero-digestive tract cancers. J Cancer Epidemiol Prev 7:131–141
32. Petridou E, Zavras AI, Lefatzis D et al (2002) The role of diet and specific micronutrients in the etiology of oral carcinoma. Cancer 94:2981–2988
33. Pisa FE, Barbone F (2002) Diet and the risk of cancers of the lung, oral cavity and pharynx, and larynx: a population-based case–control study in north-east Italy. IARC Sci Publ 156:141–143
34. Uzcudun AE, Retolaza IR, Fernandez PB et al (2002) Nutrition and pharyngeal cancer: results from a case–control study in Spain. Head Neck 24:830–840
35. Lissowska J, Pilarska A, Pilarski P et al (2003) Smoking, alcohol, diet, dentition and sexual practices in the epidemiology of oral cancer in Poland. Eur J Cancer Prev 12:25–33
36. Rajkumar T, Sridhar H, Balaram P et al (2003) Oral cancer in Southern India: the influence of body size, diet, infections and sexual practices. Eur J Cancer Prev 12:135–143
37. Sanchez MJ, Martinez C, Nieto A et al (2003) Oral and oropharyngeal cancer in Spain: influence of dietary patterns. Eur J Cancer Prev 12:49–56
38. Gaudet MM, Olshan AF, Poole C, Weissler MC, Watson M, Bell DA (2004) Diet, GSTM1 and GSTT1 and head and neck cancer. Carcinogenesis 25:735–740
39. Llewellyn CD, Linklater K, Bell J, Johnson NW, Warnakulasuriya S (2004) An analysis of risk factors for oral cancer in young people: a case–control study. Oral Oncol 40:304–313
40. Toporcov TN, Antunes JL, Tavares MR (2004) Fat food habitual intake and risk of oral cancer. Oral Oncol 40:925–931
41. De Stefani E, Boffetta P, Ronco AL et al (2005) Dietary patterns and risk of cancer of the oral cavity and pharynx in Uruguay. Nutr Cancer 51:132–139
42. Suzuki T, Wakai K, Matsuo K et al (2006) Effect of dietary antioxidants and risk of oral, pharyngeal and laryngeal squamous cell carcinoma according to smoking and drinking habits. Cancer Sci 97:760–767

43. Sapkota A, Hsu CC, Zaridze D et al (2008) Dietary risk factors for squamous cell carcinoma of the upper aerodigestive tract in central and eastern Europe. Cancer Causes Control 19:1161–1170 Epub 2008 May 30
44. Heck JE, Sapkota A, Vendhan G et al (2008) Dietary risk factors for hypopharyngeal cancer in India. Cancer Causes Control 19:1329–1337
45. Chyou PH, Nomura AM, Stemmermann GN (1995) Diet, alcohol, smoking and cancer of the upper aerodigestive tract: a prospective study among Hawaii Japanese men. Int J Cancer 60:616–621
46. Kjaerheim K, Gaard M, Andersen A (1998) The role of alcohol, tobacco, and dietary factors in upper aerogastric tract cancers: a prospective study of 10, 900 Norwegian men. Cancer Causes Control 9:99–108
47. Boeing H, Dietrich T, Hoffmann K et al (2006) Intake of fruits and vegetables and risk of cancer of the upper aero-digestive tract: the prospective EPIC-study. Cancer Causes Control 17:957–969
48. De Stefani E, Oreggia F, Boffetta P, Deneo-Pellegrini H, Ronco A, Mendilaharsu M (2000) Tomatoes, tomato-rich foods, lycopene and cancer of the upper aerodigestive tract: a case–control in Uruguay. Oral Oncol 36:47–53
49. Rogers MA, Thomas DB, Davis S, Vaughan TL, Nevissi AE (1993) A case–control study of element levels and cancer of the upper aerodigestive tract. Cancer Epidemiol Biomarkers Prev 2:305–312
50. Franceschi S, Bidoli E, Baron AE, La Vecchia C (1990) Maize and risk of cancers of the oral cavity, pharynx, and esophagus in northeastern Italy. J Natl Cancer Inst 82:1407–1411
51. Nandakumar A, Thimmasetty KT, Sreeramareddy NM et al (1990) A population-based case–control investigation on cancers of the oral cavity in Bangalore, India. Br J Cancer 62:847–851
52. Levi F, Pasche C, Lucchini F, Chatenoud L, Jacobs DR Jr, La Vecchia C (2000) Refined and whole grain cereals and the risk of oral, oesophageal and laryngeal cancer. Eur J Clin Nutr 54:487–489
53. Jacobsen BK, Bjelke E, Kvale G, Heuch I (1986) Coffee drinking, mortality, and cancer incidence: results from a Norwegian prospective study. J Natl Cancer Inst 76:823–831
54. Pintos J, Franco EL, Oliveira BV, Kowalski LP, Curado MP, Dewar R (1994) Mate, coffee, and tea consumption and risk of cancers of the upper aerodigestive tract in southern Brazil. Epidemiology 5:583–590
55. Zheng W, Sellers TA, Doyle TJ, Kushi LH, Potter JD, Folsom AR (1995) Retinol, antioxidant vitamins, and cancers of the upper digestive tract in a prospective cohort study of postmenopausal women. Am J Epidemiol 142:955–960
56. Negri E, Franceschi S, Bosetti C et al (2000) Selected micronutrients and oral and pharyngeal cancer. Int J Cancer 86:122–127
57. Rossing MA, Vaughan TL, McKnight B (1989) Diet and pharyngeal cancer. Int J Cancer 44:593–597
58. De Stefani E, Ronco A, Mendilaharsu M, Deneo-Pellegrini H (1999) Diet and risk of cancer of the upper aerodigestive tract–II. Nutrients. Oral Oncol 35:22–26
59. Marshall J, Graham S, Mettlin C, Shedd D, Swanson M (1982) Diet in the epidemiology of oral cancer. Nutr Cancer 3:145–149
60. Gridley G, McLaughlin JK, Block G, Blot WJ, Gluch M, Fraumeni JF Jr (1992) Vitamin supplement use and reduced risk of oral and pharyngeal cancer. Am J Epidemiol 135:1083–1092
61. Barone J, Taioli E, Hebert JR, Wynder EL (1992) Vitamin supplement use and risk for oral and esophageal cancer. Nutr Cancer 18:31–41
62. Pelucchi C, Talamini R, Negri E et al (2003) Folate intake and risk of oral and pharyngeal cancer. Ann Oncol 14:1677–1681
63. Marshall JR, Graham S, Haughey BP et al (1992) Smoking, alcohol, dentition and diet in the epidemiology of oral cancer. Eur J Cancer B Oral Oncol 28B:9–15
64. Rossi M, Garavello W, Talamini R et al (2007) Flavonoids and the risk of oral and pharyngeal cancer: a case–control study from Italy. Cancer Epidemiol Biomarkers Prev 16:1621–1625
65. Franceschi S, Levi F, Conti E et al (1999) Energy intake and dietary pattern in cancer of the oral cavity and pharynx. Cancer Causes Control 10:439–444

66. Soler M, Bosetti C, Franceschi S et al (2001) Fiber intake and the risk of oral, pharyngeal and esophageal cancer. Int J Cancer 91:283–287
67. Macfarlane GJ, Zheng T, Marshall JR et al (1995) Alcohol, tobacco, diet and the risk of oral cancer: a pooled analysis of three case–control studies. Eur J Cancer B Oral Oncol 31B:181–187
68. Olshan A (2006) Cancers of the larynx. In: Schottenfeld D, JFJr F (eds) Cancer epidemiology and prevention, 3rd edn. Oxford University Press, New York, pp 627–637
69. Maier H, Tisch M (1997) Epidemiology of laryngeal cancer: results of the Heidelberg case–control study. Acta Otolaryngol Suppl 527:160–164
70. Zemla B, Day N, Swiatnicka J, Banasik R (1987) Larynx cancer risk factors. Neoplasma 34:223–233
71. La Vecchia C, Negri E, D'Avanzo B, Franceschi S, Decarli A, Boyle P (1990) Dietary indicators of laryngeal cancer risk. Cancer Res 50:4497–4500
72. Zatonski W, Becher H, Lissowska J, Wahrendorf J (1991) Tobacco, alcohol, and diet in the etiology of laryngeal cancer: a population-based case–control study. Cancer Causes Control 2:3–10
73. Esteve J, Riboli E, Pequignot G et al (1996) Diet and cancers of the larynx and hypopharynx: the IARC multi-center study in southwestern Europe. Cancer Causes Control 7:240–252
74. Bosetti C, La Vecchia C, Talamini R et al (2002) Food groups and laryngeal cancer risk: a case–control study from Italy and Switzerland. Int J Cancer 100:355–360
75. De Stefani E, Correa P, Oreggia F et al (1987) Risk factors for laryngeal cancer. Cancer 60:3087–3091
76. De Stefani E, Boffetta P, Oreggia F et al (2000) Plant foods and risk of laryngeal cancer: a case–control study in Uruguay. Int J Cancer 87:129–132
77. Kapil U, Singh P, Bahadur S, Dwivedi SN, Singh R, Shukla N (2005) Assessment of risk factors in laryngeal cancer in India: a case–control study. Asian Pac J Cancer Prev 6:202–207
78. Zheng W, Blot WJ, Shu XO et al (1992) Diet and other risk factors for laryngeal cancer in Shanghai, China. Am J Epidemiol 136:178–191
79. Oreggia F, De Stefani E, Boffetta P, Brennan P, Deneo-Pellegrini H, Ronco AL (2001) Meat, fat and risk of laryngeal cancer: a case–control study in Uruguay. Oral Oncol 37:141–145
80. Mackerras D, Buffler PA, Randall DE, Nichaman MZ, Pickle LW, Mason TJ (1988) Carotene intake and the risk of laryngeal cancer in coastal Texas. Am J Epidemiol 128:980–988
81. Freudenheim JL, Graham S, Byers TE et al (1992) Diet, smoking, and alcohol in cancer of the larynx: a case–control study. Nutr Cancer 17:33–45
82. Bidoli E, Bosetti C, La Vecchia C et al (2003) Micronutrients and laryngeal cancer risk in Italy and Switzerland: a case–control study. Cancer Causes Control 14:477–484
83. Graham S, Mettlin C, Marshall J, Priore R, Rzepka T, Shedd D (1981) Dietary factors in the epidemiology of cancer of the larynx. Am J Epidemiol 113:675–680
84. Garavello W, Rossi M, McLaughlin JK et al (2007) Flavonoids and laryngeal cancer risk in Italy. Ann Oncol 18:1104–1109
85. Bosetti C, La Vecchia C, Talamini R et al (2003) Energy, macronutrients and laryngeal cancer risk. Ann Oncol 14:907–912
86. Potter JD, Steinmetz K (1996) Vegetables, fruit and phytoestrogens as preventive agents. IARC Sci Publ N 139:61–90
87. La Vecchia C, Altieri A, Tavani A (2001) Vegetables, fruit, antioxidants and cancer: a review of Italian studies. Eur J Nutr 40:261–267
88. IARC (2003) IARC Handbooks of Cancer Prevention, vol 8, Fruit and vegetables. IARC Press, Lyon
89. Garavello W, Giordano L, Bosetti C et al (2008) Diet diversity and risk of oral and pharyngeal cancer risk. Eur J Nutr 47:280–284
90. Garavello W, Lucenteforte L, Bosetti C, et al (2009) Diet diversity and the risk of laryngeal cancer: a case–control study from Italy and Switzerland. Oral Oncol 45:85–89
91. D'Avanzo B, La Vecchia C, Braga C, Franceschi S, Negri E, Parpinel M (1997) Nutrient intake according to education, smoking, and alcohol in Italian women. Nutr Cancer 28:46–51
92. Blot WJ (1992) Alcohol and cancer. Cancer Res 52:2119s–2123s

93. Blot WJ (1999) Invited commentary: more evidence of increased risks of cancer among alcohol drinkers. Am J Epidemiol 150:1138–1140 discussion 1141
94. Truswell AS (2002) Cereal grains and coronary heart disease. Eur J Clin Nutr 56:1–14
95. Giovannucci E (1995) Insulin and colon cancer. Cancer Causes Control 6:164–179
96. Bosetti C, Malvezzi M, Chatenoud L, Negri E, Levi F, La Vecchia C (2005) Trends in cancer mortality in the Americas, 1970–2000. Ann Oncol 16:489–511
97. Augustin LS, Gallus S, Franceschi S et al (2003) Glycemic index and load and risk of upper aero-digestive tract neoplasms (Italy). Cancer Causes Control 14:657–662
98. Tavani A, La Vecchia C, Gallus S et al (2000) Red meat intake and cancer risk: a study in Italy. Int J Cancer 86:425–428
99. IARC (1993) Some naturally occurring substances: food items and constituents, heterocyclic aromatic amines and mycotoxins, vol 56, IARC Monogr Eval Carcinog Risks Hum. IARC, Lyon
100. Fernandez E, Chatenoud L, La Vecchia C, Negri E, Franceschi S (1999) Fish consumption and cancer risk. Am J Clin Nutr 70:85–90
101. La Vecchia C, Tavani A (1998) Fruit and vegetables, and human cancer. Eur J Cancer Prev 7:3–8

Occupation and Other Risk Factors for Head and Neck Cancer

Andrew F. Olshan and Kimon Divaris

Introduction

In this chapter, we examine the potential role of occupational and other exposures in the etiology of head and neck cancer (most often squamous cell carcinoma, SCCHN). The focus was on factors that have been examined in multiple epidemiologic studies, including occupational exposures, gastroesophageal reflux, and oral health. We consider the study design, conduct, and analytic approach and methods that may have influenced the interpretation of results from previous studies.

SCCHN and Occupation

The relationship between occupational exposures and the risk of SCCHN have been examined in multiple studies conducted around the world. Overall, there is a less consistent pattern of associations reported for occupational exposures and the risk of oral and pharyngeal cancer than for laryngeal cancer (Table 1). Some specific occupations such as textile and leather workers, butchers, carpet workers, machinists, female electronics workers, welders, and painters, and construction workers have been found to have an elevated risk of SCCHN [1–3]. Studies that have assessed specific occupational exposures or exposure groups in relation to oropharyngeal cancer have reported associations with polycyclic aromatic hydrocarbons, formaldehyde, pesticides, and welding fumes and textile, leather, and cement dusts. However, no consistent pattern of association with specific occupations, industries, or exposures has yet emerged. As discussed below, there are methodologic issues that have to be taken into account when considering these findings.

Table 1 also presents a list of occupational exposures that have been reported to increase the risk of laryngeal cancer. The evidence for a causal relationship between

A.F. Olshan (✉) and K. Divaris
Department of Epidemiology, Gillings School of Global Public Health CB#7435, University of North Carolina, 2101B McGavran-Greenberg Hall, Chapel Hill, NC 27599, USA
e-mail: andy_olshan@unc.edu
e-mail: divarisk@DENTISRTY.UNC.EDU

A.F. Olshan (ed.), *Epidemiology, Pathogenesis, and Prevention of Head and Neck Cancer*,
DOI 10.1007/978-1-4419-1472-9_7,

Table 1 Occupational exposures and head and neck cancer: selected associations[a]

Laryngeal cancer[b]
Exposures
Formaldehyde
Asbestos
Synthetic fibers
Mustard gas
Sulfuric acid mist
Wood dust
Nickel
Hair dye
Rubber products
Organic solvents
Mineral oil
Coal dust
Hard alloy dusts
Occupations/industries
Cement workers
Asbestos miners
Shipyard workers
Building materials workers
Construction workers
Oropharyngeal cancer[c]
Exposures
Formaldehyde
Polycyclic aromatic hydrocarbons
Cement dust
Pesticides
Welding fumes
Textile dust
Leather dust
Occupations/industries
Printing
Electronics workers
Metal industry
Machinists
Petroleum industry
Painters
Furniture workers
Woodworking machine operators
Butchers
Carpet installers
Leather workers
Textile workers

[a]Selected on the basis of multiple studies reporting an elevated relative risk estimate
[b]See Olshan [5], Purdue et al. [2], Shangina et al. [6], Jayaprakash et al. [7]
[c]See Mayne et al. [1], Purdue et al. [2], Tarvainen et al. [3]

these exposures and laryngeal cancer is inconclusive. However, the International Agency for Research on Cancer (IARC) concluded that there is sufficient evidence for the carcinogenicity of inorganic acid mist and laryngeal cancer [4]. Exposure to asbestos, a known lung carcinogen, and the risk of laryngeal cancer has been extensively studied and different conclusions regarding the consistency and strength of the findings have been reached [5]. Other occupational exposures that have been associated with laryngeal cancer risk include formaldehyde, man-made mineral fibers, dusts (metal, cement, wood, and coal), mustard gas, and organic solvents [5–7]. These associations have generally been reported in more than one, but not all, epidemiologic studies.

Several methodologic issues need to be recognized when interpreting the evidence. The major threats to the validity of the findings include confounding bias and exposure misclassification. The major risk factors for SCCHN are heavy tobacco and alcohol consumption. If these factors are strongly associated with occupations and related exposures, then they may confound the association between occupation and SCCHN if not properly controlled. In the case-control studies of occupation and some cohort studies, it is typical to obtain information on history of tobacco and of alcohol use and adjust for these factors in the analysis. In other cohort studies using vital record or other sources direct data on smoking and alcohol use are not obtained. Confounding bias may influence the results of these studies to some extent.

A major concern in all occupational studies is the quality of the exposure data. In case-control studies inferences about exposure are made with varying levels of sophistication, ranging from simple determination using job title and industry to assessment by industrial hygienists using additional job duty and work environment information. The so called "job-exposure matrices" are sometimes created to provide a means to classify and assign exposure. In addition, other simple quantitative estimates of exposure dose levels and frequency of exposure may be determined. These methods have limitations based on the nature of error in self-reported data, expert review, and classification [8]. In general, these errors will lead to effect estimates that are biased towards the null (a relative risk estimate of 1.0).

Gastroesophageal Reflux

Gastroesophageal reflux is movement of gastric contents into the laryngopharynx and esophagus and is a common condition in the Western world [9–11]. Gastroesophageal reflux disease (GERD) is a more severe and chronic reflux condition that has been strongly associated with adenocarcinoma, but not squamous cell cacinoma of the esophagus [12–14]. The pathogenesis of reflux-related larynx damage is thought to involve chronic inflammation resulting in malignant transformation [15]. Studies have attempted to describe specific injurious components of reflux, reflux-associated epithelial changes, and protective mechanisms [15].

GERD has been suggested as a potential risk factor for laryngeal cancer for many years [16]. Small clinical case series studies, some including nonsmoking persons, appeared to support an association [16]. Recent clinical studies have also used more sophisticated methods to monitor pH and one reported an association although another did not [17, 18]. The clinical studies suffer from limitations such as small size, lack of a comparison group, confounding, reverse causality, and insensitive measurement [15]. A systematic review in 2003 weakly supported an association between reflux and laryngeal cancer [19].

There have been few epidemiologic studies of GERD using a comparison group. A recent study of the hospital records of 8,228 United States military veterans with laryngeal cancer and 7,648 hospital controls found that after adjustment for smoking, age, race, and alcohol use, GERD was associated with an odds ratio of 2.4 (CI=2.2–2.7) for larynx cancer [20]. The study, although large, had limitations, including ascertainment of reflux using medical records, inadequate definition of time lag between reflux and cancer diagnosis, and potential detection bias and differential referral patterns for cases and controls. A recent study used data from the Swedish inpatient registry to identify discharge diagnoses of heartburn, hiatal hernia, or esophagitis and linked this cohort with the Swedish cancer registry [21]. After exclusion of persons with a diagnosis of alcoholism, no significantly increased risk of laryngeal or pharyngeal cancer was found (RR=1.3; 0.8–2.0; RR=1.0; CI=0.5–1.6, respectively). In addition, no association was found for reflux severity or diagnostic specificity.

There is good reason to suspect that GERD and related reflux conditions can cause chronic irritation, inflammation, and tissue damage. A relationship with esophageal cancer has been supported [22]. It is noteworthy that this association is with esophageal adenocarcinoma, not squamous cell carcinoma, the latter being the predominant histologic type of oropharyngeal and laryngeal cancer.

However, the relationship with GERD and other reflux conditions with head and neck cancer is not consistent. Case series studies indicate some potential modest increase in risk one epidemiologic study reported a twofold elevated risk, while another did not. Several study design limitations have cast doubt on the validity of many of the findings. These limitations include sample size, potential error in self-reported exposure data, lack of control of smoking and alcohol, and lack of clear temporality between exposure and cancer development and diagnosis. These limitations are not insurmountable and improved future studies can be conducted to address the hypothesis.

Oral Health and SCCHN

Since as early as 1935, studies have investigated the relationship between measures of oral health and the risk of SCCHN (Table 2). Typically, these measures include tooth loss, gum bleeding, tooth brushing, general oral conditions, and frequency of dental visits. In general, some of these represent markers of periodontal disease.

Table 2 Epidemiologic studies of oral health and head and neck cancer

First author, year, location	Cancer site	Study population	Oral health measures	Covariates	Risk estimate (OR 95% CI)
Balaram (2002), India	Oral	Cases: 3 centers. 309 males and 232 females, age range: 18–87 Controls: frequency matched by center, age and gender. 292 males and 290 females.	Interviewer assessed: Number of missing teeth, general oral condition. Self-reported: tooth cleaning, denture wearing, dental checkups, gum bleeding.	Age, center, education and (men only) smoking and drinking.	Males: 3.89 (2.46, 6.17) >5 missing teeth; 4.90 (3.09, 7.78) poor oral condition; 0.89 (0.56, 1.42) ever-dental checkup. Females: 7.61 (3.89, 14.88) >5 missing teeth; 5.99 (3.00, 11.96) poor oral condition; 0.41 (0.19, 0.87) ever-dental checkup.
Bundgaard (1995), Denmark	Oral	Cases: 161 consecutive cases from one hospital. Controls: 400 (3 gender- and age-matched controls from the same geographic area, for each case.) age range: ≤45–75.	Number of teeth present, denture wearing, dental checkups.	Alcohol, tobacco, residence, marital status.	2.1 (1.1, 4.0) 5–14 teeth present; 2.4 (1.4, 4.3) 0–4 teeth present; [ref: 15–32] 2.1 (1.3, 3.3) non-regular dental checkups.
Elwood (1984), Canada	Oral, oropharyngeal, hypopharyngeal, laryngeal.	Cases: 374 continuous newly diagnosed cases Controls: 374 other-cancer patients, gender and age-matched.	Dental checkups, extraction of 5 or more teeth on one occasion, denture wearing, "special" dental work	Alcohol, tobacco, SES, marital status, special dental care, TB history	1.6 (1.1, 2.5) lack of regular dental care.
Fernandez Garrote (2001), Cuba	Oral, oropharyngeal.	Cases: 200 cases in one center (median age = 64, range: 28–91) Controls 200 admitted to the same center (unrelated diseases) frequency matched on age and gender. (median age = 62, range: 25–88 years)	Number of missing (not replaced) teeth, general oral condition upon inspection by dentist. Self-reported dental checkups, tooth brushing, gum bleeding, mouthwash use, denture wearing.	Smoking and drinking habits, gender, age, area of residence, education.	1.82 (0.76, 4.35) 6–15 missing teeth; 2.74 (1.23, 6.12) ≥16 missing teeth; [ref:≤5 missing teeth]; 1.82 (0.94, 3.53) average oral condition; 2.55 (1.24, 5.24) poor oral condition; [ref: good oral condition]; 1.61 (0.83, 3.07) ≥1 dental checkup every 5 years; 0.71 (0.6, 1.86) <1 dental checkup even 5 years; [ref: never]

(continued)

Table 2 (continued)

First author, year, location	Cancer site	Study population	Oral health measures	Covariates	Risk estimate (OR 95% CI)
Franco (1989), Brazil	Oral	Cases: 232 newly diagnosed cases referred to 3 H&N surgery centers. Controls: 464 hospital noncancer controls age, gender and residence-matched.	Frequency of dental visits, tooth brushing, denture wearing, "broken teeth"	Alcohol, tobacco, age, gender, study site, admission period.	0.6 (0.3, 1.3) <1 dental visit/year;0.6 (0.1, 2.3) ≥1 dental visit/year; [ref: never]; 2.3 (1.4, 3.7) less-than-daily tooth-brushing; 1.3 (0.9, 1.8) broken teeth.
Graham (1977), US	Oral	Cases: 584 white males in one center Controls: 1,222 white males admitted to the same center for non-neoplastic diagnoses, frequency matched (?) on age, and similar SES.	Composite index of missing, "septic", decayed teeth and need of denture repair.	None	2.26 (1.43, 3.54) anterior or posterior inadequate dentition; 4.62 (3.25, 6.58) anterior and posterior inadequate dentition. [ref: anterior and posterior adequate dentition]
Guha (2007), central Europe and Latin America	Oral, pharyngeal, laryngeal and esophageal.	Central Europe: Cases: 924 in 4 centers. Controls: 928 hospital-based, frequency matched on age and gender. (population-based controls in one center) Latin America: Cases: 2,286 in 7 centers. Controls: 1,805 hospital-based, as above.	Interviewer assessed: number of missing teeth, visible lesions, general oral health. Self-reported: both CE & LA: tooth-brushing frequency, denture use. LA only: dental checkups, gum bleeding.	Age, gender, education, center, tobacco, alcohol consum-ption, and other oral health variables (oral hygiene, missing teeth, tooth brushing (frequency, instrument, dentifrice), gum bleeding, dental checkups, mouth-wash use, denture wearing).	Central Europe: 1.09 (0.73, 1.62) 6–15 missing teeth; 0.70 (0.44, 1.11) ≥16 missing teeth; [ref: ≤5 missing teeth]; 1.68 (1.19, 2.39) average oral hygiene; 2.89 (1.74, 4.81) poor oral hygiene; [ref: good oral hygiene] Latin America: 1.28 (0.99, 1.65) 6–15 missing teeth; 1.31 (1.0, 1.72) ≥16 missing teeth; 1.08 (0.85, 1.36) average oral hygiene; 1.91 (1.49, 2.45) poor oral hygiene; 1.11 (0.80, 1.55) dental checkup every 2–5 years; 1.12 (0.83, 1.51) less than every 5 years; 1.61 (1.18, 2.20) never; [ref: every year]

Kabat (1989), US	Oral	Cases: 125 women with oral cancer participating in the American Health Foundation's study of tobacco-related cancers between 1983 and 1987 Controls: 107 women with cancers, benign neoplasms and non-neoplastic conditions unrelated to tobacco and alcohol.	Number of missing teeth, periodontal disease, mouthwash use, denture wearing, tooth brushing, gum bleeding.	Tobacco, alcohol, age and religion.	0.89 (0.32, 2.11) 1–9 missing teeth; 1.62 (0.66, 4.02) 10+ missing teeth; [ref: 0 missing teeth]; 1.12 (0.55, 2.27) gingivitis or periodontal disease; 1.12 (0.85, 1.47) gum bleeding; 0.92 (0.38, 2.08) <1 per day mouthwash use; 0.65 (0.34, 1.22) ≥ 1 per day mouthwash use; [ref: never]
Lissowska (2003), Poland	Oral, pharyngeal.	Cases: 122 cases in one center Controls: 124 hospital-based from the same geographic area, admitted for non-neoplastic or other illnesses unrelated to oral cancer risk factors, frequency matched on gender and age. Age range: 23–80	Dentist assessed: Number of missing teeth, general oral condition Self-reported: dental checkups, tooth brushing frequency, gum bleeding, denture use.	Age, gender, residence, tobacco and alcohol.	7.00 (1.68, 29.11) 6–15 missing teeth; 9.85 (2.26, 42.84) ≥ 16 missing teeth; [ref: ≤ 5 missing teeth]; 1.17 (0.53, 2.78) average oral general oral condition; 1.10 (0.49, 2.46) poor oral condition; [ref: good oral condition]; 1.94 (0.70, 5.34) every 2–5 years dental checkup; 4.67 (1.56, 14.01) less than once every 5 years dental checkup; 11.89 (3.33, 42.51) never; [ref: yearly dental checkup]
Maier (1993), Germany	Oral, oropharyngeal, laryngeal, hypopharyngeal.	Cases: 100 cases in two centers Controls 214 age and gender-matched with no known tumor status examined at the same centers. Age range: 30–75	Interviewer assessed: Gingival inflammation, number of decayed teeth, and presence of tartar.Self-reported: frequency of tooth-brushing, dental checkups.	None	2.35 (1.40, 3.95) moderate or severe gingival inflammation; [ref: no or slight gingival inflammation]; 0.31 (0.03, 1.60) less than yearly dental checkups; 0.08 (0.03, 0.19) yearly or more frequent dental checkups; [ref: never-dental visit only when in pain]

(continued)

Table 2 (continued)

First author, year, location	Cancer site	Study population	Oral health measures	Covariates	Risk estimate (OR 95% CI)
Marques (2008), Brazil	Oral, pharyngeal.	Cases: 309 cases in seven reference hospitals Controls: 468 age and gender matched patients from five of the seven reference hospitals, admitted for illnesses unrelated to oral cancer risk factors.	Self-reported: denture use, gum bleeding, frequency of dental visits, tooth-brushing and mouthwash use.	Age, gender, education, smoking, alcohol consumption and other oral health variables (denture use, dental visits, tooth-brushing, mouthwash)	0.9 (0.6, 1.5) occasional gum bleeding; 3.1 (1.2, 7.9) always/almost always gum bleeding; [ref: never]; 1.5 (0.8, 2.8) occasional (≥2 year intervals) dental visits; 2.5 (1.3, 4.8) never; [ref: annual dental visits]; 1.0 (0.6, 1.9) less than once a day mouthwash use; 3.3 (1.7, 6.1) once or more times daily mouthwash use; [ref: never]
Marshall (1992), US	Oral, oropharyngeal, pharyngeal, hypopharyngeal.	Cases: 290 cases from 20 major western NY hospitals. Controls: 290 age, gender and neighborhood-matched.	Self-reported: denture use, teeth lost but not replaced, and mouthwash use.	Age, gender, residence (matching factors), tobacco and alcohol consumption.	0.5 (0.2, 1.1) 1–2 teeth lost not replaced; 1.1 (0.6, 2.3) 3–4 teeth; 1.4 (0.7, 2.9) 5–10 teeth; 2.7 (1.1, 6.5) 11+ teeth; [ref: 0 teeth lost, not replaced]; 1.1 (0.4, 2.9) 1–5 years denture wearing; 1.3 (0.5, 3.2) 6–10 years; 0.9 (0.4, 1.9) 11–20 years; 1.3 (0.7, 2.5) 21–30 years; 2.1 (1.0, 4.5) 31+ years; [ref: <1 year denture wearing]
Michaud (2008), US	Oropharyngeal	US male health professionals' cohort: 48,375 men, median follow-up 17.7 years, age range: 40–75 years.	Self-reported: periodontal disease, number of natural teeth present.	Age, race, physical activity, diabetes, alcohol consumption, smoking history, BMI, geographical location, height, total calorific intake, red-meat intake, fruit & vegetable intake, vitamin D score.	Risk estimates are Hazard Ratios (95% CI): 1.18 (0.69, 2.01) 17–24 natural teeth; 1.60 (0.84, 3.04) 0–16 natural teeth; [ref: 25–32 natural teeth]; 1.15 (0.73, 1.81) history of periodontal disease with bone loss.

Moreno-Lopez (2000), Spain	Oral, oropharyngeal.	Cases: 75 from three hospitals. Controls: 150 healthy subjects from health care centers corresponding to those hospitals. Age range (cases): 30–84	Self reported: tooth brushing, dental visits	None	0.97 (0.42, 2.20) not regular dental checkups; 0.63 (0.14, 2.88) regular checkups; [ref: never]; 0.31 (0.18, 0.56) daily tooth brushing; [ref: less than daily]
Rosenquist (2005), Sweden	Oral, oropharyngeal.	Cases: 132 in two university hospitals Controls: 320 healthy individuals selected from population registry, matched on age, gender and country of residence. Age range (cases): 33–87	Examined: number of missing teeth, oral hygiene, gingival bleeding, tooth mobility, furcation involvement, defective teeth, denture presence/condition. Self-reported: dental checkups.	Tobacco and alcohol consumption.	3.4 (1.4, 8.5) >20 missing teeth; [ref: 0 missing teeth]; 0.4 (0.2, 0.6) regular dental checkups; [ref: not regular, >18 months interval]; 2.0 (1.1, 3.6) average oral hygiene; 5.3 (2.5, 11.3) poor oral hygiene; [ref: good oral hygiene].
Shildt (1998), Sweden	Oral, oropharyngeal.	Cases: 354 all reported to the Cancer registry of four Swedish counties, between 1980 and 1989. Controls 354 selected from the Population registry, individually matched on gender, age, county residence and alive/deceased status. Age mean: men 72.3 years, women 69.6 years.	Self-reported or kin-reported:Tooth loss, denture use, oral infections, caries, dental calculus, amalgam fillings, number of dental X-rays.	None	0.9 (0.6, 1.5) tooth loss; 1.3 (0.9, 1.9) denture use; 1.4 (0.6, 3.2) ever dental care;

(continued)

Table 2 (continued)

First author, year, location	Cancer site	Study population	Oral health measures	Covariates	Risk estimate (OR 95% CI)
Subapriya (2007), India	Oral	Cases: 388 in one hospital, between 1991 and 2003. Controls: 388 admitted relatives and friends, for diseases other than cancer, excluding tobacco and alcohol related illnesses, matched for age, gender and religion. Mean age (cases): 50.8 years	Dentist assessed: number of missing teeth, general oral condition, and oral hygiene. Self-reported: Tooth brushing frequency, dentifrice used.	Age, gender, religion, tobacco and alcohol consumption.	9.63 poor oral general conditions.
Talamini (2000), Italy	Oral, oropharyngeal.	Cases: 132 in three hospitals. Controls: 148 patients admitted to the major hospitals of the same region for illnesses unrelated to tobacco or alcohol, frequency matched with cases by age and gender. Age: median: 60 years, range: 27–86 years.	Interviewer assessed: missing non-replaced teeth, general oral condition. Self-reported: Gum bleeding, dental checkups, mouthwash use, and denture use.	Age, gender, smoking, drinking habits, fruit, and vegetable intake.	1.1 (0.5, 2.6) 6–15 missing teeth; 1.4 (0.6, 3.1) ≥16 missing teeth; [ref: ≤5 missing teeth]; 1.8 (0.9, 3.6) average oral condition; 4.5 (1.8, 10.9); [ref: good oral condition]; 1.8 (0.9, 3.6) sometimes gum bleeding; 3.9 (1.2, 12.6) always/almost always gum bleeding; [ref: never]; 0.8 (0.4, 1.6) less than or equal to once every 5 years dental checkup; 1.1 (0.5, 2.6) never dental checkup; [ref: greater than or equal to once every 5 years dental checkup].

Tezal (2005), US	Oral	NHANES III cohort, 13,798 subjects. Age > 20 years.	Periodontal disease (assessed by clinical attachment loss > 1.5 mm).	Number of filled teeth, number of decayed teeth, presence of prosthesis, age, gender, race/ethnicity, education, tobacco, alcohol, occupational hazard, and interaction term "tobacco occupational hazard".	4.57 (2.25, 9.30) CAL >1.5 mm.
Velly (1998), Brazil	Oral, pharyngeal, laryngeal.	Cases: 717 in three hospitals Controls 1,434 from the same hospital (one center) or the same catchment area (two centers), matched on gender, age, admission time and study site.	Self-reported: denture use, denture-associated sores, broken teeth, and tooth brushing frequency.	Age, gender, study center, admission period, tobacco, alcohol, dietary variables, consumption of non-alcoholic beverages, temperature of drinks, ethnicity, income, and education.	1.03 (0.61, 1.73) 1–8 years denture use; 0.80 (0.55, 1.18) 9+ years denture use; [ref: no denture use]; 0.71 (0.47, 1.06) no denture-associated sores; 1.08 (0.70, 1.66) denture-associated sores; [ref: never used dentures]; 1.79 (1.16, 2.77) infrequent brushing; [ref: daily]; 1.21 (0.85, 1.72) broken teeth present.

(continued)

Table 2 (continued)

First author, year, location	Cancer site	Study population	Oral health measures	Covariates	Risk estimate (OR 95% CI)
Winn (1991), US	Oral, pharyngeal.	Cases: 1,114 from four population-based cancer registries. Controls: 1,268 from the same geographic area, frequency matched to age, gender, race and study center, by: random digit dialing (18–4 years) and from files of Health Care Financing Administration (65–79 years). Age: median 63 years, range: 18–79 years	Self-reported: number of teeth, use of dentures, number of dental X-rays, tooth-brushing frequency, occurrence of oral diseases, gum bleeding, and mouthwash use.	Age, race, education, smoking, alcohol consumption, dietary intake of fruit, stratified by gender.	Males: 1.0 tooth loss due to gum disease; 0.8 (0.6, 1.1) periodontal disease; 0.8 (0.6, 1.2) gum bleeding; 1.1 (0.8, 1.4) denture use; 12.7 (4.8, 33.3) leukoplakia; 1.2 (0.9, 1.6) mouth sores. Females: 1.1 tooth loss due to gum disease; 1.1 (0.7, 1.6) periodontal disease; 1.0 (0.6, 1.7) gum bleeding; 1.0 (0.7, 1.5) denture use; 4.3 (1.4, 13.3) leukoplakia; 0.8 (0.5, 1.2) mouth sores.
Zheng (1990), China	Oral, oropharyngeal.	Cases: 404 in seven hospitals. Controls: 404 admitted to the same hospitals for conditions thought to be unrelated to tobacco and alcohol consumption, age, gender and study site-matched. Age range (cases): 18–80.	Dentist assessed: number of missing teeth, jagged teeth, filled teeth, decayed and septic teeth, presence of gingivitis or periodontal disease, leukoplakia, erythroplakia, and lichen planus. Self-reported: dental visits/checkups, number of years of denture-wearing, number of years elapsed between tooth loss and denture fitting.	Age, gender, education, tobacco, and alcohol.	Males: 1.3 (0.6, 2.5) 1–2 lost teeth; 4.9 (2.4, 10.1) 3–6 lost teeth; 5.9 (2.8, 12.2) 7–14 lost teeth; 5.3 (2.3, 11.9) 15–32 lost teeth; [ref: no lost teeth]; 1.2 (0.7, 1.9) 1 time/day tooth-brushing; 7.8 (2.6, 23.3) 0 times/day tooth-brushing; [ref: >1 times/day tooth-brushing]. Females: 5.2 (1.9, 14.1) 1–2 lost teeth; 8.8 (3.2, 24.6) 3–6 lost teeth; 10.4 (3.5, 30.9) 7–14 lost teeth; 7.3 (2.5, 21.6) 15–32 lost teeth; [ref: no lost teeth]; 1.1 (0.6, 2.0) 1 time/day tooth-brushing; 2.7 (0.9, 8.3) 0 times/day tooth-brushing; [ref: >1 times/day tooth-brushing].

Periodontal disease is characterized by complex interactions between predominantly Gram negative oral bacteria (found in the gingival bacterial biofilm) and immune (host) response [23, 24], resulting in inflammation of the gums (gingivitis), which if left untreated, may progress to irreversible destruction of the periodontal ligament and the tooth supporting bone (periodontitis) [25–27]. The prevalence of periodontal disease is higher among older persons and, worldwide, severe periodontal disease may be as high as 15% with milder disease found in up to 90% of individuals [24]. There are now over 30 published papers from international studies on the relationship between oral health and SCCHN. We will provide highlights of the key studies and provide an overview of the potential mechanisms and the methodologic issues involved in studying these factors.

An early study [28] reported that edentulism was more common among oral cavity cancer patients, especially among women, than other persons. Graham et al. [29] found that poor dentition, especially in combination with heavy alcohol drinking and heavy smoking was more common among cases of oral cavity cancer ($n=584$) than controls ($n=1,222$). A case-control study of oral cancer conducted in Beijing, China (404 case-control pairs) found that the number of missing teeth (OR among men for 15–32 teeth lost, compared to none lost=5.3) and no tooth brushing (OR=6.9 for men) were associated with an elevated risk [30]. In addition, an interaction between tooth loss and smoking and alcohol use was reported. A case control study in Western New York (290 cases) found an odds ratio for oral cancer of 2.7 for the loss of 11 or more teeth [31]. A Danish study (161 cases) reported that persons with less than five teeth had a tobacco and alcohol-adjusted odds ratio of 2.4 (95% CI=1.3–4.1) for oral cancer compared to persons with 15 or more teeth present [32].

A Cuban case-control study (200 cases) found that severe tooth loss (≥16 missing teeth) and poor oral condition assessed by oral inspection were associated with approximately 2.7- and 2.6-fold increased risk of oral and pharyngeal cancer, respectively [33]. A Polish case-control study (122 cases), after adjustment for alcohol and cigarette use, reported strong associations with ≥16 missing teeth (OR=9.8) and infrequent dental checkups (less than once every 5 years, OR=4.7) and tooth brushing (less than once daily, OR=3.2) for the risk of oral cancer [34]. Another small study that was carried out in Sweden (132 cases) included oral examinations, and reported associations with poor oral hygiene (OR=5.3; 95% CI=2.5–11.3) [35]. Specific dental factors included tooth loss (>20 lost teeth, OR=3.4; 95% CI=1.4–8.5), poorly fitting dentures (OR=3.8, 95% CI=1.3–11.4), whereas regular dental checkups were associated with a decreased risk of oropharyngeal cancer (OR=0.4; 95% CI=0.2–0.6). In addition, panoramic radiographs showed that markers of periodontal disease progression had an elevated, but not statistically significantly adjusted odds ratio. A study in Southern India reported an elevated risk for indicators of poor oral hygiene (gum bleeding, missing teeth, and overall oral health status [36]). One of the largest studies, including 924 cases from central Europe and 2,286 cases from Latin America included a dental examination [37]. The study reported several associations with measures of dental status and oral health, including poor general condition of the mouth (OR = 2.89, central Europe; OR = 1.89, Latin America), lack of toothbrush use (OR = 2.36, Latin America), and infrequent dental checkups (never, OR = 1.61; 95% CI = 1.18–2.20).

An analysis of data from a prospective cohort study of male health professionals (the Health Professionals Follow-up Study) included 118 cases of oropharyngeal cancer [38]. Men were asked about a history of periodontal disease with bone loss. A validation substudy was conducted using radiograph assessment. Tooth loss at baseline and in the follow-up period was also self-reported. After controlling for smoking history and other covariates the hazard ratio for oropharyngeal cancer was only 1.15 (95% CI = 0.73–1.81) for history of periodontal disease.

A study by Gillison et al. [39] assessed human papillomavirus (HPV) status in SCCHN tumors and found a different risk factor profile among persons with HPV-16-negative tumors, including a higher risk associated with increasing number of missing teeth. Fewer natural teeth (0–16) at the baseline interview were associated with a hazard ratio of 1.60 (95% CI = 0.84–3.04).

Authors have speculated on the potential mechanistic explanations for the association between oral hygiene and SCCHN [37, 38, 40]. Those include: (1) local or systemic effects through inflammation, (2) direct effect through bacterial virulence factors, and (3) direct effects from metabolic products. Hooper et al. in a systematic review concluded that there is sufficient evidence to suggest that epidemiological and etiological links between microbial infection in the oral cavity and oral cancer could exist [41]. With regard to systemic pathways, periodontal disease has been linked to a chronic systemic inflammatory response, secretion of inflammatory mediators and alteration of the overall immune condition [42–44]. This pathway is likely invoked via the elevated induction of C-reactive protein, IL-1B, IL-6, TNF-α, and matrix metalloproteinases [43, 45, 46]. Chronic inflammatory processes have been associated with an increased risk of various cancers [47, 48]. Chronic periodontal disease may also be a marker for a compromised immune condition and reduced surveillance of tumor progression [40]. It is also possible that the metabolic products of oral flora, such as acetaldehyde, are carcinogenic [49–52]. In addition, the increased production of endogenous nitrosamines may be promoted by poor oral health [53–55]. Finally, the reported interactions between tobacco and alcohol use and oral health suggest additional mechanistic complexity.

It has been argued that mouthrinse products have sufficient alcohol content to potentially increase the risk of cancer. A recent German study detected elevated salivary acetaldehyde levels after mouthwash use, in concentrations normally found after alcoholic beverage consumption [49]. Some brands contain up to 30% ethanol, and multiple studies have reported an association with mouthwash use. For example, a study of women with oropharyngeal cancer [56] found an increased risk of mouthwash use among women who did not use tobacco (OR = 1.94; 95% CI = 0.8–4.7). The large study from Europe and Latin America [37] reported that daily mouthwash use was associated with an increased risk of SCCHN (Latin America, OR = 3.40; 95% CI = 1.96, 5.89), independent of tobacco and alcohol use.

A recent Brazilian study also reported an association (OR = 3.3; 95% CI = 1.7, 6.1) with daily or more frequent mouthwash use for oral and pharyngeal cancer [57].

The epidemiologic studies of oral health and mouthrinse use face several methodologic challenges that limit definitive interpretation [58, 59]. For example, tobacco use is a strong risk factor for SCCHN and is likely associated with poor oral hygiene. Thus, the control of smoking in the analysis is critical and inadequate adjustment may lead to residual confounding. In addition, poor oral health may be associated with changes in diet and lower intake of fruits and vegetables are related to an elevated risk of oral cancer. The role of oral health may also be more subtle with oral hygiene acting as an intermediate factor between tobacco use and SCCHN. Poor oral health may also be a marker for compromised overall health and health behaviors. Finally, the usual measured markers of oral health (tooth loss, gum bleeding, tooth brushing frequency, and dental attendance) may be poor surrogates for the important underlying health condition. In addition, few studies have performed a direct observation of oral health by a trained professional, while the majority has relied on recall by study participants.

The epidemiologic studies of mouthwash use are also affected by similar concerns. It has been suggested that mouthwash is primarily used as a response to smoking. However, an elevated risk related to mouthwash use has been found among non-smokers and non-alcohol users [56, 60]. Guha et al. [37] reported a correlation between mouthwash use and the presence of visible oral lesions and suggested that the use of mouthwash may be a response to disease symptoms rather than a possible cause. Studies have also not routinely collected data on the specific mouthrinse brand and alcohol content and a refined dose-response analysis has not been possible.

Conclusions

Tobacco and alcohol use remain the most consistently reported factors associated with an elevated risk of SCCHN. However, multiple epidemiologic studies have reported associations with a variety of other factors, including occupational exposures, gastroesophageal reflux, and poor oral health. Even though most of these studies accounted for smoking and alcohol use, potential bias owing to confounding and other biases remains a concern. Future studies will be required to determine if there is sufficient evidence to suggest causality. Some of the reported associations are with factors that are relatively rare in the population (e.g., specific occupations or occupational exposures) and would have a low attributable risk, while others are more common (poor oral health, gastroesophageal reflux) with potentially larger attributable risks. Future studies can be constructed to overcome many of the limitations and should be undertaken to resolve outstanding questions about exposures, many of which are preventable.

References

1. Mayne ST, Morse DE, Winn DM (2006) Cancers of the oral cavity and pharynx. In: Schottenfeld D, Fraumeni JF (eds) Cancer epidemiology and prevention. Oxford University Press, Oxford
2. Purdue MP, Jarvholm B, Bergdahl IA, Hayes RB, Baris D (2006) Occupational exposures and head and neck cancers among Swedish construction workers. Scand J Work Environ Health 32:270–275
3. Tarvainen L, Kyyronen P, Kauppinen T, Pukkala E (2008) Cancer of the mouth and pharynx, occupation and exposure to chemical agents in Finland [in 1971–95]. Int J Cancer 123:653–659
4. (1992) Occupational exposures to mists and vapours from strong inorganic acids; and other industrial chemicals. IARC Monograph on the Evaluation of Carcinogenic Risks to Humans. IARC Monograph vol 54. Lyon, France
5. Olshan AF (2006) Laryngeal cancer. In: Schottenfeld D, Fraumeni JF (eds) Cancer epidemiology and prevention. Oxford University Press, Oxford
6. Shangina O, Brennan P, Szeszenia-Dabrowska N, Mates D, Fabiánová E, Fletcher T, t'Mannetje A, Boffetta P, Zaridze D (2006) Occupational exposure and laryngeal and hypopharyngeal cancer risk in central and eastern Europe. Am J Epidemiol 164:367–375
7. Jayaprakash V, Natarajan KK, Moysich KB, Rigual NR, Ramnath N, Natarajan N, Reid ME (2008) Wood dust exposure and the risk of upper aero-digestive and respiratory cancers in males. Occup Environ Med 65:647–654
8. Teschke K, Olshan AF, Daniels JL, De Roos AJ, Parks CG, Schulz M, Vaughan TL (2002) Occupational exposure assessment in case-control studies: opportunities for improvement. Occup Environ Med 59(9):575–593
9. Isolauri J, Laippala P (1995) Prevalence of symptoms suggestive of gastro-oesophageal reflux disease in an adult population. Ann Med 27:67–70
10. Locke GR III, Talley NJ, Fett SL, Zinsmeister AR, Melton LJ III (1997) Prevalence and clinical spectrum of gastroesophageal reflux: a population-based study in Olmsted County, Minnesota. Gastroenterology 112:1448–1456
11. Shaker R, Castell DO, Schoenfeld PS, Spechler SJ (2003) Nighttime heartburn is an under-appreciated clinical problem that impacts sleep and daytime function: the results of a Gallup survey conducted on behalf of the American Gastroenterological Association. Am J Gastroenterol 98:1487–1493
12. Boffetta P, Ye W, Adami HO, Mucci LA, Nyren O (2001) Risk of cancers of the lung, head and neck in patients hospitalized for alcoholism in Sweden. Br J Cancer 85:678–682
13. Lagergren J, Bergstrom R, Lindgren A, Nyren O (1999) Symptomatic gastroesophageal reflux as a risk factor for esophageal adenocarcinoma. N Engl J Med 340:825–831
14. Farrow DC, Vaughan TL, Sweeney C, Gammon MD, Chow WH, Risch HA, Stanford JL, Hansten PD, Mayne ST, Schoenberg JB, Rotterdam H, Ahsan H, West AB, Dubrow R, Fraumeni JF Jr, Blot WJ (2000) Gastroesophageal reflux disease, use of H2 receptor antagonists, and risk of esophageal and gastric cancer. Cancer Causes Control 11:231–238
15. Wilson JA (2005) What is the evidence that gastroesophageal reflux is involved in the etiology of laryngeal cancer? Curr Opin Otolaryngol Head Neck Surg 13:97–100
16. Assimakopoulos D, Patrikakos G (2002) The role of gastroesophageal reflux in the pathogenesis of laryngeal carcinoma. Am J Otolaryngol 23(6):351–357
17. Lewin JS, Gillenwater AM, Garrett JD, Bishop-Leone JK, Nguyen DD, Callender DL, Ayers GD, Myers JN (2003) Characterization of laryngopharyngeal reflux in patients with premalignant or early carcinomas of the larynx. Cancer 97:1010–1014
18. Geterud A, Bove M, Ruth M (2003) Hypopharyngeal acid exposure: an independent risk factor for laryngeal cancer? Laryngoscope 113:2201–2205
19. Weaver EM (2003) Association between gastroesophageal reflux and sinusitis, otitis media, and laryngeal malignancy: a systematic review of the evidence. Am J Med 115(suppl. 3A): 81S–89S

20. El-Serag HB, Hepworth EJ, Lee P, Sonnenberg A (2001) Gastroesophageal reflux disease is a risk factor for laryngeal and pharyngeal cancer. Am J Gastroenterol 96:2013–2018
21. Nilsson M, Chow WH, Lindblad M, Ye W (2005) No association between gastroesophageal reflux and cancers of the larynx and pharynx. Cancer Epidemiol Biomarkers Prev 14:1194–1197
22. Demeester SR (2009) Epidemiology and biology of esophageal cancer. Gastrointest Cancer Res 3(2 suppl.):S2–S5
23. Offenbacher S, Barros SP, Singer RE, Moss K, Williams RC, Beck JD (2007) Periodontal disease at the biofilm-gingival interface. J Periodontol 78(10):1911–1925
24. Pihlstrom BL, Michalowicz BS, Johnson NW (2005) Periodontal diseases. Lancet 366(9499):1809–1820
25. Loesche WJ, Grossman NS (2001) Periodontal disease as a specific, albeit chronic, infection: diagnosis and treatment. Clin Microbiol Rev 14(4):727–752
26. Irfan UM, Dawson DV, Bissada NF (2001) Epidemiology of periodontal disease: a review and clinical perspectives. J Int Acad Periodontol 3(1):14–21
27. Armitage GC (1999) Development of a classification system for periodontal diseases and conditions. Ann Periodontol 4(1):1–6
28. Wynder EL, Bross IJ, Feldman RM (1957) A study of the etiological factors in cancer of the mouth. Cancer 10:1300–1323
29. Graham S, Dayal H, Rohrer T, Swanson M, Sultz H, Shedd D, Fischman S (1977) Dentition, diet, tobacco, and alcohol in the epidemiology of oral cancer. J Natl Cancer Inst 59(6):1611–1618
30. Zheng TZ, Boyle P, Hu HF, Duan J, Jian PJ, Ma DQ, Shui LP, Niu SR, Scully C, MacMahon B (1990) Dentition, oral hygiene, and risk of oral cancer: a case-control study in Beijing, People's Republic of China. Cancer Causes Control 1:235–241
31. Marshall JR, Graham S, Haughey BP, Shedd D, O'Shea R, Brasure J, Wilkinson GS, West D (1992) Smoking, alcohol, dentition and diet in the epidemiology of oral cancer. Eur J Cancer B Oral Oncol 28B(1):9–15
32. Bundgaard T, Wildt J, Frydenberg M, Elbrønd O, Nielsen JE (1995) Case-control study of squamous cell cancer of the oral cavity in Denmark. Cancer Causes Control 6(1):57–67
33. Garrote LF, Herrero R, Reyes RM, Vaccarella S, Anta JL, Ferbeye L, Muñoz N, Franceschi S (2001) Risk factors for cancer of the oral cavity and oro-pharynx in Cuba. Br J Cancer 85(1):46–54
34. Lissowska J, Pilarska A, Pilarski P, Samolczyk-Wanyura D, Piekarczyk J, Bardin-Mikołłajczak A et al (2003) Smoking, alcohol, diet, dentition and sexual practices in the epidemiology of oral cancer in Poland. Eur J Cancer Prev 12(1):25–33
35. Rosenquist K (2005) Risk factors in oral and oropharyngeal squamous cell carcinoma: a population-based case-control study in southern Sweden. Swed Dent J Suppl 179:1–66
36. Subapriya R, Thangavelu A, Mathavan B, Ramachandran CR, Nagini S (2007) Assessment of risk factors for oral squamous cell carcinoma in Chidambaram, Southern India: a case-control study. Eur J Cancer Prev 16(3):251–256
37. Guha N, Boffetta P, Wünsch Filho V, Eluf Neto J, Shangina O, Zaridze D et al (2007) Oral health and risk of squamous cell carcinoma of the head and neck and esophagus: results of two multicentric case-control studies. Am J Epidemiol 166(10):1159–1173
38. Michaud DS, Liu Y, Meyer M, Giovannucci E, Joshipura K (2008) Periodontal disease, tooth loss, and cancer risk in male health professionals: a prospective cohort study. Lancet Oncol 9(6):550–558
39. Gillison ML, D'Souza G, Westra W, Sugar E, Xiao W, Begum S et al (2008) Distinct risk factor profiles for human papillomavirus type 16-positive and human papillomavirus type 16-negative head and neck cancers. J Natl Cancer Inst 100(6):407–420
40. Meyer MS, Joshipura K, Giovannucci E, Michaud DS (2008) A review of the relationship between tooth loss, periodontal disease, and cancer. Cancer Causes Control 19(9): 895–907

41. Hooper SJ, Wilson MJ, Crean SJ (2009) Exploring the link between microorganisms and oral cancer: a systematic review of the literature. Head Neck 31(9):1228–1239
42. Ebersole JL, Cappelli D, Mathys EC, Steffen MJ, Singer RE, Montgomery M, Mott GE, Novak MJ (2002) Periodontitis in humans and non-human primates: oral-systemic linkage inducing acute phase proteins. Ann Periodontol 7(1):102–111
43. Slade GD, Offenbacher S, Beck JD, Heiss G, Pankow JS (2000) Acute-phase inflammatory response to periodontal disease in the US population. J Dent Res 79(1):49–57
44. Ebersole JL, Machen RL, Steffen MJ, Willmann DE (1997) Systemic acute-phase reactants, C-reactive protein and haptoglobin, in adult periodontitis. Clin Exp Immunol 107(2):347–352
45. Noack B, Genco RJ, Trevisan M, Grossi S, Zambon JJ, De Nardin E (2001) Periodontal infections contribute to elevated systemic C-reactive protein level. J Periodontol 72(9):1221–1227
46. Page RC, Offenbacher S, Schroeder HE, Seymour GJ, Kornman KS (1997) Advances in the pathogenesis of periodontitis: summary of developments, clinical implications and future directions. Periodontol 2000 14:216–248
47. Karin M, Lawrence T, Nizet V (2006) Innate immunity gone awry: linking microbial infections to chronic inflammation and cancer. Cell 124(4):823–835
48. Coussens LM, Werb Z (2002) Inflammation and cancer. Nature 420(6917):860–867
49. Lachenmeier DW, Gumbel-Mako S, Sohnius EM, Keck-Wilhelm A, Kratz E, Mildau G (2009) Salivary acetaldehyde increase due to alcohol-containing mouthwash use: a risk factor for oral cancer. Int J Cancer 125(3):730–735
50. Kurkivuori J, Salaspuro V, Kaihovaara P, Kari K, Rautemaa R, Grönroos L, Meurman JH, Salaspuro M (2007) Acetaldehyde production from ethanol by oral streptococci. Oral Oncol 43(2):181–186
51. Homann N, Tillonen J, Rintamäki H, Salaspuro M, Lindqvist C, Meurman JH (2001) Poor dental status increases acetaldehyde production from ethanol in saliva: a possible link to increased oral cancer risk among heavy drinkers. Oral Oncol 37(2):153–158
52. Homann N, Tillonen J, Meurman JH, Rintamäki H, Lindqvist C, Rautio M, Jousimies-Somer H, Salaspuro M (2000) Increased salivary acetaldehyde levels in heavy drinkers and smokers: a microbiological approach to oral cavity cancer. Carcinogenesis 21(4):663–668
53. Abnet CC, Qiao YL, Dawsey SM, Dong ZW, Taylor PR, Mark SD (2005) Tooth loss is associated with increased risk of total death and death from upper gastrointestinal cancer, heart disease, and stroke in a Chinese population-based cohort. Int J Epidemiol 34(2):467–474
54. Badawi AF, Hosny G, el-Hadary M, Mostafa MH (1998) Salivary nitrate, nitrite and nitrate reductase activity in relation to risk of oral cancer in Egypt. Dis Markers 14(2):91–97
55. Shapiro KB, Hotchkiss JH, Roe DA (1991) Quantitative relationship between oral nitrate-reducing activity and the endogenous formation of N-nitrosoamino acids in humans. Food Chem Toxicol 29(11):751–755
56. Blot WJ, Winn DM, Fraumeni JF Jr (1983) Oral cancer and mouthwash. J Natl Cancer Inst 70(2):251–253
57. Marques LA, Eluf-Neto J, Figueiredo RA, Góis-Filho JF, Kowalski LP, Carvalho MB, Abrahão M, Wünsch-Filho V (2008) Oral health, hygiene practices and oral cancer. Rev Saude Publica 42(3):471–479
58. Cole P, Rodu B, Mathisen A (2003) Alcohol-containing mouthwash and oropharyngeal cancer: a review of the epidemiology. J Am Dent Assoc 134(8):1079–1087
59. Shapiro S, Castellana JV, Sprafka JM (1996) Alcohol-containing mouthwashes and oropharyngeal cancer: a spurious association due to underascertainment of confounders? Am J Epidemiol 144(12):1091–1095
60. Winn DM, Diehl SR, Brown LM, Harty LC, Bravo-Otero E, Fraumeni JF Jr, Kleinman DV, Hayes RB (2001) Mouthwash in the etiology of oral cancer in Puerto Rico. Cancer Causes Control 12:419–429

Host Susceptibility and Molecular Epidemiology

Li-E Wang, Guojun Li, Erich M. Sturgis, and Qingyi Wei

Genetic Susceptibility

Tobacco and alcohol exposures are major determinants of risk of squamous cell carcinoma of the head and neck (SCCHN), accounting for approximately three-fourths of all oral and pharyngeal cancers in the U.S. and an even higher attributable fraction of laryngeal cancers [1]. Other exposures include human papillomavirus, dietary, occupational, medical, and other factors that may also contribute to the etiology of this disease; however, only a fraction of exposed individuals will develop SCCHN. Therefore, the role of genetic susceptibility to carcinogenic exposures must be factored into the risk assessment process. This chapter explores some of the host factors that modulate susceptibility to epithelial carcinogenesis induced by tobacco and alcohol exposures and describes some relevant molecular epidemiology association studies of single nucleotide polymorphism (SNP) and risk of SCCHN.

Familial Aggregation of SCCHN Cancer

Epidemiologic studies of familial aggregation of SCCHN provide indirect evidence for the role of genetic predisposition in the etiology of SCCHN. Such aggregation implies shared genes, shared exposures or a combination of both. Several studies have suggested that the family history of cancer is a risk factor for SCCHN [2–5]. In a case–control study of SCCHN in a Brazil population with 754 cases and 1,507 age- and gender-matched hospital-based controls with nonmalignant diseases, it was found that the relative risk (RR) for developing SCCHN in those with family history of any cancer in first-degree relatives was twofold higher and increased to

L. Wang, G. Li, E.M. Sturgis and Q. Wei (✉)
Department of Epidemiology, The University of Texas, M. D. Anderson Cancer Center, 1515 Holcombe Blvd., Unit 1365, Houston, TX 77030, USA
e-mail: qwei@mdanderson.org

A.F. Olshan (ed.), *Epidemiology, Pathogenesis, and Prevention of Head and Neck Cancer,*
DOI 10.1007/978-1-4419-1472-9_8,

3.65 (95% confidence interval [CI] = 1.97–6.76) if the relatives also had SCCHN [3]. The same group further reported a strong association between risk for developing SCCHN and family history of SCCHN in 1,429 first degree relatives of 242 index cases of SCCHN and 934 first degree relatives of the spouses of 156 index cases in Canadian populations. The adjusted RR was 3.8 (1.1–13.0) for developing SCCHN in first-degree relatives of patients compared with the first-degree relatives of patients' spouses and 7.9 (1.5–41.6) in first-degree relatives of patients with multiple SCCHN [6].

A similar study conducted in Puerto Rico in 342 patients with carcinomas of the oral cavity and pharynx and 521 controls showed a 2.6-fold excess risk (95% CI = 1.4–4.8) in patients who reported a history of upper aerodigestive tract cancers in first degree relatives [7]. In a Japanese study of 167 patients with hypopharyngeal or cervical esophageal cancers and 167 control subjects with benign diseases, the risk for hypopharyngeal or cervical esophageal cancers associated with family history of upper aerodigestive tract cancers was 2.6-fold (1.1–6.3) [4]. A weak familial aggregation of oral and pharyngeal cancers has also been reported in another case–control investigation on 487 cases and 485 controls who reported cancer in a parent or a sibling. Risks were nonsignificantly elevated among those with a history of cancers arising from the oral cavity/pharynx (Odds Ratio [OR] = 1.2; 95% CI = 0.7–2.3) or esophagus/larynx (OR = 1.6; 95% CI = 0.7–3.8). An elevated risk of oral/pharyngeal cancers was found among those whose sisters developed other cancers (OR = 1.6; 95% CI = 1.1–2.2) [8].

Recently, a study using the Swedish Family-Cancer Database reported the familial clustering of cancer at human papillomavirus-associated sites. Site and sex-specific analysis indicated that risk of upper aerodigestive tract SCC (tumors of the lip, tongue, gums, palate, mouth, nasopharynx, oropharynx, hypopharynx, pharynx [unspecified], tonsil, and larynx) in female offspring was significantly increased in those who had siblings with cervical SCC (standardized incidence ratios [SIR] = 1.37; 95% CI = 1.03–1.79), mothers with skin SCC (1.50; 1.00–2.18), or fathers with upper aerodigestive tract SCC (1.92; 1.09–3.12); Male offsprings were at a significantly increased risk of upper aerodigestive tract SCC by having siblings with upper aerodigestive tract SCC (2.36; 1.02–5.17), mothers with vulvar (2.47; 1.41–4.02) and fathers with upper aerodigestive SCC (1.66; 1.20–2.23) [9]. A Norwegian population-based study of 127 patients diagnosed with SCCHN before the age of 45 reported nonsignificant increases in familial risk for SCCHN (OR = 2.0; 95% CI = 0.9–4.4) for both sexes, but there was a significant difference between sex (5.0 and 1.4–17.3 for women, 1.1 and 0.3–3.3 for men) [10].

Another study using the nationwide Swedish Family-Cancer Database of over 15,000 cases of upper aerodigestive tract cancers reported a nonsignificantly increased risk in children whose parents had a history of upper aerodigestive tract cancer (1.40; 0.98–1,95); however, the SIR and 95% CI were significant for offsprings with upper aerodigestive tract cancer and with all parental cancers (1.10; 1.03–1.17), especially, for offsprings with pharyngeal cancers (1.15; 1.03–1.29) [11]. In the recent pooled analysis in the International Head and Neck Cancer Epidemiology Consortium with 12 case–control studies including 8,967 SCCHN cases and 13,627 controls, the risk of SCCHN increased for those with a family history of SCCHN in first-degree relatives (OR = 1.7; 95% CI = 1.2–2.3). The risk was higher if the affected relative was a sibling (OR = 2.2; 95% CI = 1.6–3.1) rather than a parent (OR = 1.5; 95% CI = 1.1–1.8). There is a weak but significant association between risk of SCCHN and a family history of other tobacco-related neoplasms (OR = 1.1; 95% CI = 1.0–1.2), particularly of laryngeal cancer (OR = 1.3; 95% CI 1.1–1.5) [12].

Metabolic Polymorphisms

The internal dose of tobacco carcinogens to which the head and neck tissue is exposed is modulated by genetic polymorphisms in enzymes responsible for activation and detoxification of these carcinogens. These polymorphisms are frequent in the general population (>1% allelic frequency) and therefore the attributable risks may be high. Here, we focus on select genes and pathways that are involved in the metabolism of tobacco carcinogens, such as arylamines, *N*-nitrosamines, PAHs, and benzo[a]pyrene (B[a]P). A comprehensive review is beyond the scope of this chapter.

Phase I enzymes: Cytochrome P450 (CYP) 1A1, the gene that codes for aryl hydrocarbon hydroxylase (AHH), initiates a multienzyme pathway that activates polycyclic aromatic hydrocarbons (PAHs), including benzo(a)pyrene, to highly electrophilic metabolites. AHH activity levels vary by up to several thousand-fold between tissues and between individuals [13]. A higher prevalence of extensive metabolizers has been reported in oral, pharyngeal, and laryngeal cancer patients than in control subjects [14–16].

Sequencing of the *CYP1A1* gene [17, 18] identified two polymorphisms that seem to have functional relevance. A restriction fragment length polymorphism (RFLP) in the 3′ noncoding region of the gene after MspI digestion that results from a single base-pair change T>C is thought to affect the *CYP1A1* mRNA stability. The polymorphism has been associated with oral cavity cancer risk in Japanese populations [19, 20]. Individuals with the susceptible *CYP1A1* genotype contracted smoking-induced cancers at lower levels of cigarette use than did those with other *CYP1A1* genotypes [21]. Increased risk for SCCHN was also reported in two Caucasian cohorts [22, 23]. The prevalence of the C (m2) allele ranges between 0.05 and 0.30 [24, 25].

An A/G polymorphism on exon 7 results in an Ile/Val amino acid change [26] and is associated with an elevated activity of the CYP1A1 enzyme [27]. The risk genotype has a prevalence between 0.02 and 0.05 in healthy American subjects [24]. A significant association has been reported between this *CYP1A1* variant and pharyngeal, but not oral or laryngeal cancers in Japanese [28, 29] and in Caucasian populations [30]. However, a pooled analysis with 9 case–control studies with 2,334 SCCHN cases and 2,766 controls summarized a nonsignificant OR of 1.35 (95% CI = 0.95–1.82) for carrying the *CYP1A1* Val462 allele [31]. The same finding was reported from another meta-analysis on 17 published studies [32]. In a recent meta-analysis from 30 publications including 3,130 patients with oral and pharyngeal cancers and 6,267 controls, the pooled analysis showed a significant association between oral and pharyngeal cancer risk and the *CYP1A1* MspI homozygous variant (meta-OR for m2/m2 = 1.9; 95% CI = 1.4–2.7; pooled OR for m2m2 = 2.0; 95% CI = 1.3–3.1; OR for m1m2 or m2m2 = 1.3; 95% CI = 1.1–1.6). The association was also present for the *CYP1A1* (exon 7) polymorphism (OR for Val/Val = 2.2; 95% CI = 1.1–4.5) in ever smokers [33].

CYP1B1 is another phase I enzyme that catalyzes the 2- and 4-hydroxylation of 17 β-estradiol, a key reaction in hormonal carcinogenesis. Few studies have investigated its role in SCCHN [34]. Among potential functional polymorphisms, a G>A substitution in exon 3 results in an amino acid change from valine to leucine (Val432Leu) and the Val432Leu genotype was associated with a borderline elevated risk (OR = 1.41; 95% CI = 0.94–2.11) of SCCHN in a case–control study from Germany, particularly in subgroup of smokers (OR = 2.70; 95% = 1.53–4.86) [35]. However, a larger case–control analysis in non-Hispanic US whites did not find any risk association overall nor in subgroup analysis [36]. Recently, in an Indian study with 150 cases and 150 controls, haplotype analysis was done with four nonsynonymous SNPs in *CYP1B1* (Arg-Gly at codon 48, Ala-Ser at codon 119, Leu-Val at codon 432 and Asn-Ser at codon 453), Arg48Gly and Ala119Ser showed complete linkage disequilibrium (LD) in all the cases and controls. The distribution of the two haplotypes (G-T-C-A and G-T-G-A) was significantly different between cases and controls. The data also indicate modification effect of tobacco or alcohol use on the association between variant genotypes of *CYP1B1* (*CYP1B1**2 and *CYP1B1**3) and risk of SCCHN, suggesting the potential gene-environment interaction [37]. However, the findings from this relatively small study need additional validations.

A *CYP2D6* polymorphism originally described by Ayesh et al. [38] has also been evaluated as a risk factor for SCCHN. CYP2D6 metabolizes a wide range of nitrogen-containing drugs, and also the tobacco-specific nitrosamine, 4-(methylnitrosamino)-1-(3-pyridyl)-1-butanone (NNK), to mutagenic products [39]. Greater than 90% of cases of poor metabolizers can be attributed to three defective allelic *CYP2D6* variants: (1) guanine to adenine (G>A) transition at the junction of intron 3/exon 4 (G1934A), (2) a base-pair deletion in exon 5, and (3) a total gene deletion. The case–control study results for the phenotypic status have been mixed [40, 41]. With genotyping [42], null alleles, slow metabolizing alleles, and a rare, ultrarapid allele have been described [43]. It was reported that there appeared to be a significantly increased frequency of the gene duplication in laryngeal cancer patients [44], and that the *CYP2D6* 1934AA genotype was found to be associated with the development of laryngeal SCC in a Poland case–control study [45], but others reported that this association was with oral cancers only [46] but no excess in risk at all [39, 47, 48].

CYP2E1 metabolizes benzene, *N*-nitrosamines, and other low molecular weight compounds and is readily inducible. A 50-fold variation in the enzymatic activity has been observed [49]. Two RFLPs (Rsa1 and Dra1) have been suggested as genetic risk markers, and significant ethnic differences in the distribution of allele frequencies have also been documented [50] with a very low prevalence in Caucasians. Several studies have evaluated the risk for SCCHN and found an increased risk associated with the c2 homozygous or heterozygous genotype for the Rsa1 polymorphism [51–54], but not in some other studies [22, 36, 45, 47, 55–57]. Only one study that evaluated the Dra1 polymorphism reported an increased risk [51]. Recently, a German group reported that heterozygous genotype of –70G>T polymorphism (*CYP2E1*7B*) was associated with an increased risk of SCCHN in smokers in a case–control study of 312 patients and 300 cancer-free controls [58]. Given the rarity of the *CYP2E1* polymorphic genotype, as evidenced by the published studies reviewed here, future studies with a large sample size would be necessary to have the sufficient power to detect any risk association.

Phase II enzymes: Glutathione S-transferases (GSTs) catalyze the conjugation of glutathione to several electrophilic compounds, including carcinogenic polycyclic aromatic hydrocarbons and cytotoxic drugs. Such conjugated xenobiotics are rendered harmless, and their excretion is enhanced [59]. The presence or absence of the *GSTM1* gene constitutes the polymorphism, and the lack of *GSTM1* null genotype) affects approximately 50% of the Caucasian population [60]. There is a 98–100% correlation between phenotyping and genotyping for *GSTM1* [61].

In two Japanese studies of oral SCC, there appeared to be a dose–response relationship in risk with an increasing tobacco dose [23, 62], but this was not observed in a study of American whites [30]; greater risks associated with SCCHN (OR = 3.1; 95% CI = 1.1–8.5) were reported by small case–control studies [63, 64], but smaller risks (OR = 1.5; 95% CI = 1.0–2.2) were observed in a larger case–control study [65]. In our recent case–control study of 803 SCCHN patients and 839 controls with 84% non-Hispanic whites and 7% African-American and 8% Hispanic-American, the OR for *GSTM1* null genotype and risk of SCCHN was around 1 [66]. However, several meta-analyses or pooled analysis have demonstrated that *GSTM1* null genotype was associated with 1.2–1.5-fold significantly increased risk of SCCHN [31, 32, 67, 68]. In a recent review on 218 publications and three published meta-analyses, the studies on the association between *GSTM1* null genotype and risk of SCCHN, were summarized [69].

The *glutathione S-transferase theta (GSTT1)* has somewhat high activity toward epoxy and peroxide compounds [70]. GSTT1 is important in the detoxification of naturally occurring monohalomethanes as well as the industrial compounds dichloromethane and arylepoxides, such as benzo(a)pyrene found in tobacco [71]. Approximately 60–70% of the general populations are able to carry out this conjugative reaction ("conjugators"), whereas the remaining 30–40% are "nonconjugators." The conjugation is detoxifying with regard to monohalomethanes and ethylene oxide, but conjugation of dihalomethanes to formaldehyde yields a genotoxic intermediate [71].

In an early study of 105 consecutive patients with SCCHN and 99 age- and gender-matched control subjects [64], an association (OR = 2.18) with the *GSTT1* null genotype was found, which was subsequently replicated in a larger and independent frequency-matched study of 162 patients with SCCHN and 315 cancer-free controls (OR=2.27; 95% CI=1.43–3.60 for the *GSTT1* null genotype) [65]. Of great interest were the elevated risks (all above threefold) noted in the presence of combined risk genotypes [64, 65]. In a later published review of 24 studies that evaluated the risk of SCCHN in relation to the *GSTM1* and *GSTT1* null genotypes, the authors concluded that the results were inconsistent with some reporting weak or moderate associations but others reporting no association [72]. A more recent meta-analysis of 21 studies on SCCHN and the *GSTT1* null genotype suggests a borderline risk of SCCHN associated with the *GSTT1* null genotype (adjusted OR=1.2; 95% CI=1.0–1.4) [31], suggesting a possible elevated SCCHN risk associated with the *GSTT1* null genotype.

Glutathione S-transferase Pi (GSTP1) participates in the detoxification of reactive oxygen species by binding to reduced glutathione and maintaining cellular redox balance, and the *GSTP1* gene is often overexpressed in human cancers, including cancer of the esophagus, lung, stomach, colon, bladder, and cervix [32]. A *GSTP1* SNP (A313G, Ile105Val) was first described by Ali-Osman et al. [73], which results in an enzymatic product with reduced detoxification capacity and affinity for the electrophilic substrates. The *GSTP1* 105Val homozygous genotype has been estimated to be present in approximately 10% of the general population. The 105Val/Val homozygous genotype was initially found to be borderline significant in the laryngeal carcinoma subgroup (OR=2.4; 95% CI=1.0–5.9) but not other sites [29], but this finding was not confirmed in our recently published study with 803 SCCHN patients and 839 cancer-free controls (OR=0.92; 95% CI=0.75–1.12) [66] and a meta-analysis of the 105Val polymorphism and SCCHN (a summary OR of 1.1; 95% CI=0.9–1.3) [31].

N-Acetyltransferases (NAT) participate in the metabolism of xenobiotics and carcinogens through the transfer of an acetyl group. Compared with CYPs and GSTs, the involvement of NATs in detoxification is largely limited to the detoxification of amines and hydrazines [32]. The human NAT family includes a pseudogene and two functional genes, *NAT1* and *NAT2,* among these three genes, NAT2 isoenzyme is more restricted in its tissue-expression pattern, being found primarily in the intestine and liver [74]. Few studies have investigated the association between *NAT1* SNPs and SCCHN risk. One study found that the *NAT1**10 homozygous genotype was associated with a decrease in SCCHN risk (OR=0.6; 95% CI=0.2–1.9) in a study of American whites [75], whereas no such risk was found in a German study [76]. Therefore, larger studies are needed to verify these findings.

More than 30 *NAT2* alleles based on 13 SNPs have been reported [32]. The *N*-acetylation polymorphism segregates individuals into rapid, intermediate, and slow acetylator phenotypes via monogenic inheritance of the *NAT2* locus. Approximately 40–70% of Caucasians are of the "slow acetylator" phenotype and are less efficient in the metabolism of agents containing primary aromatic amine or hydrazine groups [77]. Rapid acetylation has been implicated as a risk factor for colon carcinoma. The presence of two germline copies of any of several mutant alleles of the *NAT2* gene produces a slow acetylation phenotype [77, 78]. One study reported that of 120 patients with laryngeal cancer, 84% were slow acetylators as were only 60% of the control group ($P<0.001$) [79]. Other studies also reported that slow NAT2 activity was a risk factor [47, 80], but these findings were not confirmed by several larger studies [45, 76, 81]. A recent review discussed the inconsistent finding of human *N*-Acetyltransferases polymorphisms and risk of cancers including SCCHN [82].

Epoxide Hydrolase: The *mEPHX* gene is located on the long arm of chromosome 1 and is involved in detoxification reactions, in which reactive compounds are converted into more water-soluble products. This cleavage is accomplished by the addition of water to a range of alkenes and arene oxides to form trans-dihydrodiols [83]. Although the products of hydrolysis are less reactive than the parent epoxide, the resultant diol is sometimes a precursor to a more carcinogenic form; thus hydrolysis is not strictly a detoxification pathway [84]. mEPHX has been implicated in the metabolism of B[a]P. Some reported that epoxide hydrolase was significantly less expressed in head and neck tumors than it was in the corresponding adjacent tissue [85]. There are four mEPHX alleles, resulting from the presence or absence of two point mutations in the gene. On one allele, termed the "slow allele"; tyrosine is replaced by histidine at residue 113, because C has been substituted for T with a 40–50% decrease in the enzyme activity [86].

In another allele, termed the "fast allele", arginine replaces histidine at residue 139 because G has been substituted for A, with a 25% increase in enzyme activity [86, 87]. The third allele is the wild-type allele, which has no substitutions. The fourth allele has two variants, one at residue 113 and the other at residue 139. The enzyme activity is normal in both cases [87]. One study suggested that individuals with particularly slow mEPHX activity (homozygotes) may be more susceptible to emphysema than those with more rapid activity [87]. These polymorphic sites could thus also play a role in the etiology of smoking-related cancers. In fact, a small case–control study of smoking-related cancers reported a moderate protective effect of high or intermediate enzyme activity in the heaviest smokers [84], and intermediate and high activity genotypes have been implicated in risk of laryngeal and oropharyngeal cancers [88]. In a recent report of 429 SCCHN patients and 419 healthy subjects, it was found that the 139 Arg/Arg variant of microsomal epoxide hydrolase gene was associated with a significantly higher risk of hypopharyngeal carcinoma compared with controls (OR − 4.39; 95% CI = 1.45–13.35) [89]

Alcohol Dehydrogenase: Ethanol is oxidized by alcohol dehydrogenase [90] to acetaldehyde that has mutagenic properties. Individuals having the fast metabolizing alleles for alcohol dehydrogenase (ADH), *ADH1B*2* and *ADH1C*1*, and the null allele for aldehyde dehydrogenase (ALDH), *ALDH2*2*, are shown to have increased acetylaldehyde levels and thus may have increased risk of SCCHN [91]. An early study found that the risk associated with the $ADH_3^{1\text{-}1}$ (i.e., *ADH1C*1/1*) genotype, compared with the $ADH_3^{1\text{-}2}$ (i.e., *ADH1C*1/2*) and $ADH_3^{2\text{-}2}$ (i.e., *ADH1C*2/2*) genotypes combined, was 5.3-fold (95% CI = 1.0–28.8) among drinkers [92], and a small French study also similarly reported that the $ADH_3^{1\text{-}1}$ was associated with increased risks for oropharyngeal and laryngeal cancers [93].

A later Japanese study of alcoholics found significantly higher frequencies of the variant *ALDH-2* (i.e., *ADH1B*2*) allele in alcoholics with SCCHN (52.9%)

compared with cancer-free alcoholics (9%) [94]. However, another study (229 patients and 575 controls) found no association between *ADH*$_3$ (*ADH1C*) genotype and SCCHN risk [95]. A pooled analysis examined this association using published studies on *ADH1C* [91], in which Asians were found to be most likely to have the fast *ADH1B*2* and *ADH1C*1* alleles, compared with the slow *ADH1B*1/1* and *ADH1C*1/2* genotypes in Caucasians, and the frequent *ALDH2*2* null allele among Asians was rarely observed in other populations; the pooled analysis of 1,325 cases and 1,760 controls suggested that SCCHN risk was not associated with the *ADH1C*1/2* genotype (OR = 1.00; 95% CI = 0.81–1.23) or the *ADH1C*1/1* genotype (OR = 1.14; 95% CI = 0.92–1.41), although several studies reported an increased SCCHN risk associated with the *ADH1B*1/1* and *ALDH2*1/2* genotypes. More recently, a multicenter case–control study of 811 upper aerodigestive tract cancer cases and 1,083 controls conducted in Bucharest (Romania), Lodz (Poland), Moscow (Russia), Banska Bystrika (Slovakia), and Olomouc and Prague (Czech Republic) was conducted to investigate the risk association with six SNPs in *ADH1B, ADH1C,* and *ALDH2* genes [96]. A decreased risk of 0.36 (0.17–0.77) was found to be associated with the *ADH1B* A48H + H48H (fast metabolizers) genotype for medium/heavy drinkers and 0.57 (0.36–0.91) for never/light drinkers, compared with the A48A (slow metabolizers) genotype; similarly, a significantly increased risks of 1.76 (1.13–2.75) and 5.79 (1.49–22.5) were associated with *ALDH2* 348TC and 348CC genotypes, respectively, compared with the 348TT genotype in medium/heavy drinkers; however, the stronger main effects were observed for squamous cell carcinoma of the esophagus that was included in this analysis [96].

There are accumulating effects of genetic variation on the development of SCCHN, gene–gene and gene-environment interactions especially low-penetrance genes. In a recent study with 203 oral squamous cell carcinoma (OSCC) patients and 416 cancer-free controls, the authors found that cases were more frequent with fast NAT2 acetylators (53.7%) than in controls (43.9%; OR = 1.55; 95% CI = 1.08–2.20; $P = 0.03$). Gene-gene interaction testing suggested several cancer-*NAT2* associations, with association strongest among persons without a *CYP1A1* variant (*2C or *4) allele (OR = 1.77; 95% CI = 1.20–2.60; $P = 0.03$) or with a variant *MPO* (463A) allele (OR = 2.38; 95% CI = 1.34–4.21; $P = 0.05$) [97]. In a Poland analysis on genetic polymorphisms of *CYP1A1, GSTM1, GSTP1,* and *GSTT1* in 127 head and neck cancer patients and 151 hospital controls. The authors found nonsignificant increased risk in patients with the *GSTM1* null genotype or *CYP1A1* 462Val alleles or *GSTP1* 105Val alleles and the combination of *CYP1A1* genotypes with the 462Val allele and *GSTP1* genotype with the 105Val allele, and for the combination of *CYP1A1* genotypes with the 462Val allele with the *GSTT1* null genotype.

However, the joint effect of *CYP1A1* 462Val genotypes with the *GSTM1* null genotype significantly increased the risk of SCCHN (OR = 7.15; 95% CI = 1.49–34.32), suggesting the role of metabolic genes' interactions in the development of SCCHN [98]. In a German case–control study on 312 SCCHN cases and 300 non-cancer controls, the authors found that the increased SCCHN risk was associated with *CYP1B1* (Leu432Val) CG genotype and *CYP2E1* (–70G>T) GT genotype

(OR = 10.84; 95% CI = 1.64–71.53) as well as *CYP1B1* (Leu432Val) GG genotype and *GSTM1* null genotype (OR = 11.79; 95% CI = 2.18–63.77). These findings underline the relevance of genotypes of polymorphic *CYP1B1* combined with exposures to tobacco smoke [58].

Mutagen Sensitivity as a Marker of Risk

Chromosomal analyses also have been used to study individual sensitivity to genotoxicity and cancer risk. In a cohort study of 3,182 workers who were occupationally exposed to mutagenic agents, the baseline of chromosomal aberrations were evaluated at the entry into the study, and a statistically significant increase in cancer risk (RR = 2.1) in the highest stratum of baseline aberrations was found in the follow-up [99], suggesting the potential of chromosomal aberrations in peripheral lymphocytes as markers of cancer risk.

Hsu and colleagues [100] developed a mutagen sensitivity assay based on the quantification of *in vitro* bleomycin-induced chromatid breaks in cultured lymphocytes to measure human susceptibility to environmental carcinogens. He reported that patients with SCCHN demonstrated hypersensitivity to *in vitro* bleomycin-induced chromosome breaks compared to cancer-free controls [101–104].

A multicenter meta-analysis of three case–control studies of SCCHN from MD Anderson at Houston, Memorial Sloan-Kettenng Cancer Center at New York, and the Free University Hospital at Amsterdam [105], including Dr. Hsu's studies, demonstrated that there were no differences across institutions in the distribution of mutagen sensitivity measurements and that age and use of tobacco and alcohol did not influence the mutagen sensitivity values either. Heavy smoking in the absence of the hypersensitive phenotype was associated with an OR of 11.5 (95% CI = 5.0–26.6). In heavy smokers who also exhibited mutagen hypersensitivity, OR was 44.6 (9% CI = 17.4–114).

We have modified this assay using benzo(a)pyrene diol epoxide (BPDE, an ultimate carcinogenic metabolite of benzo[a]pyrene) as the challenge mutagen. In a pilot case–control analysis of BPDE-induced mutagen sensitivity and the risk of SCCHN [106], we reported that BPDE-induced chromosome breaks were significantly higher in 60 cases than in 112 controls. On multivariate analysis, BPDE-induced sensitivity was an independent risk factor for SCCHN in a dose-response manner; however, there was no significant difference among cases by stage, site of disease, or treatment status, suggesting BPDE-induced sensitivity was a phenotypic marker of genetic susceptibility not tumor marker. BDPE sensitivity and bleomycin sensitivity have a joint effect on risk of oral premalignant lesions. The underlying mechanism for mutagen sensitivity associated with cancer proneness likely reflects more than an altered repair process [107]. In our another similar analysis with 123 newly recruited patients with SCCHN and 136 controls, using the control median as the cut-off value, high frequency of BPDE-induced chromosome breaks was associated with 1.75-fold (95% CI = 1.04–2.94) elevated risk of SCCHN [108]. These findings from the analyses of small sample sizes have been confirmed by the recently published large study of 895 SCCHN patients and 898 controls frequency-matched by age, sex, and ethnicity [109]. However, we do not know how mutagen sensitivity as measured in lymphocytes reflects the DNA repair capacity in the target tissue.

DNA Repair Phenotype as a Marker of Risk

DNA repair phenotype has been measured by several assays developed over the last decades. One is the DNA repair capacity (DRC) that can be measured by the host cell reactivation (HCR) assay in which the expression level of a damaged reporter gene as a marker of repair proficiency in the host cell can be quantitatively measured [110, 111]. This assay uses undamaged or normal cells in culture, is relatively fast, and is an objective way of measuring the repair phenotype [110]. In the assay, a damaged nonreplicating recombinant plasmid (pCMV*cat*) harboring a chloramphenicol acetyltransferase reporter gene is introduced by transfection into primary lymphocytes. Reactivated chloramphenicol acetyltransferase enzyme activity is measured as a function of nucleotide excision repair of the damaged bacterial gene [110]. Measured by this assay, both lymphocytes [112] and skin fibroblasts [113] from patients who have basal cell carcinoma but not XP have lower excision-repair rates of an UV-damaged reporter gene than individuals without cancer. This finding suggests that the repair capacity of lymphocytes can be considered a reflection of an individual's overall repair capacity.

The host-cell reactivation assay in parallel with the mutagen sensitivity assay was performed in 16 established lymphoblastoid cell lines that included three head and neck cancer cell lines [114]. In this study using ultraviolet radiation and 4 nitroquinoline oxide (4NQO) as the test mutagens, reduced cellular DNA repair capacity was significantly correlated with increased frequency of mutagen-induced chromatid breaks. In a separate study of 20 lymphoblastoid cell lines (9 from SCCHN patients and 11 from cancer-free individuals), a correlation between the host cell reactivation assay and mutagen sensitivity was also found when BPDE and bleomycin were used as the test mutagens [115].

In a pilot study of the HCR assay using BPDE as the test agent [116], the DRC of SCCHN cases ($n=55$) was found to be significantly lower than that of the controls ($P<0.001$).

Earlier epidemiologic studies have revealed the association between *in vivo* and *in vitro* BPDE-DNA adducts and smoking related cancers [117]. We have evaluated the association between levels of *in vitro* BPDE-induced adducts in peripheral blood lymphocytes (PBLs) and SCCHN risk [66, 118]. In a pilot study of 91 patients with SCCHN and 115 controls, we measured *in vitro* BPDE-induced DNA adducts in short-term cultured PBLs. BPDE-DNA adduct levels were significantly higher in the cases than in the controls. Sixty-six percentages of cases had higher levels than the mean value of controls. BPDE-induced DNA adducts was associated with 2.22-fold (95% CI = 1.22–4.04) increased risk of SCCHN, indicating that the level of *in vitro* BPDE-induced DNA-adducts was an independent risk factor for SCCHN [118]. To validate these findings, we performed another large, independent study that included 803 patients with SCCHN and 839 controls. We found that the mean BPDE-DNA adduct levels were significantly higher in the cases (77.6 ± 111.8) than in the controls (57.3 ± 98.3; $P < 0.001$). Using the median control value (29.22) as a cutoff, 63% of the cases were distributed above this level (OR = 1.71, 95% CI = 1.39–2.10, after adjustment for age, sex, smoking status, drinking status, and GST genotypes in a logistic regression model) [66].

However, it is unclear whether there is a genetic basis for the variation in these phenotypes measured in the general populations. In a recent study, we assessed the association between levels of *in vitro* BPDE-induced DNA adducts and genotypes of SNPs of the NER (nucleotide excision repair) genes *ERCC1* (rs3212986 and rs11615) and *ERCC2/XPD* (rs13181, rs1799793 and rs238406) in 707 healthy non-Hispanic whites [119]. We found that the median DNA adduct levels for the *ERCC2* rs1799793 GG, GA, and AA genotypes were 23, 29, and 30, respectively ($P_{trend} = 0.057$), but this trend was not observed for other SNPs. After adjustment for covariates, adduct values larger than the median value were significantly associated with the genotypes *ERCC1* rs3212986TT (OR = 1.89, 95% CI = 1.03–3.48), *ERCC2/XPD* rs238406AA (OR = 0.64, 95% CI = 0.41–0.99), and rs238406CA (OR = 0.63, 95% CI = 0.45–0.89) compared with their corresponding wild-type homozygous genotypes. These results suggest that the genotypes in DNA repair genes may have an effect on the measured DNA repair phenotypes.

It is well known that at least 150 genes participate in various DNA repair pathways, and thus the alteration of the key gene expression in RNA or protein levels may have an influence on DNA repair functions and lead to the altered cancer risk. In two previous pilot case–control studies of SCCHN, we found that lower mRNA expression levels of several DNA repair genes of both the mismatch repair pathway [120] and the NER pathway [121] measured by multiplex reverse transcription-PCR assays were associated with an increased risk of SCCHN. Recently, we quantified NER protein levels in the cell extracts of lymphocytes using a reverse-phase protein microarray [122]. The results suggested that XPF may be a crucial rate-limiting factor in DNA repair and that the reverse-protein microarray assay may be a useful tool for measuring protein markers of susceptibility to cancer [122]. Taken together, these results suggest that individuals with low expression levels of DNA repair genes may be at a higher risk of developing SCCHN.

DNA Repair Gene Polymorphisms

Genetic polymorphisms of DNA repair genes may also contribute to individual variation in DNA repair capacity. Tobacco carcinogen BPDE-induced DNA damage is effectively removed by the NER pathway that involves more than 20 proteins, but only 8 of which are considered the core NER proteins (i.e., ERCC1, XPA, XPB, XPC, XPD, XPE, XPF and XPG) [123], and mutations in any of these genes encoding the proteins, except for ERCC1, cause the well-known XP disease phenotype that is associated with more than 1,000-fold increased risk of skin cancer [124].

To date, the entire coding regions of several NER genes have been re-sequenced, and numerous single nucleotide polymorphisms (SNPs) have been identified to date in the eight core genes (i.e., *ERCC1*, *XPA*, *XPB*, *XPC*, *XPD*, *XPE*, *XPF*, and *XPG*) of the NER pathway http://www.ncbi.nlm.nih.gov/SNP/ (http://egp.gs.washington.edu/directory.html). In these identified SNPs, there are a total of 40 nonsynonymous SNPs (nsSNPs), but only five are confirmed as common (i.e., minor allele frequency >=0.05) nsSNPs (i.e., *XPC* Ala499Val [rs2228000] and Lys939Gln [rs2228001], *XPD* Asp312Asn [rs1799793] and Lys751Gln [rs13181], and *XPG* His1104Asp [rs17655]) and have been studied for their association with cancer risk. Other than these nsSNPs, two common regulatory SNPs located at the 3′UTR region of *ERCC1* (C8092A, rs3212986) and 5′UTR region of *XPA* (G23A, rs1800975) were also suggested to be associated with cancer risk [125]. Most studies of the association between these SNPs and risk of SCCHN and the effects of NER genotypes on the DRC phenotype have been summarized in a recent review [125]. Here, we present only those newer studies that were not included in this review.

One study investigated both *XRCC1* and *XPD* polymorphisms in 110 oral carcinoma cases, 84 leukoplakia and 110 controls in the Travancore South Indian population and found that the variant alleles of *XRCC1* codon 399 and *XPD* codon 751 were associated with higher risk of oral cancer in smokers and betel quid chewers than in nonsmokers and nonchewers [126]. Another study of 106 cases and 164 healthy controls in Thailand found that the variant genotypes of *XPD* exon 6 were associated with increased risk of OSCC in females (OR = 3.93; 95% CI = 1.14–13.6) but not in males [127], whereas one Japanese case–control study with 122 patients with OSCC and 241 controls evaluated five SNPs, each in one of the *XPA*, *XPC*, *XPC*, *XPF*, and *ERCC1* genes and found that only the *XPA* 5′UTR AG and *ERCC1* 3′UTR GA heterozygotes had significantly altered risk of OSCC [128]. In a Taiwanese study of 154 oral cancer patients and 105 age-matched controls, *XPA* 5′ UTR G23A and *XPD* Lys751Gln polymorphisms and smoking status were found to have a synergistic effect on oral cancer risk [129]. In the recent German case–control study on 312 SCCHN cases and 300 cancer-free controls, it also showed the effect of *XPD* Lys751Gln polymorphism on risk of SCCHN in never smokers [58]. We performed a large study of 829 SCCHN cases and 854 cancer-free controls by genotyping for seven selected common nonsynonymous and regulatory variants in the NER core genes, i.e., 5 nsSNPs (*XPC* Ala499Val and Lys939Gln, *XPD* Asp312Asn and Lys751Gln, and *XPG* His1104Asp) and two common regulatory SNPs located at the 3′UTR region of *ERCC1* C8092A and 5′UTR region of *XPA*; we found that only carriers of the *XPC* 499Val/Val genotype had a significantly increased SCCHN risk (OR = 1.65; 95% CI = 1.16–2.36).

In an analysis of the joint effects, however, the number of observed risk genotypes was associated with SCCHN risk in a dose-response manner ($P = 0.017$) [130]. It is clear that the SNPs in the NER pathway may play a role in the etiology of SCCHN, but large, population-based, preferably prospective studies are needed to confirm published data to date. A recent meta-analysis of *XPC* polymorphisms suggested that *XPC* pat+ allele might increase risk of SCCHN [131]. A recent review summarized the association between genetic polymorphisms of genes involved in DNA repair, cell cycle, xenobiotic metabolism, and growth factor pathway and outcomes of SCCHN [132]. Three genetic polymorphisms *CCND1* A870G, *XRCC1* Arg399Gln, and *FGFR4* Gly388Arg, which are well-known polymorphisms implicating prognosis in other cancers, were suggested to be validated for their associations with survival outcomes in large studies [132].

Cigarette smoke consists of hundreds of carcinogens that can cause reactive oxygen species, resulting in single-base lesions and single and double-strand breaks in DNA that can lead to cancer [133]. The base lesions and single strand breaks are repaired mainly by the base-excision repair (BER) pathway that includes a number of DNA repair enzymes, of which APE1, ADPRT, and XRCC1 proteins play key roles [134], whereas two other pathways exist to repair double-strand breaks, i.e., the homologous recombination repair (HHR), involving a number of proteins including RAD51, XRCC2, XRCC3, RAD51B, RAD51C, and RAD51D [135], and the nonhomologous end-joining (NHEJ), involving the DNA-dependent protein kinase complex (DNA-PK) including KU70 and KU80 proteins encoded by the *XRCC6* and *XRCC5* genes, respectively [136].

In a small study conducted in India, the variant allele of *XRCC1* Arg399Gln was found to be associated with higher risk of oral cancer in smokers and betel quid chewers than in nonsmokers and nonchewers [126], while the variant *XRCC3* 241Met was associated with increased risk of OSCC in a Thailand study [127]. In a US study of 279 OSCC patients with genotyping data on *XRCC1* Arg399Gln, *XRCC3* Thr241Met, *XPD* Lys751Gln, and *MGMT* Leu84Phe and Val143Ile, it was found that *XRCC3* 241Met allele was associated with an increased risk of second neoplasms, whereas the *XRCC1* 399Gln allele was associated with a decreased risk of all-cause mortality [137]. In an early US study of *XRCC1* SNPs and SCCHN risk, a markedly decreased OR for the Gln/Gln genotype among whites (OR=0.1; 95% CI=0.04–0.6) and blacks (OR=0.01; 95% CI=0.0004–0.3) was found as well as a suggestive interaction between the Arg194Trp and Arg399Gln polymorphisms and tobacco use [138]. However, in a study of 305 SCCHN cases and 319 controls of non-Hispanic whites, we did not find evidence of risk associated with the *XRCC1* Arg399Gln and *APE* Asp148Glu polymorphisms or with the *XRCC3* 241Met allele [139] in a much larger study of 853 SCCHN patients and 854 controls of non-Hispanic white subjects, but we found that a significantly decreased risk of SCCHN was associated with the *ADPRT762* Ala/Ala (OR=0.51; 95% CI=0.27–0.97), compared with the *ADPRT762* Val/Val genotype [140].

In a French study of *XRCC2* Arg188His and *XRCC3* Thr241Met polymorphisms in 121 oral/pharynx cancer cases, 129 larynx cancer cases, and 172 noncancer controls, all Caucasians were smokers, only the *XRCC2* His-allele was found to be associated with an increased risk of pharyngeal cancer (OR=2.9; 95% CI=1.3–6.2), whereas a reduced risk of supraglottic cancer was found for carriers of the *XRCC3*Met variant allele (OR = 0.3; 95% CI = 0.2–0.7) [141]. A Belgian research group performed a case–control study with 152 Caucasian SCCHN patients and 157 healthy controls matched for age, gender, and ethnicity [142]. It was found that significant positive association between the *XRCC3* Thr241Met polymorphism was significantly associated with increased risk of SCCHN with an adjusted OR of 1.96 (P = 0.02). However, the *LIG4* Thr9Ile and the *RAD51* 5′_UTR-135 G>C polymorphisms were associated with a significant reduced risk for SCCHN (OR = 0.43, P = 0.01; OR = 0.43, P = 0.05, respectively), especially among the heavy smokers for the *RAD51* −135G>C polymorphism [142]. In our another published study of *RAD51* and *p53* SNPs and risk of SCCHN in 716 SCCHN patients and 719 matched controls (all non-Hispanic whites), we reported a significantly decreased SCCHN risk (OR = 0.66; 95% CI = 0.50–0.87) associated with *RAD51* 172TT homozygotes compared with carriers of other genotypes, particularly among *p53* Arg72Arg homozygotes (OR = 0.60; 95% CI = 0.41–0.89) (homogeneity test P = 0.047) [143]. Recently, a Taiwanese research group reported that polymorphisms of *XRCC4* and *ERCC6* are associated with increased risk of oral cancer in Taiwanese [144, 145]. Another research group in Taiwan also reported the combined effect of *XRCC1-4* SNPs on oral cancer risk [146].

Another important gene, human *OGG1* (*hOGG1*), encodes a DNA glycosylase that is involved in the excision repair of 8-hydroxy-2′-deoxyguanine (8-OH-dG) from oxidatively-damaged DNA. One study of 169 Caucasian orolaryngeal cancer cases and 338 controls found that a significantly increased risk for orolaryngeal cancer was associated with both the *hOGG1* 326(Ser)/326(Cys) (OR = 1.6; 95% CI = 1.04–2.6) and *hOGG1* 326(Cys)/326(Cys) (OR = 4.1; 95% CI = 1.3–13) genotypes [147]. In another Japanese study of 192 SCCHN patients, an association between the Cys/Cys genotype and HNSCC with heavy smoking (>40 pack-years) was reported (OR = 8.10, 95% CI = 1.06–61.73) [148]. However, these finding was not confirmed by our larger study of 706 SCCHN cases and 1,196 controls of non-Hispanic whites [149].

Finally, we recently published a study on *NEIL1* and *NEIL2* common variants and risk of squamous cell carcinomas of the oral cavity and oropharynx (SCCOOP) [150] Human DNA glycosylases NEIL1 and NEIL2 participate in oxidized base excision repair and protect cells from DNA damage. We genotyped and estimated haplotypes of the *NEIL1* rs7182283 G>T and rs4462560 C>G and *NEIL2* rs804270 C>G polymorphisms for 872 patients with SCCOOP and 1,044 cancer-free non-Hispanic white control subjects frequency-matched by age and sex. We found no overall differences in the frequencies of alleles, genotypes, and haplotypes of *NEIL1* rs7182283 G>T and rs4462560 C>G polymorphisms between cases and controls. However, the *NEIL2* rs804270 CC genotype was associated with a significantly increased risk of SCCOOP (adjusted OR = 1.30; 95% CI = 1.02–1.65) [150].

Overall, it appeared that there is a publication bias in the early reports for an elevated SCCHN risk associated with SNPs of DNA repair genes in small case–control studies that tended not to be confirmed by the later large studies. Therefore, large, population-based, preferably prospective studies are needed to confirm published data, although such large studies may be a challenge because SCCHN cancers are relatively rare.

Polymorphisms of Genes Involved in One-Carbon Metabolic Pathway

Folate, one of the constituents of vegetables and fruits, provides methyl groups required for intracellular methylation reactions and DNA synthesis. Several key enzymes are involved in folate-related metabolism. These enzymes include methylenetetrahydrofolate reductase (MTHFR), which catalyzes folate metabolic transformation to 5-methyltetrahydrofolate that converts methionine to S-adenosylmethionine, the universal methyl donor; thymidylate synthase (TYMS) is involved in the use of methyl group in pyrimidine synthesis; and methionine synthase (MTR) and methionine synthase reductase (MTRR) are involved in the use of methyl group in the methylation of macromolecules [151]. The serine hydroxymethyltransferase (SHMT) catalyses the reversible conversion of serine and tetrahydrofolate to glycine and 5,10-methylene tetrahydrofolate [152–154]. Human SHMT genes code for two different isoforms of proteins: the cytosolic SHMT (cSHMT or SHMT1) and the mitochondrial SHMT (mSHMT or SHMT2) [155].

As shown in Table 1, there are numerous SNPs reported for the *MTHFR*, *TYMS*, *MTR*, *MTRR*, and *SHMT1* genes (reported in http://www.ncbi.nlm.nih.gov/sites/entrez), but only a few are common, putatively functional and have been studied for their associations with SCCHN risk. In a series of published studies of over 700 cases and over 1,000 controls, we investigated the role of selected SNPs in these genes in the etiology of SCCHN. As summarized in Table 1, among the SNPs investigated, we found that the AC heterozygous and CC homozygous genotypes of the *MTHFR* 1298A>C SNP [156], the 0bp/0bp genotype of the *TYMS* 3′UTR variant [157], and the AA genotype of the *MTRR* 66G>A SNP [158] were associated with statistically lower risk of SCCHN compared with their wild-type homozygous genotypes, respectively. The combination of variant alleles of SNPs in each gene showed certain significant associations with risk of SCCHN (Table 1). The associations between *MTHFR*, *MTR*, *MTRR* SNPs, and risk of SCCHN have also been reported by a Japanese and an Italian research groups even though with smaller sample sizes [159, 160].

Polymorphisms of Genes Involved in Cell Cycle Control and Apoptosis

Because carcinogenesis of the head and neck also involves abnormalities in cell cycle control [161], polymorphisms of cell cycle genes are good candidates for investigations of genetic susceptibility to SCCHN. Normal cell-cycle control

Table 1 Associations of genetic variants in genes involved in folate metabolism and risk of SCCHN

Gene/ polymorphism rs#	Genotype (No. of cases/ controls)	OR (95% CI)[a]	No. of variant alleles (No. of cases/controls)	OR (95% CI)[a]	Reference
MTHFR	CC (258/278)	1.00	0–1[b] (97/158)	1.00	[156]
677C>T	CT (244/216)	1.21 (0.9–1.6)	2 (233/197)	1.85 (1.3–2.5)	
rs1801133	TT (35/51)	0.72 (0.5–1.2)	3 (170/143) ≥	1.93 (1.4–2.7)	
MTHFR	AA (328/274)	1.00	4 (37/47)	1.25 (0.8–2.1)	
1298A>C	AC (199/240)	0.69 (0.5–0.9)			
rs1801131	CC (10/31)	0.28 (0.1–0.6)			
MTHFR	GG (490/507)	1.00			
1793G>A	GA (47/37)	1.35 (0.9–2.1)			
rs2274976	AA (0/1)	–			
MTR	AA (472/876)	1.00	0[c] (76/200)	1.00	[158]
2756A>G	AG (232/327)	1.31 (1.07–1.60)	1 (281/486)	1.47 (1.08–1.99)	
rs1805087	GG (17/31)	1.00 (0.55–1.84)	2 (276/420)	1.67 (1.23–2.27)	
MTRR 66G>A	GG (231/369)	1.00	3 or 4 (88/128)	1.74 (1.18–2.54)	
rs1801394	GA (376/589)	1.02 (0.82–1.26)			
	AA (114/276)	0.68 (0.52–0.90)			
SHMT1	CC (330/575)	1.00	0[d] (265/553)	1.00	[189]
34761C>T	CT (294/522)	0.99 (0.81–1.20)	1–3 (355/537)	1.39 (1.14–1.70)	
rs1979277	TT (97/137)	1.22 (0.91–1.64)	4–6 (101/144)	1.49 (1.09–1.97)	
SHMT1	CC (337/585)	1.00			
34840C>G	CG (303/516)	1.03 (0.84–1.25)			
rs3783	GG (81/133)	1.05 (0.77–1.43)			
SHMT1	CC (315/569)	1.00			
34859C>T	CT (323/528)	1.11 (0.91–1.35)			
rs1979276	TT (83/137)	1.10 (0.81–1.49)			
TYMS	3R3R (184/313)	1.00	0[e] (109/173)	1.00	[157]
TSER	2R3R (374/526)	1.23 (0.98–1.55)	1 (209/310)	1.08 (0.80–1.46)	
rs34743033	2R2R (146/246)	1.01 (0.77–1.33)	2 (236/354)	1.08 (0.80–1.56)	
TYMS	6bp/6bp	1.00	3 (120/168)	1.11 (0.79–1.56)	
TS3′UTR	(339/517)	1.07 (0.87–1.31)	4 (30/80)	0.60 (0.37–0.98)	
rs34489327	6bp/0bp	0.67 (0.47–0.94)			
	(311/446)				
	0bp/0bp (54/122)				

[a]Adjusted for age, sex, smoking status and drinking status

[b]The numbers 0 to ≥4 represent the numbers of variants within the haplotype genotypes, i.e., 0 = no variant and 1 to ≥ 4 = 1 to ≥4 variants; the variant (risk) alleles used for the calculation were 677T, 1298A and 1793A

[c]The combined *MTR AA* and *MTRR AA* genotype had zero risk allele of either gene; the *MTR AA* and *MTRR GA* or *MTR AG/MTRR AA* genotype had only one risk allele; the *MTR AA* and *MTRR GG* or *MTR AG* and *MTRR GA* or *MTR GG* and *MTRR AA* had two risk alleles; and *MTR AG* and *MTRR GG* or *MTR GG* and *MTRR GA* or *MTR GG/MTRR GG* had three or four risk alleles

[d]The numbers 0–6 represent the number of variants within the 22 haplotype genotypes (i.e. 0 = no variant and 1–6 = 1–6 variants); the variant (risk) alleles used for the calculation were 34761T, 34840G and 34859T

[e]The combined *TSER* 2R2R and *TS3′ UTR* 6bp/6bp genotype had zero protective alleles of *TS* gene; the *TSER* 2R3R and *TS3_UTR* 6bp/6bp or *TSER* 2R2R and *TS3_UTR* 6bp/0bp had one protective allele; *TSER* 3R3R and *TS3_UTR* 6bp/6bp or *TSER* 2R3R and *TS3_UTR* 6bp/0bp or *TSER* 2R2R and *TS3_UTR* 0bp/0bp had two protective alleles; *TSER* 3R3R and *TS3_UTR* 6bp/0bp or *TSER* 2R3R and *TS3_UTR* 0bp/0bp had three protective alleles; and *TSER* 3R3R and *TS3_UTR* 0bp/0bp had four protective alleles

ensures a delay in the cell cycle allowing DNA damage to be repaired before the cell begins the process of growth, mitosis, and division. Those cells with unrepairable DNA damage will undergo apoptosis, a process also called programmed cell death [162].

The transition through G1 to S phase of the cell cycle is regulated by cyclin dependent kinases (CDKs). Cyclin D1 (CCND1) is a key regulatory protein, playing a critical role in the transition from the G1 phase to the S phase of the cell cycle [163]. Activation and overexpression of CCND1 have been found in a variety of tumors, including head and neck cancers [164]. There is something missing here that creates an alternative splice site in its mRNA, encoding a protein with an altered C-terminal domain. Our early study found that a G→A polymorphism (870G>A) in exon 4 of the *CCND1* modulates individual susceptibility to SCCHN in 233 SCCHN patients and 248 controls [165]. In a Poland study of 63 patients with larynx cancer and 102 healthy controls, the genotypes with A allele were associated with an over twofold increased risk of larynx cancer compared to the GG genotype [166]. The cyclin-dependent kinase inhibitor gene p21 (Waf1/Cip1) induces cellular growth arrest, terminal differentiation, and apoptosis. Polymorphisms that cause amino acid change may lead to alterations in the gene function and therefore may affect the regulation of cell cycle and increase susceptibility for cancer.

In another study, Ralhan et al. [167] described a novel polymorphism in the *p21* (*Waf1/Cip1*) gene identified in an Indian population. An A→G transition at codon 149 resulted in an amino acid substitution from aspartate to glycine in the proliferating cell nuclear antigen binding COOH-terminal domain of p21 (Waf1/Cip1) that may affect PCNA-p21 (Waf1/Cip1) interactions, thereby affecting the regulation of cellular proliferation. They found that this codon 149 polymorphism variant was identified in 11 of 30 (37%) premalignant lesions (7 of 19 hyperplastic lesions and 4 of 11 dysplastic lesions) and 11 of 30 (37%) squamous cell carcinomas (SCCs), whereas only 7 of 50 (14%) unrelated age- and gender-matched healthy subjects had this variant allele. This *p21* variant was more likely to be identified in those patients, whose tumors did not have p53 mutations, suggesting a p53-independent role for this p21 variant in the pathogenesis of oral cancer.

In a series of published studies of over 700 cases and over 1,000 controls, we investigated the role of selected SNPs in these genes in the etiology of SCCHN. As summarized in Table 2, among other SNPs investigated, we found that variant genotypes of the *p73* GC/AT [168], *p21* 70TC and 98AC [169], *FAS* −1377G>A (but not *FAS* −670 A>G, *FASLG* −844 C>T and *FASLG* IVS2nt −124 A>G) [170], and *CASP3* rs4647601:G>T (but not *CASP3* rs4647602:C>A and *CASP3* rs4647603:G>A) [171] were associated with risks of SCCHN compared with their wild-type homozygous genotypes, respectively.

p27 (also known as CDKN1B), a cyclin-dependent kinase inhibitor, regulates progression from G1 to S phase, plays an important role in modulating cell-cycle control, apoptosis, and cell growth. Abnormalities in p27 may affect cell cycle delay required for DNA repair in response to exposure to carcinogens. Because reduced DNA repair is associated with risk of SCCHN, *p27* variants may play a role in the development of SCCHN. A coding exon 1 polymorphism at codon 109 (T→G)

Table 2 Risk of SCCHN associated with polymorphisms of genes involved in cell cycle control and apoptosis

Gene/SNP/Variant	SCCHN cases *n*	SCCHN cases %	Controls *n*	Controls %	Adjusted OR[a] (95% CI)
Cell-cycle control regulation					
p73 rs2273953-rs1801173 G4C14>A4T14	708	100	1,229	100	
GC/GC	399	56.4	773	62.9	1.00
GC/AT	271	38.3	387	31.5	1.36 (1.12–1.66)
AT/AT	38	5.4	69	5.6	1.11 (0.73–1.69)
p21 rs1059234 70C>T	712	100	1,222	100	
CC	596	84	1,080	88	1.00
TC	110	15	136	11	1.47 (1.12–1.93)
TT	6	1	6	1	2.01 (0.64–6.31)
p21 rs1801270 98C>A	712	100	1,222	100	
CC	599	84	1,074	88	1.00
AC	104	15	141	11	1.32 (1.00–1.73)
AA	9	1	7	1	2.50 (0.92–6.81)
Apoptosis pathways					
FAS rs2234767 −1377G>A	721	100	1,234	100	
GG	562	78	957	78	1.00
AG	142	20	264	21	0.91 (0.73–1.15)
AA	17	2	13	1	2.23 (1.07–4.64)
CASP3 rs4647601:G>T	930	100	993	100	
GG	314	34	365	37	1.00
GT	435	47	463	47	1.08 (0.88–1.33)
TT	181	19	165	16	1.32 (1.00–1.73)

[a]Adjusted for age, sex, smoking status, and drinking status [168–171]

in *p27* was identified and may have an effect on the functions of its protein. We tested the association of this polymorphism with the risk of SCCHN in a hospital-based case–control study of 713 non-Hispanic white patients newly diagnosed with SCCHN and 1,189 cancer-free controls frequency matched to the cases by age (±5 years), sex, and smoking status. We found that the variant *p27* 109GG was associated with a non-statistically significantly increased risk of SCCHN compared with the *p27* 109VV (crude OR = 1.29; 95% CI = 0.88–1.90; adjusted OR = 1.20; 95% CI = 0.81–1.77), but this risk was significantly increased among male subjects (adjusted OR = 1.55, 95% CI = 1.00–2.42), current alcohol users (adjusted OR = 1.68, 95% CI = 1.01–2.82) and limited to oral cavity cancer (adjusted OR = 1.77, 95% CI = 1.03–3.04). The risk was also associated with tumor stage and increased with the progression of OSCC. These findings suggest that the *p27* variant 109GG genotype may not play a major role in the etiology of SCCHN but may contribute to a subset of SCCHN [172].

Among many cell cycle regulatory genes (cyclins, cyclin dependent kinases, cyclin dependent kinase inhibitors, various tumor suppressors), perhaps the two most critical tumor suppressor genes are *p53* and *Rb*. The Rb protein is a critical effector of DNA damage checkpoint function by eliciting G1-phase cell cycle arrest, while *p53* controls cell cycle progression via regulation of several important genes including *p21*, *MDM2*, *GADD45*, *BAX*, *c-Myc*, and *BCL2* [173] and induces apoptosis or G_1 cell-cycle arrest [174]. The loss of function of the p53 pathway or the Rb pathway results in the loss of cell cycle control, leading to the loss of checkpoint integrity, allowing unchecked progression through the cell cycle, toward proliferation, instead of being arrested to repair DNA damage or to undergo apoptosis [175]. This loss of homeostatic control is the basis for human malignancies including SCCHN. Smoking and alcohol are necessary but may not be sufficient to cause SCCHN development, individual differences in individual variations of genes in cell cycle checkpoint control may play a critical role in determining the fate of such exposures and understanding susceptibility to SCCHN.

p53 alterations may result from both somatic mutations and germline variations [176, 177]. Mutant p53 protein and processed mutant peptide may alter the cellular and humoral immunity in SCCHN [178]. A common SNP of *p53* at codon 72 in exon 4 results in a substitution of Pro for Arg in the transactivation domain [179]. The common Arg variant allele may alter the susceptibility of p53 to oncogenic proteins, such as HPV E6 and *MDM2*, for its degradation [180, 181]. In case–control analyses, the polymorphism of p53 codon 72 has been reported to be associated with HPV-associated oropharynx [182–184]. In our recent analysis on 814 SCCHN non-Hispanic white patients and 934 cancer-free controls, while there was no evidence of associations between *BAX* (−248 G>A), *BCL2* (−938 C>A) or *p53* codon 72 SNPs and SCCHN risk in single-locus analyses, further analyses showed that, among *p53* heterozygotes after adjustment for age, sex and smoking and alcohol status, the *BAX* AA genotype was associated with an elevated risk of SCCHN (OR = 6.60; 95% CI = 1.38–31.50) compared with the *BAX* GG genotype or OR = 6.58; 95% CI = 1.38–31.49 compared with the combined genotypes (GG + AG), whereas *BCL2* A variant genotypes were associated with a decreased risk of SCCHN (adjusted OR = 0.68; 95% CI = 0.47–0.98 for CA vs. CC and OR = 0.67; 95% CI = 0.48–0.95 for AA vs. CA + CC). These altered risks appeared to be consistent with the roles of the antiapoptotic BCL2 and the pro-apoptotic BAX. Our data suggest that the risk of SCCHN may be associated with these two SNPs of *BAX* and *BCL2* promoter regions, particularly among *p53* heterozygotes [185]. In another analysis, we reported that *p53BP1* (*p53* binding protein 1) variants may have protective effects on SCCHN risk, but such effects were confined to *p53* variant allele/haplotype carriers [186].

p73, a member of the p53 family, activates the promoters of several p53-responsive genes participating in cell-cycle control, DNA repair, and apoptosis, and p73 inhibits cell growth in a p53-like manner by inducing apoptosis or G_1 cell cycle arrest [174]. It is possible that *p73* germ-line variants could possess similar function to that of p53 in modifying the risk for SCCHN. As expected, the two linked non-coding exon 2 polymorphisms of *p73* at positions 4 (G>A) and 14 (C>T) are thought to affect p73 function by altering gene expression, perhaps by altering the efficiency of translational initiation (Kaghad et al., 1997), and is associated with a statistically significantly increased risk for SCCHN (OR = 1.33; 95% CI = 1.10–1.60). The significantly increased risk was more pronounced in younger individuals (younger than 50 years), women, and smokers [168].

Because of limited space for this review, many other relevant studies could not be included here. However, there are several other recent review articles that may provide additional detailed information about the role of genetic variants in the etiology of SCCHN [32, 69, 132, 187].

Risk Prediction Model and Genome-Wide Association Studies

Although smoking tobacco and alcohol use are clearly the dominant risk factors for SCCHN, evaluation of these known risk factors with host-specific risk factors is of great importance in defining the risk. SCCHN occurs largely in the exposed individuals who are susceptible to that exposure. Therefore, host factors involved in the metabolism of tobacco and alcohol related carcinogens and DNA damage and repair are critical in the risk assessment. In particular, phenotype assessment of biological pathways and genotype assessment of genes involved in these biological pathways are of great value in building the risk assessment model. It is now feasible to perform whole genome association studies that aim at identifying new genes or SNPs that are disease specific so that the gene-environment interactions can be evaluated more precisely. However, it is most likely that multiple susceptibility factors must be accounted for to represent the true dimensions of gene-environment interactions in the etiology of SCCHN.

The ability to identify smokers or drinkers with the highest risks of developing SCCHN has substantial preventive implications. These subgroups could be targeted for the most intensive smoking and drinking cessation interventions, could be enrolled into chemoprevention trials, and might be suitable for more aggressive screening programs not appropriate for the general population. Finally, studying susceptibility to common cancers and widely prevalent exposures may provide further insights into the basic mechanisms of carcinogenesis. This knowledge is essential for the design of future epidemiologic and intervention studies.

As we described in a recent review [188], several published genome-wide association studies of lung cancer provide us additional opportunities to correlate genotypes and phenotypes of DNA repair. In addition, genome-wide association studies of SCCHN are currently ongoing. Therefore, the combination of the new high-throughput techniques such as genome-wide scans, epigenetic profiling, transcriptional profiling, and proteomics studies will provide powerful approaches for molecular epidemiological association studies in predicting SCCHN risk.

Acknowledgements This work was supported in part by National Institutes of Health grants R01 CA100264 (Q. Wei), R01 ES11740 (Q. Wei), and R01 CA131274 (Q. Wei).

References

1. Blot WJ, McLaughlin JK, Winn DM, Austin DF, Greenberg RS, Preston-Martin S, Bernstein L, Schoenberg JB, Stemhagen A, Fraumeni JF Jr (1988) Smoking and drinking in relation to oral and pharyngeal cancer. Cancer Res 48:3282–3287
2. Ankathil R, Mathew A, Joseph F, Nair MK (1996) Is oral cancer susceptibility inherited? Report of five oral cancer families. Eur J Cancer B Oral Oncol 32B:63–67
3. Foulkes WD, Brunet JS, Kowalski LP, Narod SA, Franco EL (1995) Family history of cancer is a risk factor for squamous cell carcinoma of the head and neck in Brazil: a case–control study. Int J Cancer 63:769–773
4. Morita M, Kuwano H, Nakashima T, Taketomi A, Baba H, Saito T, Tomoda H, Egashira A, Kawaguchi H, Kitamura K, Sugimachi K (1998) Family aggregation of carcinoma of the hypopharynx and cervical esophagus: special reference to multiplicity of cancer in upper aerodigestive tract. Int J Cancer 76:468–471
5. Morita M, Saeki H, Mori M, Kuwano H, Sugimachi K (2002) Risk factors for esophageal cancer and the multiple occurrence of carcinoma in the upper aerodigestive tract. Surgery 131:S1–S6
6. Foulkes WD, Brunet JS, Sieh W, Black MJ, Shenouda G, Narod SA (1996) Familial risks of squamous cell carcinoma of the head and neck: retrospective case–control study. BMJ 313:716–721
7. Brown LM, Gridley G, Diehl SR, Winn DM, Harty LC, Otero EB, Fraumeni JF Jr, Hayes RB (2001) Family cancer history and susceptibility to oral carcinoma in Puerto Rico. Cancer 92:2102–2108
8. Goldstein AM, Blot WJ, Greenberg RS, Schoenberg JB, Austin DF, Preston Martin S, Winn DM, Bernstein L, McLaughlin JK, Fraumeni JF Jr (1994) Familial risk in oral and pharyngeal cancer. Eur J Cancer B Oral Oncol 30B:319–322
9. Hussain SK, Sundquist J, Hemminki K (2008) Familial clustering of cancer at human papillomavirus-associated sites according to the Swedish Family-Cancer Database. Int J Cancer 122:1873–1878
10. Mork J, Moller B, Glattre E (1999) Familial risk in head and neck squamous cell carcinoma diagnosed before the age of 45: a population-based study. Oral Oncol 35:360–367
11. Li X, Hemminki K (2003) Familial upper aerodigestive tract cancers: incidence trends, familial clustering and subsequent cancers. Oral Oncol 39:232–239
12. Negri E, Boffetta P, Berthiller J, Castellsague X, Curado MP, Maso LD, Daudt AW, Fabianova E, Fernandez L, Wunsch-Filho V, Franceschi S, Hayes RB, Herrero R, Koifman S, Lazarus P, Lence JJ, Levi F, Mates D, Matos E, Menezes A, Muscat J, Eluf-Neto J, Olshan AF, Rudnai P, Shangina O, Sturgis EM, Szeszenia-Dabrowska N, Talamini R, Wei Q, Winn DM, Zaridze D, Lissowska J, Zhang ZF, Ferro G, Brennan P, La Vecchia C, Hashibe M (2008) Family history of cancer: pooled analysis in the International Head and Neck Cancer Epidemiology Consortium. Int J Cancer 124:394–401
13. Shields PG, Caporaso NE, Falk RT, Sugimura H, Trivers GE, Trump BF, Hoover RN, Weston A, Harris CC (1993) Lung cancer, race, and a CYP1A1 genetic polymorphism. Cancer Epidemiol Biomarkers Prev 2:481–485
14. Andreasson L, Bjorlin G, Hocherman M, Korsgaard R, Trell E (1987) Laryngeal cancer, aryl hydrocarbon hydroxylase inducibility and smoking. A follow-up study. ORL J Otorhinolaryngol Relat Spec 49:187–192
15. Andreasson L, Bjorlin G, Laurell P, Trell E, Korsgaard R (1985) Oral and oropharyngeal cancer, aryl hydrocarbon hydroxylase inducibility and smoking. A follow-up study. ORL J Otorhinolaryngol Relat Spec 47:131–138
16. Brandenburg JH, Kellermann G (1978) Aryl hydrocarbon hydroxylase inducibility in laryngeal carcinoma. Arch Otolaryngol 104:151–152
17. Jaiswal AK, Gonzalez FJ, Nebert DW (1985) Human P1–450 gene sequence and correlation of mRNA with genetic differences in benzo[a]pyrene metabolism. Nucleic Acids Res 13:4503–4520

18. Petersen DD, McKinney CE, Ikeya K, Smith HH, Bale AE, McBride OW, Nebert DW (1991) Human CYP1A1 gene: cosegregation of the enzyme inducibility phenotype and an RFLP. Am J Hum Genet 48:720–725
19. Sato M, Sato T, Izumo T, Amagasa T (1999) Genetic polymorphism of drug-metabolizing enzymes and susceptibility to oral cancer. Carcinogenesis 20:1927–1931
20. Tanimoto K, Hayashi S, Yoshiga K, Ichikawa T (1999) Polymorphisms of the CYP1A1 and GSTM1 gene involved in oral squamous cell carcinoma in association with a cigarette dose. Oral Oncol 35:191–196
21. Nakachi K, Imai K, Hayashi S, Kawajiri K (1993) Polymorphisms of the CYP1A1 and glutathione S-transferase genes associated with susceptibility to lung cancer in relation to cigarette dose in a Japanese population. Cancer Res 53:2994–2999
22. Matthias C, Bockmuhl U, Jahnke V, Jones PW, Hayes JD, Alldersea J, Gilford J, Bailey L, Bath J, Worrall SF, Hand P, Fryer AA, Strange RC (1998) Polymorphism in cytochrome P450 CYP2D6, CYP1A1, CYP2E1 and glutathione S-transferase, GSTM1, GSTM3, GSTT1 and susceptibility to tobacco-related cancers: studies in upper aerodigestive tract cancers. Pharmacogenetics 8:91–100
23. Oude Ophuis MB, van Lieshout EM, Roelofs HM, Peters WH, Manni JJ (1998) Glutathione S-transferase M1 and T1 and cytochrome P4501A1 polymorphisms in relation to the risk for benign and malignant head and neck lesions. Cancer 82:936–943
24. Hirvonen A, Husgafvel-Pursiainen K, Karjalainen A, Anttila S, Vainio H (1992) Point-mutational MspI and Ile-Val polymorphisms closely linked in the CYP1A1 gene: lack of association with susceptibility to lung cancer in a Finnish study population. Cancer Epidemiol Biomarkers Prev 1:485–489
25. Sugimura H, Suzuki I, Hamada GS, Iwase T, Takahashi T, Nagura K, Iwata H, Watanabe S, Kino I, Tsugane S (1994) Cytochrome P-450 IA1 genotype in lung cancer patients and controls in Rio de Janeiro, Brazil. Cancer Epidemiol Biomarkers Prev 3:145–148
26. Hayashi S, Watanabe J, Kawajiri K (1992) High susceptibility to lung cancer analyzed in terms of combined genotypes of P450IA1 and Mu-class glutathione S-transferase genes. Jpn J Cancer Res 83:866–870
27. Cosma G, Crofts F, Taioli E, Toniolo P, Garte S (1993) Relationship between genotype and function of the human CYP1A1 gene. J Toxicol Environ Health 40:309–316
28. Katoh T, Kaneko S, Kohshi K, Munaka M, Kitagawa K, Kunugita N, Ikemura K, Kawamoto T (1999) Genetic polymorphisms of tobacco- and alcohol-related metabolizing enzymes and oral cavity cancer. Int J Cancer 83:606–609
29. Morita S, Yano M, Tsujinaka T, Akiyama Y, Taniguchi M, Kaneko K, Miki H, Fujii T, Yoshino K, Kusuoka H, Monden M (1999) Genetic polymorphisms of drug-metabolizing enzymes and susceptibility to head-and-neck squamous-cell carcinoma. Int J Cancer 80:685–688
30. Park JY, Muscat JE, Ren Q, Schantz SP, Harwick RD, Stern JC, Pike V, Richie JP Jr, Lazarus P (1997) CYP1A1 and GSTM1 polymorphisms and oral cancer risk. Cancer Epidemiol Biomarkers Prev 6:791–797
31. Hashibe M, Brennan P, Strange RC, Bhisey R, Cascorbi I, Lazarus P, Oude Ophuis MB, Benhamou S, Foulkes WD, Katoh T, Coutelle C, Romkes M, Gaspari L, Taioli E, Boffetta P (2003) Meta- and pooled analyses of GSTM1, GSTT1, GSTP1, and CYP1A1 genotypes and risk of head and neck cancer. Cancer Epidemiol Biomarkers Prev 12:1509–1517
32. Ho T, Wei Q, Sturgis EM (2007) Epidemiology of carcinogen metabolism genes and risk of squamous cell carcinoma of the head and neck. Head Neck 29:682–699
33. Varela-Lema L, Taioli E, Ruano-Ravina A, Barros-Dios JM, Anantharaman D, Benhamou S, Boccia S, Bhisey RA, Cadoni G, Capoluongo E, Chen CJ, Foulkes W, Goloni-Bertollo EM, Hatagima A, Hayes RB, Katoh T, Koifman S, Lazarus P, Manni JJ, Mahimkar M, Morita S, Park J, Park KK, Pavarino Bertelli EC, de Souza Fonseca Ribeiro EM, Roy B, Spitz MR, Strange RC, Wei Q, Ragin CC (2008) Meta-analysis and pooled analysis of GSTM1 and CYP1A1 polymorphisms and oral and pharyngeal cancers: a HuGE-GSEC review. Genet Med 10:369–384

34. Bartsch H, Nair U, Risch A, Rojas M, Wikman H, Alexandrov K (2000) Genetic polymorphism of CYP genes, alone or in combination, as a risk modifier of tobacco-related cancers. Cancer Epidemiol Biomarkers Prev 9:3–28
35. Ko Y, Abel J, Harth V, Brode P, Antony C, Donat S, Fischer HP, Ortiz-Pallardo ME, Thier R, Sachinidis A, Vetter H, Bolt HM, Herberhold C, Bruning T (2001) Association of CYP1B1 codon 432 mutant allele in head and neck squamous cell cancer is reflected by somatic mutations of p53 in tumor tissue. Cancer Res 61:4398–4404
36. Li G, Liu Z, Sturgis EM, Chamberlain RM, Spitz MR, Wei Q (2005) CYP2E1 G1532C, NQO1 Pro187Ser, and CYP1B1 Val432Leu polymorphisms are not associated with risk of squamous cell carcinoma of the head and neck. Cancer Epidemiol Biomarkers Prev 14:1034–1036
37. Singh AP, Shah PP, Mathur N, Buters JT, Pant MC, Parmar D (2007) Genetic polymorphisms in Cytochrome P4501B1 and susceptibility to Head and Neck Cancer. Mutat Res 639(1–2):11–9
38. Ayesh R, Idle JR, Ritchie JC, Crothers MJ, Hetzel MR (1984) Metabolic oxidation phenotypes as markers for susceptibility to lung cancer. Nature 312:169–170
39. Crespi CL, Penman BW, Gelboin HV, Gonzalez FJ (1991) A tobacco smoke-derived nitrosamine, 4-(methylnitrosamino)-1-(3-pyridyl)-1-butanone, is activated by multiple human cytochrome P450s including the polymorphic human cytochrome P4502D6. Carcinogenesis 12:1197–1201
40. Caporaso NE, Tucker MA, Hoover RN, Hayes RB, Pickle LW, Issaq HJ, Muschik GM, Green-Gallo L, Buivys D, Aisner S et al (1990) Lung cancer and the debrisoquine metabolic phenotype. J Natl Cancer Inst 82:1264–1272
41. Roots I, Drakoulis N, Ploch M, Heinemeyer G, Loddenkemper R, Minks T, Nitz M, Otte F, Koch M (1988) Debrisoquine hydroxylation phenotype, acetylation phenotype, and ABO blood groups as genetic host factors of lung cancer risk. Klin Wochenschr 66(Suppl 11):87–97
42. Heim M, Meyer UA (1990) Genotyping of poor metabolisers of debrisoquine by allele-specific PCR amplification. Lancet 336:529–532
43. Spina E, Campo GM, Avenoso A, Caputi AP, Zuccaro P, Pacifici R, Gatti G, Strada G, Bartoli A, Perucca E (1994) CYP2D6-related oxidation polymorphism in Italy. Pharmacol Res 29:281–289
44. Agundez JA, Gallardo L, Ledesma MC, Lozano L, Rodriguez-Lescure A, Pontes JC, Iglesias-Moreno MC, Poch J, Ladero JM, Benitez J (2001) Functionally active duplications of the CYP2D6 gene are more prevalent among larynx and lung cancer patients. Oncology 61:59–63
45. Gajecka M, Rydzanicz M, Jaskula-Sztul R, Kujawski M, Szyfter W, Szyfter K (2005) CYP1A1, CYP2D6, CYP2E1, NAT2, GSTM1 and GSTT1 polymorphisms or their combinations are associated with the increased risk of the laryngeal squamous cell carcinoma. Mutat Res 574:112–123
46. Worrall SF, Corrigan M, High A, Starr D, Matthias C, Wolf CR, Jones PW, Hand P, Gilford J, Farrell WE, Hoban P, Fryer AA, Strange RC (1998) Susceptibility and outcome in oral cancer: preliminary data showing an association with polymorphism in cytochrome P450 CYP2D6. Pharmacogenetics 8:433–439
47. Gonzalez MV, Alvarez V, Pello MF, Menendez MJ, Suarez C, Coto E (1998) Genetic polymorphism of *N*-acetyltransferase-2, glutathione S-transferase-M1, and cytochromes P450IIE1 and P450IID6 in the susceptibility to head and neck cancer. J Clin Pathol 51:294–298
48. Gronau S, Koenig-Greger D, Jerg M, Riechelmann H (2003) Gene polymorphisms in detoxification enzymes as susceptibility factor for head and neck cancer? Otolaryngol Head Neck Surg 128:674–680
49. Lieber CS (1999) Microsomal ethanol-oxidizing system (MEOS): the first 30 years (1968–1998) – a review. Alcohol Clin Exp Res 23:991–1007
50. Stephens EA, Taylor JA, Kaplan N, Yang CH, Hsieh LL, Lucier GW, Bell DA (1994) Ethnic variation in the CYP2E1 gene: polymorphism analysis of 695 African-Americans, European-Americans and Taiwanese. Pharmacogenetics 4:185–192
51. Bouchardy C, Hirvonen A, Coutelle C, Ward PJ, Dayer P, Benhamou S (2000) Role of alcohol dehydrogenase 3 and cytochrome P-4502E1 genotypes in susceptibility to cancers of the upper aerodigestive tract. Int J Cancer 87:734–740

52. Gattas GJ, de Carvalho MB, Siraque MS, Curioni OA, Kohler P, Eluf-Neto J, Wunsch-Filho V (2006) Genetic polymorphisms of CYP1A1, CYP2E1, GSTM1, and GSTT1 associated with head and neck cancer. Head Neck 28:819–826
53. Hung HC, Chuang J, Chien YC, Chern HD, Chiang CP, Kuo YS, Hildesheim A, Chen CJ (1997) Genetic polymorphisms of CYP2E1, GSTM1, and GSTT1; environmental factors and risk of oral cancer. Cancer Epidemiol Biomarkers Prev 6:901–905
54. Tan W, Song N, Wang GQ, Liu Q, Tang HJ, Kadlubar FF, Lin DX (2000) Impact of genetic polymorphisms in cytochrome P450 2E1 and glutathione S-transferases M1, T1, and P1 on susceptibility to esophageal cancer among high-risk individuals in China. Cancer Epidemiol Biomarkers Prev 9:551–556
55. Boccia S, Cadoni G, Sayed-Tabatabaei FA, Volante M, Arzani D, De Lauretis A, Cattel C, Almadori G, van Duijn CM, Paludetti G, Ricciardi G (2008) CYP1A1, CYP2E1, GSTM1, GSTT1, EPHX1 exons 3 and 4, and NAT2 polymorphisms, smoking, consumption of alcohol and fruit and vegetables and risk of head and neck cancer. J Cancer Res Clin Oncol 134:93–100
56. Marques CF, Koifman S, Koifman RJ, Boffetta P, Brennan P, Hatagima A (2006) Influence of CYP1A1, CYP2E1, GSTM3 and NAT2 genetic polymorphisms in oral cancer susceptibility: results from a case–control study in Rio de Janeiro. Oral Oncol 42:632–637
57. Rydzanicz M, Wierzbicka M, Gajecka M, Szyfter W, Szyfter K (2005) The impact of genetic factors on the incidence of multiple primary tumors (MPT) of the head and neck. Cancer Lett 224:263–278
58. Harth V, Schafer M, Abel J, Maintz L, Neuhaus T, Besuden M, Primke R, Wilkesmann A, Thier R, Vetter H, Ko YD, Bruning T, Bolt HM, Ickstadt K (2008) Head and neck squamous-cell cancer and its association with polymorphic enzymes of xenobiotic metabolism and repair. J Toxicol Environ Health A 71:887–897
59. Zhong S, Wyllie AH, Barnes D, Wolf CR, Spurr NK (1993) Relationship between the GSTM1 genetic polymorphism and susceptibility to bladder, breast and colon cancer. Carcinogenesis 14:1821–1824
60. Seidegard J, Vorachek WR, Pero RW, Pearson WR (1988) Hereditary differences in the expression of the human glutathione transferase active on trans-stilbene oxide are due to a gene deletion. Proc Natl Acad Sci U S A 85:7293–7297
61. Roots I, Brockmoller J, Drakoulis N, Loddenkemper R (1992) Mutant genes of cytochrome P-450IID6, glutathione S-transferase class Mu, and arylamine *N*-acetyltransferase in lung cancer patients. Clin Investig 70:307–319
62. Nomura T, Noma H, Shibahara T, Yokoyama A, Muramatusu T, Ohmori T (2000) Aldehyde dehydrogenase 2 and glutathione S-transferase M 1 polymorphisms in relation to the risk for oral cancer in Japanese drinkers. Oral Oncol 36:42–46
63. Park LY, Muscat JE, Kaur T, Schantz SP, Stern JC, Richie JP Jr, Lazarus P (2000) Comparison of GSTM polymorphisms and risk for oral cancer between African-Americans and Caucasians. Pharmacogenetics 10:123–131
64. Trizna Z, Clayman GL, Spitz MR, Briggs KL, Goepfert H (1995) Glutathione s-transferase genotypes as risk factors for head and neck cancer. Am J Surg 170:499–501
65. Cheng L, Sturgis EM, Eicher SA, Char D, Spitz MR, Wei Q (1999) Glutathione-S-transferase polymorphisms and risk of squamous-cell carcinoma of the head and neck. Int J Cancer 84:220–224
66. Li D, Wang LE, Chang P, El-Naggar AK, Sturgis EM, Wei Q (2007) In vitro benzo[a]pyrene diol epoxide-induced DNA adducts and risk of squamous cell carcinoma of head and neck. Cancer Res 67:5628–5634
67. Lohmueller KE, Pearce CL, Pike M, Lander ES, Hirschhorn JN (2003) Meta-analysis of genetic association studies supports a contribution of common variants to susceptibility to common disease. Nat Genet 33:177–182
68. Tripathy CB, Roy N (2006) Meta-analysis of glutathione S-transferase M1 genotype and risk toward head and neck cancer. Head Neck 28:217–224

69. Hiyama T, Yoshihara M, Tanaka S, Chayama K (2008) Genetic polymorphisms and head and neck cancer risk (Review). Int J Oncol 32:945–973
70. Meyer DJ, Coles B, Pemble SE, Gilmore KS, Fraser GM, Ketterer B (1991) Theta, a new class of glutathione transferases purified from rat and man. Biochem J 274(Pt 2):409–414
71. Pemble S, Schroeder KR, Spencer SR, Meyer DJ, Hallier E, Bolt HM, Ketterer B, Taylor JB (1994) Human glutathione S-transferase theta (GSTT1): cDNA cloning and the characterization of a genetic polymorphism. Biochem J 300(Pt 1):271–276
72. Geisler SA, Olshan AF (2001) GSTM1, GSTT1, and the risk of squamous cell carcinoma of the head and neck: a mini-HuGE review. Am J Epidemiol 154:95–105
73. Ali-Osman F, Akande O, Antoun G, Mao JX, Buolamwini J (1997) Molecular cloning, characterization, and expression in Escherichia coli of full-length cDNAs of three human glutathione S-transferase Pi gene variants. Evidence for differential catalytic activity of the encoded proteins. J Biol Chem 272:10004–10012
74. Boukouvala S, Sim E (2005) Structural analysis of the genes for human arylamine *N*-acetyltransferases and characterisation of alternative transcripts. Basic Clin Pharmacol Toxicol 96:343–351
75. Olshan AF, Weissler MC, Watson MA, Bell DA (2000) GSTM1, GSTT1, GSTP1, CYP1A1, and NAT1 polymorphisms, tobacco use, and the risk of head and neck cancer. Cancer Epidemiol Biomarkers Prev 9:185–191
76. Fronhoffs S, Bruning T, Ortiz-Pallardo E, Brode P, Koch B, Harth V, Sachinidis A, Bolt HM, Herberhold C, Vetter H, Ko Y (2001) Real-time PCR analysis of the *N*-acetyltransferase NAT1 allele *3, *4, *10, *11, *14 and *17 polymorphism in squamous cell cancer of head and neck. Carcinogenesis 22:1405–1412
77. Blum M, Demierre A, Grant DM, Heim M, Meyer UA (1991) Molecular mechanism of slow acetylation of drugs and carcinogens in humans. Proc Natl Acad Sci U S A 88:5237–5241
78. Deguchi T (1992) Sequences and expression of alleles of polymorphic arylamine *N*-acetyltransferase of human liver. J Biol Chem 267:18140–18147
79. Drozdz M, Gierek T, Jendryczko A, Pilch J, Piekarska J (1987) *N*-acetyltransferase phenotype of patients with cancer of the larynx. Neoplasma 34:481–484
80. Katoh T, Kaneko S, Boissy R, Watson M, Ikemura K, Bell DA (1998) A pilot study testing the association between *N*-acetyltransferases 1 and 2 and risk of oral squamous cell carcinoma in Japanese people. Carcinogenesis 19:1803–1807
81. Chen C, Ricks S, Doody DR, Fitzgibbons ED, Porter PL, Schwartz SM (2001) *N*-Acetyltransferase 2 polymorphisms, cigarette smoking and alcohol consumption, and oral squamous cell cancer risk. Carcinogenesis 22:1993–1999
82. Agundez JA (2008) Polymorphisms of human *N*-acetyltransferases and cancer risk. Curr Drug Metab 9:520–531
83. Lancaster JM, Brownlee HA, Bell DA, Futreal PA, Marks JR, Berchuck A, Wiseman RW, Taylor JA (1996) Microsomal epoxide hydrolase polymorphism as a risk factor for ovarian cancer. Mol Carcinog 17:160–162
84. Heckbert SR, Weiss NS, Hornung SK, Eaton DL, Motulsky AG (1992) Glutathione S-transferase and epoxide hydrolase activity in human leukocytes in relation to risk of lung cancer and other smoking-related cancers. J Natl Cancer Inst 84:414–422
85. Janot F, Massaad L, Ribrag V, de Waziers I, Beaune PH, Luboinski B, Parise O Jr, Gouyette A, Chabot GG (1993) Principal xenobiotic-metabolizing enzyme systems in human head and neck squamous cell carcinoma. Carcinogenesis 14:1279–1283
86. Hassett C, Aicher L, Sidhu JS, Omiecinski CJ (1994) Human microsomal epoxide hydrolase: genetic polymorphism and functional expression in vitro of amino acid variants. Hum Mol Genet 3:421–428
87. Smith CA, Harrison DJ (1997) Association between polymorphism in gene for microsomal epoxide hydrolase and susceptibility to emphysema. Lancet 350:630–633
88. Jourenkova-Mironova N, Mitrunen K, Bouchardy C, Dayer P, Benhamou S, Hirvonen A (2000) High-activity microsomal epoxide hydrolase genotypes and the risk of oral, pharynx, and larynx cancers. Cancer Res 60:534–536

89. Lacko M, Roelofs HM, Te Morsche RH, Voogd AC, Oude Ophuis MB, Peters WH, Manni JJ (2008) Microsomal epoxide hydrolase genotypes and the risk for head and neck cancer. Head Neck 30:836–844
90. Chung KY, Mukhopadhyay T, Kim J, Casson A, Ro JY, Goepfert H, Hong WK, Roth JA (1993) Discordant p53 gene mutations in primary head and neck cancers and corresponding second primary cancers of the upper aerodigestive tract. Cancer Res 53:1676–1683
91. Brennan P, Lewis S, Hashibe M, Bell DA, Boffetta P, Bouchardy C, Caporaso N, Chen C, Coutelle C, Diehl SR, Hayes RB, Olshan AF, Schwartz SM, Sturgis EM, Wei Q, Zavras AI, Benhamou S (2004) Pooled analysis of alcohol dehydrogenase genotypes and head and neck cancer: a HuGE review. Am J Epidemiol 159:1–16
92. Harty LC, Caporaso NE, Hayes RB, Winn DM, Bravo-Otero E, Blot WJ, Kleinman DV, Brown LM, Armenian HK, Fraumeni JF Jr, Shields PG (1997) Alcohol dehydrogenase 3 genotype and risk of oral cavity and pharyngeal cancers. J Natl Cancer Inst 89:1698–1705
93. Coutelle C, Ward PJ, Fleury B, Quattrocchi P, Chambrin H, Iron A, Couzigou P, Cassaigne A (1997) Laryngeal and oropharyngeal cancer, and alcohol dehydrogenase 3 and glutathione S-transferase M1 polymorphisms. Hum Genet 99:319–325
94. Yokoyama A, Muramatsu T, Ohmori T, Yokoyama T, Okuyama K, Takahashi H, Hasegawa Y, Higuchi S, Maruyama K, Shirakura K, Ishii H (1998) Alcohol-related cancers and aldehyde dehydrogenase-2 in Japanese alcoholics. Carcinogenesis 19:1383–1387
95. Sturgis EM, Dahlstrom KR, Guan Y, Eicher SA, Strom SS, Spitz MR, Wei Q (2001) Alcohol dehydrogenase 3 genotype is not associated with risk of squamous cell carcinoma of the oral cavity and pharynx. Cancer Epidemiol Biomarkers Prev 10:273–275
96. Hashibe M, Boffetta P, Zaridze D, Shangina O, Szeszenia-Dabrowska N, Mates D, Janout V, Fabianova E, Bencko V, Moullan N, Chabrier A, Hung R, Hall J, Canzian F, Brennan P (2006) Evidence for an important role of alcohol- and aldehyde-metabolizing genes in cancers of the upper aerodigestive tract. Cancer Epidemiol Biomarkers Prev 15:696–703
97. Buch SC, Nazar-Stewart V, Weissfeld JL, Romkes M (2008) Case–control study of oral and oropharyngeal cancer in whites and genetic variation in eight metabolic enzymes. Head Neck 30:1139–1147
98. Reszka E, Czekaj P, Adamska J, Wasowicz W (2008) Relevance of glutathione S-transferase M1 and cytochrome P450 1A1 genetic polymorphisms to the development of head and neck cancers. Clin Chem Lab Med 46(8):1090–1096
99. Hagmar L, Brogger A, Hansteen IL, Heim S, Hogstedt B, Knudsen L, Lambert B, Linnainmaa K, Mitelman F, Nordenson I et al (1994) Cancer risk in humans predicted by increased levels of chromosomal aberrations in lymphocytes: Nordic study group on the health risk of chromosome damage. Cancer Res 54:2919–2922
100. Hsu TC, Cherry LM, Samaan NA (1985) Differential mutagen susceptibility in cultured lymphocytes of normal individuals and cancer patients. Cancer Genet Cytogenet 17:307–313
101. Hsu TC, Spitz MR, Schantz SP (1991) Mutagen sensitivity: a biological marker of cancer susceptibility. Cancer Epidemiol Biomarkers Prev 1:83–89
102. Schantz SP, Hsu TC (1989) Mutagen-induced chromosome fragility within peripheral blood lymphocytes of head and neck cancer patients. Head Neck 11:337–342
103. Schantz SP, Hsu TC, Ainslie N, Moser RP (1989) Young adults with head and neck cancer express increased susceptibility to mutagen-induced chromosome damage. JAMA 262:3313–3315
104. Schantz SP, Spitz MR, Hsu TC (1990) Mutagen sensitivity in patients with head and neck cancers: a biologic marker for risk of multiple primary malignancies. J Natl Cancer Inst 82:1773–1775
105. Cloos J, Spitz MR, Schantz SP, Hsu TC, Zhang ZF, Tobi H, Braakhuis BJ, Snow GB (1996) Genetic susceptibility to head and neck squamous cell carcinoma. J Natl Cancer Inst 88:530–535
106. Wang LE, Sturgis EM, Eicher SA, Spitz MR, Hong WK, Wei Q (1998) Mutagen sensitivity to benzo(a)pyrene diol epoxide and the risk of squamous cell carcinoma of the head and neck. Clin Cancer Res 4:1773–1778

107. Wu X, Lippman SM, Lee JJ, Zhu Y, Wei QV, Thomas M, Hong WK, Spitz MR (2002) Chromosome instability in lymphocytes: a potential indicator of predisposition to oral premalignant lesions. Cancer Res 62:2813–2818
108. Xiong P, Hu Z, Li C, Wang LE, El-Naggar AK, Sturgis EM, Wei Q (2007) In vitro benzo[a] pyrene diol epoxide-induced DNA damage and chromosomal aberrations in primary lymphocytes, smoking, and risk of squamous cell carcinoma of the head and neck. Int J Cancer 121:2735–2740
109. Wang LE, Xiong P, Zhao H, Spitz MR, Sturgis EM, Wei Q (2008) Chromosome instability and risk of squamous cell carcinomas of head and neck. Cancer Res 68:4479–4485
110. Athas WF, Hedayati MA, Matanoski GM, Farmer ER, Grossman L (1991) Development and field-test validation of an assay for DNA repair in circulating human lymphocytes. Cancer Res 51:5786–5793
111. Slebos RJ, Taylor JA (2001) A novel host cell reactivation assay to assess homologous recombination capacity in human cancer cell lines. Biochem Biophys Res Commun 281:212–219
112. Wei Q, Matanoski GM, Farmer ER, Hedayati MA, Grossman L (1993) DNA repair and aging in basal cell carcinoma: a molecular epidemiology study. Proc Natl Acad Sci U S A 90:1614–1618
113. Alcalay J, Freeman SE, Goldberg LH, Wolf JE (1990) Excision repair of pyrimidine dimers induced by simulated solar radiation in the skin of patients with basal cell carcinoma. J Invest Dermatol 95:506–509
114. Wei Q, Spitz MR, Gu J, Cheng L, Xu X, Strom SS, Kripke ML, Hsu TC (1996) DNA repair capacity correlates with mutagen sensitivity in lymphoblastoid cell lines. Cancer Epidemiol Biomarkers Prev 5:199–204
115. Sturgis EM, Clayman GL, Guan Y, Guo Z, Wei Q (1999) DNA repair in lymphoblastoid cell lines from patients with head and neck cancer. Arch Otolaryngol Head Neck Surg 125:185–190
116. Cheng L, Eicher SA, Guo Z, Hong WK, Spitz MR, Wei Q (1998) Reduced DNA repair capacity in head and neck cancer patients. Cancer Epidemiol Biomarkers Prev 7:465–468
117. Wiencke JK (2002) DNA adduct burden and tobacco carcinogenesis. Oncogene 21:7376–7391
118. Li D, Firozi PF, Chang P, Wang LE, Xiong P, Sturgis EM, Eicher SA, Spitz MR, Hong WK, Wei Q (2001) In vitro BPDE-induced DNA adducts in peripheral lymphocytes as a risk factor for squamous cell carcinoma of the head and neck. Int J Cancer 93:436–440
119. Zhao H, Wang LE, Li D, Chamberlain RM, Sturgis EM, Wei Q (2008) Genotypes and haplotypes of ERCC1 and ERCC2/XPD genes predict levels of benzo[a]pyrene diol epoxide-induced DNA adducts in cultured primary lymphocytes from healthy individuals: a genotype–phenotype correlation analysis. Carcinogenesis 29:1560–1566
120. Wei Q, Eicher SA, Guan Y, Cheng L, Xu J, Young LN, Saunders KC, Jiang H, Hong WK, Spitz MR, Strom SS (1998) Reduced expression of hMLH1 and hGTBP/hMSH6: a risk factor for head and neck cancer. Cancer Epidemiol Biomarkers Prev 7:309–314
121. Cheng L, Sturgis EM, Eicher SA, Spitz MR, Wei Q (2002) Expression of nucleotide excision repair genes and the risk for squamous cell carcinoma of the head and neck. Cancer 94:393–397
122. Wei Q, Wang LE, Sturgis EM, Mao L (2005) Expression of nucleotide excision repair proteins in lymphocytes as a marker of susceptibility to squamous cell carcinomas of the head and neck. Cancer Epidemiol Biomarkers Prev 14:1961–1966
123. Sancar A (1996) DNA excision repair. Annu Rev Biochem 65:43–81
124. Kraemer KH, Lee MM, Andrews AD, Lambert WC (1994) The role of sunlight and DNA repair in melanoma and nonmelanoma skin cancer. The xeroderma pigmentosum paradigm. Arch Dermatol 130:1018–1021
125. Neumann AS, Sturgis EM, Wei Q (2005) Nucleotide excision repair as a marker for susceptibility to tobacco-related cancers: a review of molecular epidemiological studies. Mol Carcinog 42:65–92

126. Ramachandran S, Ramadas K, Hariharan R, Rejnish Kumar R, Radhakrishna Pillai M (2006) Single nucleotide polymorphisms of DNA repair genes XRCC1 and XPD and its molecular mapping in Indian oral cancer. Oral Oncol 42:350–362
127. Kietthubthew S, Sriplung H, Au WW, Ishida T (2006) Polymorphism in DNA repair genes and oral squamous cell carcinoma in Thailand. Int J Hyg Environ Health 209:21–29
128. Sugimura T, Kumimoto H, Tohnai I, Fukui T, Matsuo K, Tsurusako S, Mitsudo K, Ueda M, Tajima K, Ishizaki K (2006) Gene-environment interaction involved in oral carcinogenesis: molecular epidemiological study for metabolic and DNA repair gene polymorphisms. J Oral Pathol Med 35:11–18
129. Bau DT, Tsai MH, Huang CY, Lee CC, Tseng HC, Lo YL, Tsai Y, Tsai FJ (2007) Relationship between polymorphisms of nucleotide excision repair genes and oral cancer risk in Taiwan: evidence for modification of smoking habit. Chin J Physiol 50:294–300
130. An J, Liu Z, Hu Z, Li G, Wang LE, Sturgis EM, El-Naggar AK, Spitz MR, Wei Q (2007) Potentially functional single nucleotide polymorphisms in the core nucleotide excision repair genes and risk of squamous cell carcinoma of the head and neck. Cancer Epidemiol Biomarkers Prev 16:1633–1638
131. Zhang D, Chen C, Fu X, Gu S, Mao Y, Xie Y, Huang Y, Li Y (2008) A meta-analysis of DNA repair gene XPC polymorphisms and cancer risk. J Hum Genet 53:18–33
132. Hopkins J, Cescon DW, Tse D, Bradbury P, Xu W, Ma C, Wheatley-Price P, Waldron J, Goldstein D, Meyer F, Bairati I, Liu G (2008) Genetic polymorphisms and head and neck cancer outcomes: a review. Cancer Epidemiol Biomarkers Prev 17:490–499
133. Hoeijmakers JH (2001) Genome maintenance mechanisms for preventing cancer. Nature 411:366–374
134. Hung RJ, Hall J, Brennan P, Boffetta P (2005) Genetic polymorphisms in the base excision repair pathway and cancer risk: a HuGE review. Am J Epidemiol 162:925–942
135. Kurumizaka H, Ikawa S, Nakada M, Enomoto R, Kagawa W, Kinebuchi T, Yamazoe M, Yokoyama S, Shibata T (2002) Homologous pairing and ring and filament structure formation activities of the human Xrcc2*Rad51D complex. J Biol Chem 277:14315–14320
136. Lieber MR, Ma Y, Pannicke U, Schwarz K (2003) Mechanism and regulation of human non-homologous DNA end-joining. Nat Rev Mol Cell Biol 4:712–720
137. Gal TJ, Huang WY, Chen C, Hayes RB, Schwartz SM (2005) DNA repair gene polymorphisms and risk of second primary neoplasms and mortality in oral cancer patients. Laryngoscope 115:2221–2231
138. Olshan AF, Watson MA, Weissler MC, Bell DA (2002) XRCC1 polymorphisms and head and neck cancer. Cancer Lett 178:181–186
139. Duan Z, Shen H, Lee JE, Gershenwald JE, Ross MI, Mansfield PF, Duvic M, Strom SS, Spitz MR, Wei Q (2002) DNA repair gene XRCC3 241Met variant is not associated with risk of cutaneous malignant melanoma. Cancer Epidemiol Biomarkers Prev 11:1142–1143
140. Li C, Hu Z, Lu J, Liu Z, Wang LE, El-Naggar AK, Sturgis EM, Spitz MR, Wei Q (2007) Genetic polymorphisms in DNA base-excision repair genes ADPRT, XRCC1, and APE1 and the risk of squamous cell carcinoma of the head and neck. Cancer 110:867–875
141. Benhamou S, Tuimala J, Bouchardy C, Dayer P, Sarasin A, Hirvonen A (2004) DNA repair gene XRCC2 and XRCC3 polymorphisms and susceptibility to cancers of the upper aerodigestive tract. Int J Cancer 112:901–904
142. Werbrouck J, De Ruyck K, Duprez F, Van Eijkeren M, Rietzschel E, Bekaert S, Vral A, De Neve W, Thierens H (2008) Single-nucleotide polymorphisms in DNA double-strand break repair genes: association with head and neck cancer and interaction with tobacco use and alcohol consumption. Mutat Res 656:74–81
143. Lu J, Wang LE, Xiong P, Sturgis EM, Spitz MR, Wei Q (2007) 172G>T variant in the 5′ untranslated region of DNA repair gene RAD51 reduces risk of squamous cell carcinoma of the head and neck and interacts with a P53 codon 72 variant. Carcinogenesis 28:988–994
144. Chiu CF, Tsai MH, Tseng HC, Wang CL, Tsai FJ, Lin CC, Bau DT (2008) A novel single nucleotide polymorphism in ERCC6 gene is associated with oral cancer susceptibility in Taiwanese patients. Oral Oncol 44:582–586

145. Tseng HC, Tsai MH, Chiu CF, Wang CH, Chang NW, Huang CY, Tsai CW, Liang SY, Wang CL, Bau DT (2008) Association of XRCC4 codon 247 polymorphism with oral cancer susceptibility in Taiwan. Anticancer Res 28:1687–1691
146. Yen CY, Liu SY, Chen CH, Tseng HF, Chuang LY, Yang CH, Lin YC, Wen CH, Chiang WF, Ho CH, Chen HC, Wang ST, Lin CW, Chang HW (2008) Combinational polymorphisms of four DNA repair genes XRCC1, XRCC2, XRCC3, and XRCC4 and their association with oral cancer in Taiwan. J Oral Pathol Med 37:271–277
147. Elahi A, Zheng Z, Park J, Eyring K, McCaffrey T, Lazarus P (2002) The human OGG1 DNA repair enzyme and its association with orolaryngeal cancer risk. Carcinogenesis 23:1229–1234
148. Hashimoto T, Uchida K, Okayama N, Imate Y, Suehiro Y, Hamanaka Y, Ueyama Y, Yamashita H, Hinoda Y (2006) Interaction of OGG1 Ser326Cys polymorphism with cigarette smoking in head and neck squamous cell carcinoma. Mol Carcinog 45:344–348
149. Zhang Z, Shi Q, Wang LE, Sturgis EM, Spitz MR, El-Naggar AK, Hong WK, Wei Q (2004) No Association between hOGG1 Ser326Cys polymorphism and risk of squamous cell carcinoma of the head and neck. Cancer Epidemiol Biomarkers Prev 13:1081–1083
150. Zhai X, Zhao H, Liu Z, Wang LE, El-Naggar AK, Sturgis EM, Wei Q (2008) Functional variants of the NEIL1 and NEIL2 genes and risk and progression of squamous cell carcinoma of the oral cavity and oropharynx. Clin Cancer Res 14:4345–4352
151. Ulrich CM (2005) Nutrigenetics in cancer research – folate metabolism and colorectal cancer. J Nutr 135:2698–2702
152. Herbig K, Chiang EP, Lee LR, Hills J, Shane B, Stover PJ (2002) Cytoplasmic serine hydroxymethyltransferase mediates competition between folate-dependent deoxyribonucleotide and S-adenosylmethionine biosyntheses. J Biol Chem 277:38381–38389
153. Schirch L, Peterson D (1980) Purification and properties of mitochondrial serine hydroxymethyltransferase. J Biol Chem 255:7801–7806
154. Shane B (1989) Folylpolyglutamate synthesis and role in the regulation of one-carbon metabolism. Vitam Horm 45:263–335
155. Girgis S, Nasrallah IM, Suh JR, Oppenheim E, Zanetti KA, Mastri MG, Stover PJ (1998) Molecular cloning, characterization and alternative splicing of the human cytoplasmic serine hydroxymethyltransferase gene. Gene 210:315–324
156. Neumann AS, Lyons HJ, Shen H, Liu Z, Shi Q, Sturgis EM, Shete S, Spitz MR, El-Naggar A, Hong WK, Wei Q (2005) Methylenetetrahydrofolate reductase polymorphisms and risk of squamous cell carcinoma of the head and neck: a case–control analysis. Int J Cancer 115:131–136
157. Zhang Z, Shi Q, Sturgis EM, Spitz MR, Hong WK, Wei Q (2004) Thymidylate synthase 5′- and 3′-untranslated region polymorphisms associated with risk and progression of squamous cell carcinoma of the head and neck. Clin Cancer Res 10:7903–7910
158. Zhang Z, Shi Q, Liu Z, Sturgis EM, Spitz MR, Wei Q (2005) Polymorphisms of methionine synthase and methionine synthase reductase and risk of squamous cell carcinoma of the head and neck: a case–control analysis. Cancer Epidemiol Biomarkers Prev 14:1188–1193
159. Capaccio P, Ottaviani F, Cuccarini V, Cenzuales S, Cesana BM, Pignataro L (2005) Association between methylenetetrahydrofolate reductase polymorphisms, alcohol intake and oropharyngolaryngeal carcinoma in northern Italy. J Laryngol Otol 119:371–376
160. Suzuki T, Matsuo K, Hasegawa Y, Hiraki A, Wakai K, Hirose K, Saito T, Sato S, Ueda R, Tajima K (2007) One-carbon metabolism-related gene polymorphisms and risk of head and neck squamous cell carcinoma: case–control study. Cancer Sci 98:1439–1446
161. Scully C, Field JK, Tanzawa H (2000) Genetic aberrations in oral or head and neck squamous cell carcinoma (SCCHN): 1. Carcinogen metabolism, DNA repair and cell cycle control. Oral Oncol 36:256–263
162. Vogelstein B, Kinzler KW (2004) Cancer genes and the pathways they control. Nat Med 10:789–799
163. Sherr CJ (1996) Cancer cell cycles. Science 274:1672–1677
164. Nakahara Y, Shintani S, Mihara M, Kiyota A, Ueyama Y, Matsumura T (2000) Alterations of Rb, p16(INK4A) and cyclin D1 in the tumorigenesis of oral squamous cell carcinomas. Cancer Lett 160:3–8

165. Zheng Y, Shen H, Sturgis EM, Wang LE, Eicher SA, Strom SS, Frazier ML, Spitz MR, Wei Q (2001) Cyclin D1 polymorphism and risk for squamous cell carcinoma of the head and neck: a case–control study. Carcinogenesis 22:1195–1199
166. Rydzanicz M, Golusinski P, Mielcarek-Kuchta D, Golusinski W, Szyfter K (2006) Cyclin D1 gene (CCND1) polymorphism and the risk of squamous cell carcinoma of the larynx. Eur Arch Otorhinolaryngol 263:43–48
167. Ralhan R, Agarwal S, Mathur M, Wasylyk B, Srivastava A (2000) Association between polymorphism in p21(Waf1/Cip1) cyclin-dependent kinase inhibitor gene and human oral cancer. Clin Cancer Res 6:2440–2447
168. Li G, Sturgis EM, Wang LE, Chamberlain RM, Amos CI, Spitz MR, El-Naggar AK, Hong WK, Wei Q (2004) Association of a p73 exon 2 G4C14-to-A4T14 polymorphism with risk of squamous cell carcinoma of the head and neck. Carcinogenesis 25:1911–1916
169. Li G, Liu Z, Sturgis EM, Shi Q, Chamberlain RM, Spitz MR, Wei Q (2005) Genetic polymorphisms of p21 are associated with risk of squamous cell carcinoma of the head and neck. Carcinogenesis 26:1596–1602
170. Zhang Z, Wang LE, Sturgis EM, El-Naggar AK, Hong WK, Amos CI, Spitz MR, Wei Q (2006) Polymorphisms of FAS and FAS ligand genes involved in the death pathway and risk and progression of squamous cell carcinoma of the head and neck. Clin Cancer Res 12:5596–5602
171. Chen K, Zhao H, Hu Z, Wang LE, Zhang W, Sturgis EM, Wei Q (2008) CASP3 polymorphisms and risk of squamous cell carcinoma of the head and neck. Clin Cancer Res 14:6343–6349
172. Li G, Sturgis EM, Wang LE, Chamberlain RM, Spitz MR, El-Naggar AK, Hong WK, Wei Q (2004) Association between the V109G polymorphism of the p27 gene and the risk and progression of oral squamous cell carcinoma. Clin Cancer Res 10:3996–4002
173. Scully C, Field JK, Tanzawa H (2000) Genetic aberrations in oral or head and neck squamous cell carcinoma 3: clinico-pathological applications. Oral Oncol 36:404–413
174. Yang A, Walker N, Bronson R, Kaghad M, Oosterwegel M, Bonnin J, Vagner C, Bonnet H, Dikkes P, Sharpe A, McKeon F, Caput D (2000) p73-deficient mice have neurological, pheromonal and inflammatory defects but lack spontaneous tumours. Nature 404:99–103
175. Street D, Delgado G (1995) The role of p53 and HPV in cervical cancer. Gynecol Oncol 58:287–288
176. Andersson S, Rylander E, Strand A, Sallstrom J, Wilander E (2001) The significance of p53 codon 72 polymorphism for the development of cervical adenocarcinomas. Br J Cancer 85:1153–1156
177. Zehbe I, Voglino G, Wilander E, Genta F, Tommasino M (1999) Codon 72 polymorphism of p53 and its association with cervical cancer. Lancet 354:218–219
178. Couch ME, Ferris RL, Brennan JA, Koch WM, Jaffee EM, Leibowitz MS, Nepom GT, Erlich HA, Sidransky D (2007) Alteration of cellular and humoral immunity by mutant p53 protein and processed mutant peptide in head and neck cancer. Clin Cancer Res 13:7199–7206
179. Kawajiri K, Nakachi K, Imai K, Watanabe J, Hayashi S (1993) Germ line polymorphisms of p53 and CYP1A1 genes involved in human lung cancer. Carcinogenesis 14:1085–1089
180. Storey A, Thomas M, Kalita A, Harwood C, Gardiol D, Mantovani F, Breuer J, Leigh IM, Matlashewski G, Banks L (1998) Role of a p53 polymorphism in the development of human papillomavirus-associated cancer. Nature 393:229–234
181. Tu HF, Chen HW, Kao SY, Lin SC, Liu CJ, Chang KW (2008) MDM2 SNP 309 and p53 codon 72 polymorphisms are associated with the outcome of oral carcinoma patients receiving postoperative irradiation. Radiother Oncol 87:243–252
182. Brant O, Hoffmann M, Kanappilly A, Gorogh T, Gottschlich S (2007) P53 codon 72 polymorphism in squamous cell carcinoma of the head and neck region. Anticancer Res 27:3301–3305
183. Ji X, Neumann AS, Sturgis EM, Adler-Storthz K, Dahlstrom KR, Schiller JT, Wei Q, Li G (2008) p53 codon 72 polymorphism associated with risk of human papillomavirus-associated squamous cell carcinoma of the oropharynx in never-smokers. Carcinogenesis 29:875–879

184. Perrone F, Mariani L, Pastore E, Orsenigo M, Suardi S, Marcomini B, DaRiva L, Licitra L, Carbone A, Pierotti MA, Pilotti S (2007) p53 codon 72 polymorphisms in human papillomavirus-negative and human papillomavirus-positive squamous cell carcinomas of the oropharynx. Cancer 109:2461–2465
185. Chen K, Hu Z, Wang LE, Sturgis EM, El-Naggar AK, Zhang W, Wei Q (2007) Single-nucleotide polymorphisms at the TP53-binding or responsive promoter regions of BAX and BCL2 genes and risk of squamous cell carcinoma of the head and neck. Carcinogenesis 28:2008–2012
186. Chen K, Hu Z, Wang LE, Zhang W, El-Naggar AK, Sturgis EM, Wei Q (2007) Polymorphic TP53BP1 and TP53 gene interactions associated with risk of squamous cell carcinoma of the head and neck. Clin Cancer Res 13:4300–4305
187. Huang WY, Olshan AF, Schwartz SM, Berndt SI, Chen C, Llaca V, Chanock SJ, Fraumeni JF Jr, Hayes RB (2005) Selected genetic polymorphisms in MGMT, XRCC1, XPD, and XRCC3 and risk of head and neck cancer: a pooled analysis. Cancer Epidemiol Biomarkers Prev 14:1747–1753
188. Li C, Wang LE, Wei Q (2008) DNA repair phenotype and cancer susceptibility – a mini review. Int J Cancer
189. Zhang Z, Shi Q, Sturgis EM, Spitz MR, Wei Q (2005) Polymorphisms and haplotypes of serine hydroxymethyltransferase and risk of squamous cell carcinoma of the head and neck: a case–control analysis. Pharmacogenet Genomics 15:557–564
190. Kaghad M, Bonnet H et al (1997) Monoallelically expressed gene related to p53 at 1p36, a region frequently deleted in neuroblastoma and other human cancers. Cell 90(4):809–819

Chemoprevention of Head and Neck Cancers

William N. William Jr., Christopher H. Lieu, and Scott M. Lippman

Introduction

The term "chemoprevention" in reference to cancer was introduced by Sporn in 1976 and was defined as the use of natural, synthetic, or biologic compounds to halt, reverse, or prevent the initial phase of carcinogenesis or the progression of neoplastic cells to cancer [1]. The following three key biologic features of malignant transformation support the development of chemopreventive strategies: it involves the multipath, multistep, and multifocal disruption of normal cellular function.

The multiple steps of carcinogenesis involve accumulation of genetic and epigenetic changes that lead to abnormalities in several functional pathways leading to the cell's acquisition of a malignant phenotype. The malignant phenotype, as described by Hanahan and Weinberg, is characterized by independence of growth signals, resistance to antigrowth signals, avoidance of apoptosis, limitless replicative potential, angiogenesis, and ability to invade adjacent tissues and metastasize [2]. The genetic and epigenetic abnormalities pertaining specifically to head and neck carcinogenesis have been described elsewhere in this book. It is particularly relevant for chemoprevention, however, that these abnormalities are multifocal and occur both in a clonal or multiclonal fashion.

The concept of field cancerization, or carcinogenesis, was proposed by Slaughter et al. in 1953 [3]. In the aerodigestive tract, field cancerization is characterized, for example, by diffuse genetic damage resulting from exposure of the entire epithelial surface to tobacco-related carcinogens [4]. Field carcinogenesis translates clinically into an increased risk of second primary tumors in patients with curatively treated head and neck cancers. These tumors arise not only in the head and neck but also in other sites such as the lungs, esophagus, and bladder exposed to the same carcinogens with a frequency ranging from 10 to 40% [5–10]. Cytogenetic and

W.N. William, C.H. Lieu, and S.M. Lippman (✉)
Department of Thoracic/Head and Neck Medical Oncology, The University of Texas M. D. Anderson Cancer Center, 1515 Holcombe Blvd., Unit 432, Houston, TX 77030, USA
e-mail: slippman@mdanderson.org

A.F. Olshan (ed.), *Epidemiology, Pathogenesis, and Prevention of Head and Neck Cancer*, DOI 10.1007/978-1-4419-1472-9_9, © Springer Science+Business Media, LLC 2010 genetic analyses have provided evidence that second primary tumors in the head and neck region may be clonally related to the primary tumor (and thus result from clonal expansion and spreading of premalignant or transformed cells from the index lesion) or may be genetically independent of the primary tumor (and thus arise synchronously or metachronously with it in the same field of defects) [4, 11–15]. Regardless of the clonal origin of second primary malignant (or premalignant) cells, these field-carcinogenesis-related studies call for a systemic approach to eliminate these clones, given that a large portion of the aerodigestive tract epithelium (if not its entirety) may be at risk for cancer following exposure to carcinogens. The concept of diffuse epithelial injury is further illustrated by a recent finding of Bhutani et al. demonstrating a high correlation of methylation indexes in the promoter region of tumor suppressor genes (a marker of cancer risk) in oral and bronchial tissues of smokers [16].

Head and neck cancers (particularly of the oral cavity) provide an excellent opportunity for the development of chemopreventive interventions since this region is easily accessible for biopsies and thus facilitates translational studies that can inform the design and improve the interpretation of clinical trial results. Furthermore, premalignant lesions of the oral cavity (e.g., leukoplakia and erythroleukoplakia) have been identified and characterized for their natural history and histopathologic and molecular abnormalities, all increasing their utility as clinical model systems.

Although tobacco and alcohol use leads to an increased population-wide incidence of head and neck cancers, exposure to these carcinogens alone may not confer a high enough cancer risk for individuals to justify implementation of chemopreventive measures. As discussed in detail elsewhere by William et al. [17], the maximum success of a given chemopreventive intervention depends on applying it to individuals with elevated baseline cancer risk, using agents with a favorable therapeutic index (i.e., high efficacy with low likelihood of adverse events), and incorporating biomarkers that predict drug sensitivity and resistance and allow an early readout of long-term outcome (surrogate [intermediate] endpoint biomarkers).

The following sections of this chapter discuss recent advances in head and neck cancer risk assessment and describe the most relevant chemoprevention clinical trials completed to date. The chapter will conclude with a brief summary of major future directions of this field.

Risk Assessment

Cancer risk assessment is intimately related to chemoprevention, since it allows for the identification of a population most suitable for consideration for preventive interventions.

In 2002, the American Association for Cancer Research issued guidelines recommending the development of chemoprevention strategies focusing on intra-epithelial neoplasias. Intra-epithelial neoplasias are lesions on the causal pathway leading from normal epithelial to cancers. Three key features justify the use of intra-epithelial neoplasias as a central component in chemoprevention research: they are near obligate cancer precursors, constitute a risk marker for cancer, and often represent, in themselves, a disease or condition requiring surveillance and treatment [18]. In 2006, the American Association for Cancer Research updated its guidelines and recognized the importance of "molecular" intra-epithelial neoplasias, i.e., molecular abnormalities that may occur not only in histopathologically abnormal tissue, but also in microscopically normal-appearing cells, that contribute to the carcinogenic process and could be targeted for chemoprevention [19].

In oral cancers, intra-epithelial neoplasias may be clinically characterized as oral leukoplakia or erythroplakia. While these lesions do not necessarily precede cancers, and only undergo full transformation to invasive lesions in the minority of cases, they are generally associated with increased cancer risk (when compared to the overall population). Thus, they are considered oral premalignant lesions and constitute excellent platforms for head and neck cancer chemoprevention research.

Oral Leukoplakia/Erythroplakia and Cancer Risk

The term oral leukoplakia has been defined as white plaques in the oral cavity of questionable cancer risk having excluded other known diseases or disorders that carry no increased risk for cancer [20]. Oral leukoplakia is a clinical term with no specific histological abnormality. Microscopically, it may show atrophy, hyperplasia, and may or may not show dysplasia. Clinically, two major types of leukoplakia have been characterized: homogeneous (uniformly flat, thin, and with shallow cracks of the surface keratin) and non-homogeneous (including speckled, nodular, and verrucous varieties). Mixed white and red plaques are termed erythroleukoplakia. Erythroplakia is defined as a fiery red patch that cannot be characterized clinically or pathologically as any other definable disease [20]. Tobacco use is the most common predisposing factor for the development of these oral pre-malignant lesions.

The natural history of oral premalignant lesions varies according to several factors, including the type of exposure to tobacco, location of the lesion, and elimination of the causative agent. In an observational study in Mumbai, India, for example, 42.5% of untreated leukoplakias naturally disappeared in 5 years, while 41.5% remained unchanged [21]. Similarly, in a study involving 57,518 industrial workers in Gujarat, India, the 2-year rate of disease shrinkage/disappearance, and disease stabilization was 31.6% and 57.3% [22]. Regression in leukoplakias was more frequent in tobacco chewers and pipe smokers than in individuals who smoked cigarettes in a third study in India [23]. In a study in Denmark involving 138 patients, reduction or abstinence (for 3 months) of tobacco consumption was associated with a reduction in the size of leukoplakia in 56% of the patients, and after total abstinence for 1 year, there was an 80% rate of reduction or disappearance of the premalignant lesions [24]. In Hungary, 520 patients were followed after attempted elimination of the causative agent – the lesions completely disappeared in 33.8%, improved in 25.3%, remained unchanged in 26%, and progressed in 9% of patients. The lesions in the tongue and floor of the mouth seemed to have a higher likelihood of progression than the lesions in the buccal mucosa and commissures [25].

In regards to the rate of malignant transformation (i.e., development of oral cancer), longitudinal studies have different results according to the region of the world where they were performed. In community-based surveys in developing countries (e.g. India), transformation rates as low as 0.06% per year have been reported [23]. This figure seems to be lower than what is found in studies in Western countries – in an observational study in the US ($N=257$), 17.5% of the individuals with oral leukoplakia developed invasive cancer with a mean follow-up of 8.1 years [26]. The geographic differences are largely attributed to two factors: possibility of under-reporting of invasive cancers in developing countries and bias toward selection of a worse prognosis, "hospital-based" population in the studies in developed countries. Nonetheless, in a pooled analysis of the literature, Petti et al. estimated a global malignant transformation rate for oral premalignant lesions of 1.36% per year (95% confidence interval 0.69–2.03%) [27]. This figure reflects the cancer incidence in patients at varying degrees of risk for malignant transformation, and underscores the importance of identifying factors that may differentiate high from low risk cohorts within the group of patients with leukoplakia, in order to personalize follow-up strategies and develop chemopreventive interventions based on each person's individual cancer risk.

Besides demographics, the following clinical criteria have also been described as prognostic factors for development of invasive cancers: age, gender, anatomical site, clinical appearance and size, causative agent, and histology.

The influence of age in the rate of malignant transformation is illustrated by Swedish and Hungarian studies. In Sweden, the maximal incidence of oral cancer developing in areas of leukoplakia occurred between the ages of 70–89 (7.5%), as opposed to 1% in individuals less than 50 years [28]. Similarly, in Hungary, the frequency of malignant transformation was higher when leukoplakias were diagnosed in the eighth decade (8.2%) when compared to the fourth decade (2.9%) [29].

Women with leukoplakia appear to be at higher risk to develop invasive cancer then men in several studies [26, 30–33], with a reported frequency of malignant transformation of 5.8% versus 2.1% in a study involving 331 individuals in Denmark [30].

The anatomic site of premalignant lesions has also been correlated with malignant transformation in some studies [26, 30, 31, 34] but not others [32, 35]. Banoczy demonstrated that 13% of the leukoplakias in the floor of the mouth progressed to cancer, compared to 2.9% and 1.1% of the leukoplakias in the buccal mucosa and buccal commissures, respectively [31]. Similarly, Kramer et al. demonstrated that 24% of patients with leukoplakia on the floor of the mouth and/or ventral tongue developed oral cancer [34]. Nonetheless, more recently, Schepman et al. did not demonstrate differences in leukoplakia malignant transformation rates according to anatomical site [32].

An approximate four-to-five-times higher risk of malignant transformation is observed in nonhomogeneous leukoplakia compared to their homogeneous counterpart [36]. In 520 Hungarian patients with leukoplakia, for example, none of the "leukoplakia simplex" progressed to invasive cancer, compared to 4.6% and 28% of the "verrucosa" and "erosiva" subtypes, respectively [29]. A similar pattern (i.e., higher cancer risk in lesions with nodular and/or verrucous components, as well as in lesions with red areas – erythroleukoplakias) was observed in several other studies in the US, Europe, and Asia [26, 32–35, 37–39]. Despite the fact that homogenous lesions carry a low cancer risk, they should still be monitored, since in the study of Silverman et al., for example, the frequency of transformation during the follow-up period was still clinically significant (6.5%) [26]. Besides clinical appearance, size and extent of oral premalignant lesions have also been shown to be directly correlated with cancer risk in multiples studies [30, 35, 40, 41]. Additionally, a clinically distinct subtype of leukoplakia, termed proliferative verrucous leukoplakia, has been characterized as persistent, multifocal leukoplakia, which progresses from a flat appearance at initial presentation through increasing degrees of thickness, fissuring and warty proliferation, until invariable transformation to invasive cancer in 60–100% of cases, despite surgical intervention [42–45].

While exposure to tobacco is the most important environmental factor associated with the development of premalignant lesions, leukoplakias that arise in individuals with no obvious etiologic factor seem to have a higher risk for malignant transformation [26, 28–32]. Silverman et al., for example, reported a 24% frequency of malignant transformation in nonsmokers, compared to 16% and 12% in individuals who continued to smoke and quit smoking after the diagnosis of leukoplakia, respectively [26]. Additionally, some nonsmoke tobacco habits (e.g., snuff) carry a lesser risks of oral cancer than others (e.g., quids) [36].

The use of histological criteria of oral premalignant lesions to assess cancer risk has been problematic. On one hand, epithelial dysplasia is more often recognized in nonhomogeneous leukoplakias than in homogenous leukoplakias [37, 46–48], and there is an obvious congruence between the risk of malignant transformation and (clinically) nonhomogeneous, (histologically) dysplastic lesions [26]. On the other hand, leukoplakias without evidence of dysplasia may still progress to cancer [49]. Moreover, a correlation between degree of dysplasia and cancer risk has been found in some [50, 51], but not all, studies [52]. Additionally, although criteria for the diagnosis of dysplasia have been described, there is a high inter- and intra-examiner discordance between the presence or absence, and grade of dysplasia [53–55]. Hence, although dysplasia may be generally considered a poor prognostic factor in patients with oral premalignant lesions, the correlation with clinical criteria, and, more recently, molecular criteria (as discussed in the next section) will provide a better picture of each individual's cancer risk [51].

Molecular Markers of Cancer Risk

In 2000, Lee et al. published the first comprehensive and mature cancer risk model involving translational molecular studies collected within the context of a randomized phase III study of patients with oral leukoplakia. While that risk assessment model was not designed to be generalized and has not yet been validated, the authors convincingly demonstrated that incorporation of molecular markers to clinical and demographic criteria may improve the ability to predict development of cancers of the aerodigestive tract. Specifically, a biomarker score characterized by high chromosome polysomy, high p53 protein accumulation in the parabasal layer, and loss of heterozygosity (LOH) at 3p or 9p improved cancer risk prediction when added to clinical information (i.e., prior history of cancer and degree of dysplasia – the two most important clinical risk factors identified in that cohort of patients) [51]. Similarly, in lung cancer, risk models that include molecular data have recently been shown to have higher accuracy than risk models based on clinical-demographic information alone [56]. These studies justify the incorporation of a translational component of biomarker discovery in chemoprevention clinical trials, in order to identify, not only better molecular predictors of cancer risk, but also markers relevant to the carcinogenic process, which may become possible targets for future chemopreventive interventions. Two molecular markers stand out as very promising for head and neck cancer risk assessment: chromosomal allelic imbalances and cyclin D1.

Chromosomal Allelic Imbalances

Allelic imbalances in multiple chromosomal loci have been identified early on in the process of head and neck carcinogenesis [4]. Mao et al. demonstrated that LOH in regions of the genome harboring tumor suppressor genes (i.e., 3p14 and/or 9p21) occur in up to 51% of patients with oral leukoplakia, and are associated with a risk of invasive cancer of 37%, compared to 6% in patients without LOH ($P=0.039$) [57]. The importance of LOH in the carcinogenic process is further underscored by the findings of allelic imbalances in large areas of mucosa, illustrating the concept of field cancerization [4].

Following the publication of the work by Mao et al., other groups confirmed the prognostic implications of LOH in oral premalignant lesions. Partridge et al. demonstrated allelic imbalances at 3p21, 8p21–23, and/or 9p21 in 77% of patients with oral leukoplakia or erythroplakia with histological evidence of dysplasia, and microsatellite instability at a frequency of 55%. The estimated 5-year cancer risk of patients with allelic imbalances at two or more loci was 75%, compared to 30% in patients with allelic imbalance in less than two loci ($P=0.008$) [58]. In a subsequent case–control study, 95% of patients who developed cancer had two or more allelic imbalances at 5 key chromosomal regions in the precursor lesions (i.e., 3p 8p21–23, 9p13–24, and 13q13–31), compared to 41% of the matched controls [59].

In the largest retrospective study performed to date, Rosin et al. analyzed 116 cases or oral premalignant lesions for LOH at 19 microsatellite loci on seven chromosome arms (3p, 4q, 8p, 9p, 11q, 13q, and 17p). Individuals with LOH at 3p and/or 9p but at no other chromosome arm had a 3.8-fold increase in the relative risk for developing carcinoma in situ or invasive cancer (5-year risk of 26%, compared to 2% in patients without LOH at 3p and 9p). In patients with LOH at 3p and/or 9p and another chromosome arm, there was a 33-fold increase in the relative risk for cancer, translating into a 5-year risk of 47% [60].

In addition to predicting progression of leukoplakia to cancer, LOH is also associated with increased risk of second primary tumors in patients with curatively treated oral cancer who subsequently develop an area of premalignant lesion at the site of the surgical resection. In this context, patients with LOH at 3p and/or 9p have a 5-year cancer risk of 72%, compared to 6% in patients without LOH at 3p and 9p [61].

Although promising, the prognostic value of chromosomal allelic imbalances has never been evaluated in a prospective study. However, an ongoing randomized controlled trial of erlotinib for prevention of oral cancer includes LOH as a criterion for selection of a high risk cohort [17] and might be able to validate the aforementioned findings.

Cyclin D1

Cyclin D1 is a key protein involved in the G1-S phase transition, thus serving as a regulator of the cell cycle. It influences cell proliferation and differentiation, and its expression is controlled by intracellular signaling events in response to extracellular stimuli [62]. It has been shown to promote genetic instability in vitro and promote tumorigenesis in vivo [63, 64].

In a single arm, phase II study of biochemoprevention with 13-*cis*-retinoic acid, interferon-alpha, and alpha-tocopherol, cyclin D1 expression dysregulation detected at last follow-up after the intervention was correlated with histological progression of upper aerodigestive tract pre-malignant lesions and cancer development [65]. Additionally, in the same study, cyclin D1 A allele of the polymorphism located at nucleotide 870 of exon 4 was associated with resistance to downregulation of cyclin D1 protein expression by treatment and a higher likelihood of progression to cancer [66]. Of note, the cyclin D1 gene G/A870 polymorphism results in both a normally spliced and an alternatively spliced transcript that encodes a protein lacking the ubiquitnation destruction box. As a result, this alternate protein is resistant to proteolysis and has an increased half life, stimulating cell proliferation, thus supporting the more aggressive clinical course of lesions of A/A or G/A genotype compared to the G/G genotype [67–69]. A second biochemoprevention phase II study in patients with laryngeal dysplasia confirmed the aforementioned findings – a shorter cancer-free survival was observed in patients harboring the cyclin D1 A/A or G/A genotype. Furthermore, high cyclin D1 protein expression in each genotype subgroups was also associated with decreased cancer-free survival [70].

These results are intriguing, as cyclin D1 not only participates in the carcinogenic process of and confers an increased risk of progression of premalignant lesions to head and neck cancer but may also serve as a therapeutic target for chemoprevention. Although direct inhibitors of cyclin D1 are not yet in clinical use, drugs directed at upstream regulators of this protein (such as the epidermal growth factor receptor inhibitors erlotinib and cetuximab) are currently being evaluated in patients with oral premalignant lesions.

Chemoprevention Clinical Trials

A number of clinical trials for chemoprevention of cancers of the head and neck have been completed to date and are discussed in the next sections of this chapter. These trials either targeted a population with premalignant lesions (e.g., leukoplakia, erythroplakia), or attempted at preventing second primary tumors in patients with a curatively treated head and neck cancer. While none of these studies resulted in drug approvals specifically for head and neck cancer prevention, they set the stage for the development of novel clinical trial designs with a strong translational research component that will inform the next generation of studies.

Clinical Trials for Premalignant Lesions

Clinical trials for head and neck premalignancies have often focused on reducing the size of clinical lesions and/or reversing histological abnormalities. While many drugs have been shown to be able to elicit a clinical or histological response, to our knowledge, there has never been a trial which used the more clinically relevant and definitive primary endpoint of reduction of cancer incidence. The use of clinical, histological, and molecular surrogate intermediary endpoints in cancer chemoprevention trials is not without its challenges, as reviewed elsewhere [17, 19, 71]. In the setting or oral premalignancies, problems with using clinical response as an endpoint include: (1) a merely marginal correlation of responses with cancer-free survival in one of the largest and longest term chemoprevention trials performed to date [72], and (2) the persistence of molecular abnormalities, despite clinical resolution of the lesions after chemoprevention intervention, indicating a continuing risk of malignant transformation of the epithelium [73]. Hence, the results of the clinical trials presented below should be interpreted in light of these limitations. Nonetheless, use of surrogate intermediary endpoints may still be useful in early phase chemoprevention clinical trials to select agents to be more definitively tested in a phase III setting [71].

In 1986, Hong et al. published the results of a pivotal, randomized, placebo controlled trial of 13-*cis*-retinoic acid 1–2 mg/kg/day for 3 months in 44 patients with leukoplakia. There was a statistically significant difference in the clinical response rate (67% versus 10%) and the rates of reversal of dysplasia (54% versus 10%) favoring the experimental arm. However, after 2–3 months of treatment, relapses occurred in 56% of the patients. Typical retinoid-induced toxicities (cheilitis, facial erythema, dryness and peeling of the skin, conjunctivitis, and hypertriglyceridemia) were observed [74].Around the same time, Stitch et al. demonstrated that vitamin A (200,000 IU/week) for 6 months was more effective than placebo (57% versus 3%) in producing complete remissions in 54 tobacco/betel nut chewers in Kerala, India with well-developed oral leukoplakias [75]. Additionally, the same group also demonstrated, in a separate trial with a similar patient population, higher 6-month leukoplakia remission rates in patients treated for 6 months with beta-carotene (180 mg/week), or beta-carotene (180 mg/week) plus vitamin A (100,000 IU/week), compared to placebo (15%, 28%, and 3%, respectively) [76]. Later studies confirmed the superiority of vitamin A (300,000 IU/week) or beta-carotene (360 mg/week) for 12 months compared to placebo in producing complete responses (52%, 33%, and 10%, respectively), but 50–66% of the patients relapsed after stopping the supplementation [77].

To address the toxicity issues and the high relapse rate after treatment discontinuation observed in the trial of Hong et al. [74], Lippman et al. treated 70 patients with leukoplakia with an induction regimen of 13-*cis*-retinoic acid (1.3 mg/kg/day) for 3 months. Patients with stable disease or clinical response (55%, $N=59$) were then randomized to 9-month maintenance therapy with low-dose 13-*cis*-retinoic acid (0.5 mg/kg/day) or beta-carotene (30 mg/day). There was a statistically significant higher rate of disease stabilization or clinical responses in the group that received 13-*cis*-retinoic acid (92% versus 45%), which also had greater toxicity [78]. Nonetheless, on long term follow-up (median of 66 months), the incidence of in situ or invasive cancer was not different between the two arms (23% for low-dose 13-*cis*-retinoic acid versus 27% for the beta-carotene) [79].

A follow-up trial evaluated a longer, 3-year treatment period with 13-*cis*-retinoic acid at lower doses (0.5 mg/kg/day for 1 year followed by 0.25 mg/kg/day orally for 2 years), or beta-carotene (50 mg/day) plus vitamin A (in the form of retinyl palmitate 25,000 IU/day) in 162 patients with leukoplakia. The rationale for the treatment groups was to use, in the control arm, 13-*cis*-retinoic acid at more tolerable doses for long term treatment, and compare it to an experimental arm of a combination of two active drugs (beta-carotene and retinyl palmitate, based on the work by Stich et al. [75, 76]) in a noninferiority trial design. When the study was conducted, beta-carotene had to be dropped from the experimental arm owing to emerging data demonstrating an increased risk of lung cancer incidence and mortality in other ongoing chemoprevention trials at that time. The main results of the study were: an inferior 3-month response rate in the vitamin A alone arm, a lack of statistical significance in the test for noninferiority between the control and the experimental arm(s), and more importantly, a similar oral-cancer-free survival across all groups with only a marginal correlation of 3-month clinical response and long-term oral cancer free survival [72]. The major implications of this study, one of the longest-term performed to date in this setting, are that 13-*cis*-retinoic acid is still not well tolerated for long-term treatment, even at reduced doses, and that better tolerated regimens (i.e., vitamin A alone) are largely ineffective. Furthermore, an impact in oral cancer incidence is yet to be demonstrated with any of these regimens.

Strategies to improve the tolerability and efficacy of retinoid-based regimens have included the use of synthetic retinoids. To this end, Chiesa et al. randomized 170 patients operated on for leukoplakias with benign histology to receive fenretinide 200 mg/day or placebo for 1 year. The trial was discontinued prematurely owing to slow accrual. However, the experimental arm exhibited a lower incidence of relapses, new leukoplakias or carcinomas [80]. Similarly, Lippman et al. demonstrated activity of fenretinide 200 mg/day in retinoid-resistant leukoplakias in a single-arm, phase II study, although responses were short-lived and correlated with previous response to retinoid therapy [81]. In a follow-up phase II trial of fenretinide 900 mg/m^2 twice daily (days 1–7 for four 3-week cycles), the high dose regimen was found to be ineffective, and related pre-clinical data in an in vitro model of oral pre-malignancy favored the use of low-dose regimens in this setting [82].

Besides retinoids, other agents have been studied in phase I/II trials involving patients with oral premalignant lesions, including cyclooxygenase inhibitors (ketorolac and celecoxib), mutated p53 targeted agents (ONYX-015), and the protease inhibitor Bowman-Birk Inhibitor. Oral rinse with ketorolac did not increase 3-month response rates compared to placebo (30% versus 32%, respectively), and potential explanations for the lack of effect included issues with tissue penetration after topic exposure to the drug [83]. A pilot study of various doses of celecoxib in oral leukoplakia also failed to demonstrate significant activity [84]. A mouthwash with ONYX-015 (an attenuated adenovirus cytotoxic to cells with dysfunction p53-dependant signaling pathways) elicited histologic resolution of dysplasia in 37% of 19 patients, but the majority of the responses were transient [85]. In the phase II trial of the Bowman-Birk Inhibitor, promising results were observed, with a response rate of 31% among 32 subjects [86].

Taken together, the literature on patients with oral premalignant lesions does not indicate, so far, the availability of an optimal agent that should be recommended routinely for chemoprevention of head and neck cancers or treatment of leukoplakia/erythroplakia, either due to toxicity concerns (such as high dose 13-*cis*-reitnoic acid, which hinders its long-term use) or lack of efficacy. Nonetheless, trials continue to be performed in order to identify drugs with a better therapeutic index, as well as predictive markers of activity. Promising agents in this setting include the epidermal growth factor receptor inhibitors, peroxisome proliferator-activated receptor-gamma agonists, and green tea extract, among others.

Clinical Trials for Prevention of Second Primary Tumors

The distinction between second primary tumors of the head and neck and loco-regional recurrence is somewhat debatable. Nonetheless, regardless of the clonal origin of the cells, head and neck cancers arising after potentially curative treatment of an index cancer are not infrequent and carry significant morbidity and mortality. Hence, there is a rationale for developing chemopreventive strategies in this setting.

Following the initial results of studies using retinoids in patients with premalignant lesions, Hong et al. designed a trial evaluating a 12-month treatment with 13-*cis*-retinoic acid (50–100 mg/m^2/day) or placebo in 103 patients with head and neck cancer after potentially curative treatment with surgery and/or radiotherapy. There were no differences in local, nodal or distant recurrences between the groups, but the rate of second primary tumors was significantly lower in the 13-*cis*-retinoic acid arm (4% versus 24%, $P=0.005$) [87]. On long term follow-up (54.5 months), the difference between the groups remained statistically significant, albeit smaller [88].

Bolla et al. randomized 316 patients with early stage head and neck cancer to receive the second-generation retinoid etretinate (50 mg/day for 1 month followed by 25 mg/day for 23 months) or placebo in the adjuvant setting. No differences in disease-free survival, overall survival and incidence of second primary tumors were observed between the arms [89].

The European Organization of Research and Treatment of Cancer conducted the largest randomized study for prevention of second primary tumors performed to date (the European Study on Chemoprevention with Vitamin A and N-Acetylcysteine – EUROSCAN). In this trial, 2,592 patients (60% with head and neck cancer and 40% with lung cancer) were randomly assigned, in a 2×2 factorial design, to receive no intervention, retinyl palmitate (300,000 IU/day for 1 year followed by 150,000 IU for 2 year), N-acetylcysteine (600 mg/day), or both. After a median follow-up of 49 months, 919 patients had an event (recurrence, second primary tumor or death), and there were no statistically significant differences in recurrence-free survival, overall survival or incidence of second primary tumors in any of the arms [90].

Another large trial involving 1,190 patients with squamous cell carcinomas of the head and neck (stage I or II) evaluated the effects of 3-year treatment with low dose 13-*cis*-retinoic acid (30 mg/day) or placebo and failed to demonstrate any benefit from the intervention in terms of overall survival or incidence of second primary tumors [91]. Other smaller scale, phase III chemoprevention studies to prevent second primary tumors within the context of head and neck cancers using beta-carotene ($N=264$) [92], and alpha-tocopherol and beta-carotene ($N=540$) [93] were also negative.

Conclusions and Future Directions

The field of head and neck cancer chemoprevention has been evolving rapidly over the past several years. Advances in cancer risk models that integrate molecular data with already established clinical, demographic, and histological criteria will improve the ability to identify a population at the highest risk of head and neck cancer and thus in greatest need for chemopreventive interventions. In parallel, development of novel, particularly molecular-targeted, agents with established activity in advanced disease, better characterized mechanisms of action, and a more favorable toxicity profile will increase the options of available drugs to be tested for chemoprevention. Identification of molecules that may serve as predictive markers of benefit, toxicity and long-term outcome will streamline chemoprevention clinical research and potentially accelerate the transition of experimental agents to clinical practice.

A model of modern chemoprevention clinical trial design is the ongoing randomized, double-blind, placebo-controlled, multi-institutional Erlotinib Prevention of Oral Cancer (EPOC) trial. Patients with oral premalignant lesions with or without a history of curatively treated oral cancer are selected for EPOC based on high risk determined by LOH profile of the lesion. Patients are randomized (1:1) to receive 1-year treatment with placebo or the epidermal growth factor receptor inhibitor erlotinib. The choice of intervention has been carefully selected based on preclinical data and clinical activity of this class of drugs in the setting of advanced disease. Serial biopsies are being collected in order to study biomarkers with potential prognostic value and that may predict erlotinib activity. With this careful design in a very high-risk population, EPOC requires only 150 patients to be randomized between the two treatment arms to demonstrate a potential benefit from the intervention, and EPOC will be the first trial in oral premalignancy patients to have the definitive primary endpoint of cancer incidence and thus, the ability to establish whether an agent is efficacious in preventing cancer in the selected patient population [17].

The EPOC trial is a personalized prevention in so far as it selects people at the highest risk and thus greatest need for the intervention, screening out individuals at less risk and need and thus with less reason to risk potential side effects of the drug. Incorporating some features of the EPOC design may help streamline future definitive chemoprevention trials by reducing, via high-risk populations, their sample sizes, and durations. A primary future goal of cancer chemoprevention is a standard personalized medicine, as it already takes place in the treatment setting of advanced disease.

References

1. Sporn MB, Dunlop NM, Newton DL et al (1976) Prevention of chemical carcinogenesis by vitamin A and its synthetic analogs (retinoids). Fed Proc 35:1332–1338
2. Hanahan D, Weinberg RA (2000) The hallmarks of cancer. Cell 100:57–70
3. Slaughter DP, Southwick HW, Smejkal W (1953) Field cancerization in oral stratified squamous epithelium; clinical implications of multicentric origin. Cancer 6:963–968
4. Califano J, van der Riet P, Westra W et al (1996) Genetic progression model for head and neck cancer: implications for field cancerization. Cancer Res 56:2488–2492
5. Olsen JH (1985) Second cancer following cancer of the respiratory system in Denmark, 1943–80. Natl Cancer Inst Monogr 68:309–324

6. Cooper JS, Pajak TF, Rubin P et al (1989) Second malignancies in patients who have head and neck cancer: incidence, effect on survival and implications based on the RTOG experience. Int J Radiat Oncol Biol Phys 17:449–456
7. Licciardello JT, Spitz MR, Hong WK (1989) Multiple primary cancer in patients with cancer of the head and neck: second cancer of the head and neck, esophagus, and lung. Int J Radiat Oncol Biol Phys 17:467–476
8. Christensen PH, Joergensen K, Munk J et al (1987) Hyperfrequency of pulmonary cancer in a population of 415 patients treated for laryngeal cancer. Laryngoscope 97:612–614
9. Tepperman BS, Fitzpatrick PJ (1981) Second respiratory and upper digestive tract cancers after oral cancer. Lancet 2:547–549
10. Ecimovic P, Pompe-Kirn V (2002) Second primary cancers in laryngeal cancer patients in Slovenia, 1961–1996. Eur J Cancer 38:1254–1260
11. Jang SJ, Chiba I, Hirai A et al (2001) Multiple oral squamous epithelial lesions: are they genetically related? Oncogene 20:2235–2242
12. Worsham MJ, Wolman SR, Carey TE et al (1995) Common clonal origin of synchronous primary head and neck squamous cell carcinomas: analysis by tumor karyotypes and fluorescence in situ hybridization. Hum Pathol 26:251–261
13. Bedi GC, Westra WH, Gabrielson E et al (1996) Multiple head and neck tumors: evidence for a common clonal origin. Cancer Res 56:2484–2487
14. Scholes AG, Woolgar JA, Boyle MA et al (1998) Synchronous oral carcinomas: independent or common clonal origin? Cancer Res 58:2003–2006
15. Lydiatt WM, Anderson PE, Bazzana T et al (1998) Molecular support for field cancerization in the head and neck. Cancer 82:1376–1380
16. Bhutani M, Pathak AK, Fan YH et al (2008) Oral epithelium as a surrogate tissue for assessing smoking-induced molecular alterations in the lungs. Cancer Prev Res (Phila Pa) 1:39–44
17. William WN, Heymach JV, Kim ES et al (2009) Molecular targets for cancer chemoprevention. Nat Rev Drug Discov 8(3):213–225
18. O'Shaughnessy JA, Kelloff GJ, Gordon GB et al (2002) Treatment and prevention of intraepithelial neoplasia: an important target for accelerated new agent development. Clin Cancer Res 8:314–346
19. Kelloff GJ, Lippman SM, Dannenberg AJ et al (2006) Progress in chemoprevention drug development: the promise of molecular biomarkers for prevention of intraepithelial neoplasia and cancer – a plan to move forward. Clin Cancer Res 12:3661–3697
20. Warnakulasuriya S, Johnson NW, van der Waal I (2007) Nomenclature and classification of potentially malignant disorders of the oral mucosa. J Oral Pathol Med 36:575–580
21. Mehta FS, Shroff BC, Gupta PC et al (1972) Oral leukoplakia in relation to tobacco habits. A ten-year follow-up study of Bombay policemen. Oral Surg Oral Med Oral Pathol 34:426–433
22. Silverman S, Bhargava K, Smith LW et al (1976) Malignant transformation and natural history of oral leukoplakia in 57,518 industrial workers of Gujarat, India. Cancer 38:1790–1795
23. Gupta PC, Mehta FS, Daftary DK et al (1980) Incidence rates of oral cancer and natural history of oral precancerous lesions in a 10-year follow-up study of Indian villagers. Community Dent Oral Epidemiol 8:283–333
24. Pindborg JJ, Roed-Peterson B, Renstrup G (1972) Role of smoking in floor of the mouth leukoplakias. J Oral Pathol 1:22–29
25. Banoczy J, Sugar L (1975) Progressive and regressive changes in Hungarian oral leukoplakias in the course of longitudinal studies. Community Dent Oral Epidemiol 3:194–197
26. Silverman S Jr, Gorsky M, Lozada F (1984) Oral leukoplakia and malignant transformation. A follow-up study of 257 patients. Cancer 53:563–568
27. Petti S (2003) Pooled estimate of world leukoplakia prevalence: a systematic review. Oral Oncol 39:770–780
28. Einhorn J, Wersall J (1967) Incidence of oral carcinoma in patients with leukoplakia of the oral mucosa. Cancer 20:2189–2193
29. Banoczy J, Sugar L (1972) Longitudinal studies in oral leukoplakias. J Oral Pathol 1:265–272

30. Roed-Peterson B (1971) Cancer development in oral leukoplakia follow-up of 331 patients. J Dent Res 50:711 (abstract 720)
31. Banoczy J (1977) Follow-up studies in oral leukoplakia. J Maxillofac Surg 5:69–75
32. Schepman KP, van der Meij EH, Smeele LE et al (1998) Malignant transformation of oral leukoplakia: a follow-up study of a hospital-based population of 166 patients with oral leukoplakia from The Netherlands. Oral Oncol 34:270–275
33. Lind PO (1987) Malignant transformation in oral leukoplakia. Scand J Dent Res 95:449–455
34. Kramer IR, El-Labban N, Lee KW (1978) The clinical features and risk of malignant transformation in sublingual keratosis. Br Dent J 144:171–180
35. Holmstrup P, Vedtofte P, Reibel J et al (2006) Long-term treatment outcome of oral premalignant lesions. Oral Oncol 42:461–474
36. Reibel J (2003) Prognosis of oral pre-malignant lesions: significance of clinical, histopathological, and molecular biological characteristics. Crit Rev Oral Biol Med 14:47–62
37. Pindborg JJ, Jolst O, Renstrup G et al (1968) Studies in oral leukoplakia: a preliminary report on the period pervalence of malignant transformation in leukoplakia based on a follow-up study of 248 patients. J Am Dent Assoc 76:767–771
38. Pindborg JJ, Renstrup G, Poulsen HE et al (1963) Studies in oral leukoplakias. V. Clinical and histologic signs of malignancy. Acta Odontol Scand 21:407–414
39. Gupta PC, Bhonsle RB, Murti PR et al (1989) An epidemiologic assessment of cancer risk in oral precancerous lesions in India with special reference to nodular leukoplakia. Cancer 63:2247–2252
40. Saito T, Yamashita T, Notani K et al (1995) Flow cytometric analysis of nuclear DNA content in oral leukoplakia: relation to clinicopathologic findings. Int J Oral Maxillofac Surg 24:44–47
41. Napier SS, Cowan CG, Gregg TA et al (2003) Potentially malignant oral lesions in Northern Ireland: size (extent) matters. Oral Dis 9:129–137
42. Bagan JV, Jimenez Y, Sanchis JM et al (2003) Proliferative verrucous leukoplakia: high incidence of gingival squamous cell carcinoma. J Oral Pathol Med 32:379–382
43. Hansen LS, Olson JA, Silverman S Jr (1985) Proliferative verrucous leukoplakia. A long-term study of thirty patients. Oral Surg Oral Med Oral Pathol 60:285–298
44. Silverman S Jr, Gorsky M (1997) Proliferative verrucous leukoplakia: a follow-up study of 54 cases. Oral Surg Oral Med Oral Pathol Oral Radiol Endod 84:154–157
45. Zakrzewska JM, Lopes V, Speight P et al (1996) Proliferative verrucous leukoplakia: a report of ten cases. Oral Surg Oral Med Oral Pathol Oral Radiol Endod 82:396–401
46. Shafer WG, Waldron CA (1961) A clinical and histopathologic study of oral leukoplakia. Surg Gynecol Obstet 112:411–420
47. Mehta FS, Pindborg JJ, Gupta PC et al (1969) Epidemiologic and histologic study of oral cancer and leukoplakia among 50,915 villagers in India. Cancer 24:832–849
48. Kaugars GE, Burns JC, Gunsolley JC (1988) Epithelial dysplasia of the oral cavity and lips. Cancer 62:2166–2170
49. Pindborg JJ, Daftary DK, Mehta FS (1977) A follow-up study of sixty-one oral dysplastic precancerous lesions in Indian villagers. Oral Surg Oral Med Oral Pathol 43:383–390
50. Burkhardt A, Maerker R (1978) Dysplasieklassifikation oraler leukoplakien und präkanzerosen. Bedeutung für prognose und therapie. Dtsch Z Mund Kiefer Gesichtschir 2:199–205
51. Lee JJ, Hong WK, Hittelman WN et al (2000) Predicting cancer development in oral leukoplakia: ten years of translational research. Clin Cancer Res 6:1702–1710
52. Cruz IB, Snijders PJ, Meijer CJ et al (1998) p53 expression above the basal cell layer in oral mucosa is an early event of malignant transformation and has predictive value for developing oral squamous cell carcinoma. J Pathol 184:360–368
53. Pindborg JJ, Reibel J, Holmstrup P (1985) Subjectivity in evaluating oral epithelial dysplasia, carcinoma in situ and initial carcinoma. J Oral Pathol 14:698–708
54. Abbey LM, Kaugars GE, Gunsolley JC et al (1995) Intraexaminer and interexaminer reliability in the diagnosis of oral epithelial dysplasia. Oral Surg Oral Med Oral Pathol Oral Radiol Endod 80:188–191

55. Karabulut A, Reibel J, Therkildsen MH et al (1995) Observer variability in the histologic assessment of oral premalignant lesions. J Oral Pathol Med 24:198–200
56. Spitz MR, Etzel CJ, Dong Q et al (2008) An expanded risk prediction model for lung cancer. Cancer Prev Res (Phila Pa) 1:250–254
57. Mao L, Lee JS, Fan YH et al (1996) Frequent microsatellite alterations at chromosomes 9p21 and 3p14 in oral premalignant lesions and their value in cancer risk assessment. Nat Med 2:682–685
58. Partridge M, Emilion G, Pateromichelakis S et al (1998) Allelic imbalance at chromosomal loci implicated in the pathogenesis of oral precancer, cumulative loss and its relationship with progression to cancer. Oral Oncol 34:77–83
59. Partridge M, Pateromichelakis S, Phillips E et al (2000) A case-control study confirms that microsatellite assay can identify patients at risk of developing oral squamous cell carcinoma within a field of cancerization. Cancer Res 60:3893–3898
60. Rosin MP, Cheng X, Poh C et al (2000) Use of allelic loss to predict malignant risk for low-grade oral epithelial dysplasia. Clin Cancer Res 6:357–362
61. Rosin MP, Lam WL, Poh C et al (2002) 3p14 and 9p21 loss is a simple tool for predicting second oral malignancy at previously treated oral cancer sites. Cancer Res 62:6447–6450
62. Donnellan R, Chetty R (1998) Cyclin D1 and human neoplasia. Mol Pathol 51:1–7
63. Zhou P, Jiang W, Weghorst CM et al (1996) Overexpression of cyclin D1 enhances gene amplification. Cancer Res 56:36–39
64. Wang TC, Cardiff RD, Zukerberg L et al (1994) Mammary hyperplasia and carcinoma in MMTV-cyclin D1 transgenic mice. Nature 369:669–671
65. Papadimitrakopoulou VA, Izzo J, Mao L et al (2001) Cyclin D1 and p16 alterations in advanced premalignant lesions of the upper aerodigestive tract: role in response to chemoprevention and cancer development. Clin Cancer Res 7:3127–3134
66. Izzo JG, Papadimitrakopoulou VA, Liu DD et al (2003) Cyclin D1 genotype, response to biochemoprevention, and progression rate to upper aerodigestive tract cancer. J Natl Cancer Inst 95:198–205
67. Alt JR, Cleveland JL, Hannink M et al (2000) Phosphorylation-dependent regulation of cyclin D1 nuclear export and cyclin D1-dependent cellular transformation. Genes Dev 14:3102–3114
68. Diehl JA, Cheng M, Roussel MF et al (1998) Glycogen synthase kinase-3beta regulates cyclin D1 proteolysis and subcellular localization. Genes Dev 12:3499–3511
69. Diehl JA, Zindy F, Sherr CJ (1997) Inhibition of cyclin D1 phosphorylation on threonine-286 prevents its rapid degradation via the ubiquitin-proteasome pathway. Genes Dev 11:957–972
70. Papadimitrakopoulou V, Izzo JG, Liu DD et al (2009) Cyclin D1 and cancer development in laryngeal premalignancy patients. Cancer Prev Res (Phila Pa) 2:14–21
71. Szabo E (2008) Assessing efficacy in early-phase cancer prevention trials: the case of oral premalignancy. Cancer Prev Res (Phila Pa) 1:312–315
72. Papadimitrakopoulou VA, Lee JJ, William WN Jr et al (2009) Randomized trial of 13-cis retinoic acid compared with retinyl palmitate with or without beta-carotene in oral premalignancy. J Clin Oncol 27:599–604
73. Mao L, El-Naggar AK, Papadimitrakopoulou V et al (1998) Phenotype and genotype of advanced premalignant head and neck lesions after chemopreventive therapy. J Natl Cancer Inst 90:1545–1551
74. Hong WK, Endicott J, Itri LM et al (1986) 13-cis-retinoic acid in the treatment of oral leukoplakia. N Engl J Med 315:1501–1505
75. Stich HF, Hornby AP, Mathew B et al (1988) Response of oral leukoplakias to the administration of vitamin A. Cancer Lett 40:93–101
76. Stich HF, Rosin MP, Hornby AP et al (1988) Remission of oral leukoplakias and micronuclei in tobacco/betel quid chewers treated with beta-carotene and with beta-carotene plus vitamin A. Int J Cancer 42:195–199
77. Sankaranarayanan R, Mathew B, Varghese C et al (1997) Chemoprevention of oral leukoplakia with vitamin A and beta carotene: an assessment. Oral Oncol 33:231–236

78. Lippman SM, Batsakis JG, Toth BB et al (1993) Comparison of low-dose isotretinoin with beta carotene to prevent oral carcinogenesis. N Engl J Med 328:15–20
79. Papadimitrakopoulou VA, Hong WK, Lee JS et al (1997) Low-dose isotretinoin versus beta-carotene to prevent oral carcinogenesis: long-term follow-up. J Natl Cancer Inst 89:257–258
80. Chiesa F, Tradati N, Grigolato R et al (2005) Randomized trial of fenretinide (4-HPR) to prevent recurrences, new localizations and carcinomas in patients operated on for oral leukoplakia: long-term results. Int J Cancer 115:625–629
81. Lippman SM, Lee JJ, Martin JW et al (2006) Fenretinide activity in retinoid-resistant oral leukoplakia. Clin Cancer Res 12:3109–3114
82. William WN Jr, Lee JJ, Lippman SM et al (2009) High-dose fenretinide in oral leukoplakia. Cancer Prev Res (Phila Pa) 2:22–26
83. Mulshine JL, Atkinson JC, Greer RO et al (2004) Randomized, double-blind, placebo-controlled phase IIb trial of the cyclooxygenase inhibitor ketorolac as an oral rinse in oropharyngeal leukoplakia. Clin Cancer Res 10:1565–1573
84. Papadimitrakopoulou VA, William WN Jr, Dannenberg AJ et al (2008) Pilot randomized phase II study of celecoxib in oral premalignant lesions. Clin Cancer Res 14:2095–2101
85. Rudin CM, Cohen EE, Papadimitrakopoulou VA et al (2003) An attenuated adenovirus, ONYX-015, as mouthwash therapy for premalignant oral dysplasia. J Clin Oncol 21:4546–4552
86. Armstrong WB, Kennedy AR, Wan XS et al (2000) Clinical modulation of oral leukoplakia and protease activity by Bowman-Birk inhibitor concentrate in a phase IIa chemoprevention trial. Clin Cancer Res 6:4684–4691
87. Hong WK, Lippman SM, Itri LM et al (1990) Prevention of second primary tumors with isotretinoin in squamous-cell carcinoma of the head and neck. N Engl J Med 323:795–801
88. Benner SE, Pajak TF, Lippman SM et al (1994) Prevention of second primary tumors with isotretinoin in patients with squamous cell carcinoma of the head and neck: long-term follow-up. J Natl Cancer Inst 86:140–141
89. Bolla M, Lefur R, Van Ton J et al (1994) Prevention of second primary tumours with etretinate in squamous cell carcinoma of the oral cavity and oropharynx. Results of a multicentric double-blind randomised study. Eur J Cancer 30A:767–772
90. van Zandwijk N, Dalesio O, Pastorino U et al (2000) EUROSCAN, a randomized trial of vitamin A and N-acetylcysteine in patients with head and neck cancer or lung cancer. For the EUropean Organization for Research and Treatment of Cancer Head and Neck and Lung Cancer Cooperative Groups. J Natl Cancer Inst 92:977–986
91. Khuri FR, Lee JJ, Lippman SM et al (2006) Randomized phase III trial of low-dose isotretinoin for prevention of second primary tumors in stage I and II head and neck cancer patients. J Natl Cancer Inst 98:441–450
92. Mayne ST, Cartmel B, Baum M et al (2001) Randomized trial of supplemental beta-carotene to prevent second head and neck cancer. Cancer Res 61:1457–1463
93. Bairati I, Meyer F, Gelinas M et al (2005) A randomized trial of antioxidant vitamins to prevent second primary cancers in head and neck cancer patients. J Natl Cancer Inst 97:481–488

Index